Study and Review Guide for
Applied Anatomy & Physiology for Manual Therapists

Study and Review Guide for Applied Anatomy & Physiology for Manual Therapists

Pat Archer, MS, AT ret, LMT
Educational Liaison
Discoverypoint School of Massage
Seattle, Washington

Lisa Nelson, BA, AT/R, LMT
Director of Education
Discoverypoint School of Massage
Seattle, Washington

Wolters Kluwer | Lippincott Williams & Wilkins
Health
Philadelphia · Baltimore · New York · London
Buenos Aires · Hong Kong · Sydney · Tokyo

Acquisitions Editor: Kelley Squazzo
Product Manager: Linda G. Francis
Marketing Manager: Shauna Kelley
Design Coordinator: Joan Wendt
Compositor: SPi Global

Copyright © 2013 Patricia A. Archer and Lisa A. Nelson

Lippincott Williams & Wilkins—A Wolters Kluwer Business

351 West Camden Street
Baltimore, MD 21201

Two Commerce Square
2001 Market Street
Philadelphia, PA 19103

Printed in South Korea

All rights reserved. This book is protected by copyright. No part of this book may be reproduced or transmitted in any form or by any means, including as photocopies or scanned-in or other electronic copies, or utilized by any information storage and retrieval system without written permission from the copyright owner, except for brief quotations embodied in critical articles and reviews. Materials appearing in this book prepared by individuals as part of their official duties as U.S. government employees are not covered by the above-mentioned copyright. To request permission, please contact Lippincott Williams & Wilkins at Two Commerce Square, 2001 Market Street, Philadelphia, PA 19103, via email at permissions@lww.com, or via website at lww.com (products and services).

ISBN-13: 978-1-60547-750-3
ISBN-10: 1-60547-750-8

DISCLAIMER

Care has been taken to confirm the accuracy of the information present and to describe generally accepted practices. However, the authors, editors, and publisher are not responsible for errors or omissions or for any consequences from application of the information in this book and make no warranty, expressed or implied, with respect to the currency, completeness, or accuracy of the contents of the publication. Application of this information in a particular situation remains the professional responsibility of the practitioner; the clinical treatments described and recommended may not be considered absolute and universal recommendations.

The authors, editors, and publisher have exerted every effort to ensure that drug selection and dosage set forth in this text are in accordance with the current recommendations and practice at the time of publication. However, in view of ongoing research, changes in government regulations, and the constant flow of information relating to drug therapy and drug reactions, the reader is urged to check the package insert for each drug for any change in indications and dosage and for added warnings and precautions. This is particularly important when the recommended agent is a new or infrequently employed drug.

Some drugs and medical devices presented in this publication have Food and Drug Administration (FDA) clearance for limited use in restricted research settings. It is the responsibility of the health care provider to ascertain the FDA status of each drug or device planned for use in their clinical practice.

To purchase additional copies of this book, call Books of Discovery's customer service department at (800) 775-9227 or fax orders to (720) 479-9322.

Visit Books of Discovery at BooksofDiscovery.com.

10 9 8 7 6

Introduction

ABOUT THIS STUDY AND REVIEW GUIDE

This *Study and Review Guide* was written to help you (the student) organize, experience, think about, and connect to the essential A&P details and concepts of *Applied Anatomy and Physiology for Manual Therapists*. While some learning activities are simply blank illustrations from the textbook to help you review or quiz your recall, other exercises provide new and different ways of looking at the information to deepen your understanding. For example, the crossword puzzles and fill-in exercises will help you focus on the simple declarative information such as names, locations, and definitions. Other activities like the games and model building provide more active kinesthetic learning opportunities, while coloring, charting, and mind mapping exercises can help you visually and mentally organize the information in several different ways. Additionally, unit quizzes that blend questions from several chapters challenge you to integrate information and help you test your knowledge in a more comprehensive manner. Finally, if you know you do well in a study group, the group activities will provide your group some fun and active review exercises.

USER TIPS AND SUGGESTIONS

Whether you choose to work through every exercise in order, jump around, or pick and choose just a few exercises from a chapter, here are some tips and suggestions to help you maximize the use of this guide:

- *Use the learning objectives chart* at the beginning of each chapter to identify and choose the specific learning exercises and/or group activities that cover the information you want to review.
- *Try different types of exercises* both to help you identify the ones that work best for you and to challenge your mind to look at the information in different ways.
- *Note activities you like* that are introduced in the first few chapters, and adapt them to the content in other chapters. Several examples of these adaptable exercises include
  - Charts and tables
  - Mind maps, Venn diagrams, and other graphic organizers
  - Concept maps
  - Flash cards (including several creative ways to make and use them)
  - Games

Finally, if you are looking for more exercises or study tips, please visit http://thePoint.lww.com/Archer-Nelson or contact us through our Web site, www.mtaed.com.

    Happy studying!

    Lisa and Pat

Table of Contents

Unit I • Introduction to Anatomy, Physiology, and the Manual Therapies

Chapter 1: Applying A&P to the Practice of Manual Therapy 1
Chapter 2: The Body and Its Terminology 16
Unit I Practice Exam 29

Unit II • Cells, Tissues, and Membranes

Chapter 3: Chemistry, Cells, and Tissues 34
Chapter 4: Body Membranes and the Integumentary System 43
Unit II Practice Exam 52

Unit III • Framework and Movement

Chapter 5: The Skeletal System 57
Chapter 6: The Skeletal Muscle System 71
Unit III Practice Exam 90

Unit IV • Communication and Control

Chapter 7: The Nervous System 95
Chapter 8: Neuromuscular and Myofascial Connections 113
Chapter 9: The Endocrine System 125
Unit IV Practice Exam 136

Unit V • Circulation and Body Defense

Chapter 10: The Cardiovascular System 141
Chapter 11: The Lymphatic System 158
Chapter 12: Immunity and Healing 169
Unit V Practice Exam 177

Unit VI • Metabolic Processes, Elimination, and Reproduction

Chapter 13: The Respiratory System 181
Chapter 14: The Digestive System 190
Chapter 15: The Urinary System 199
Chapter 16: The Reproductive System 206
Unit VI Practice Exam 214
Answer Key 219

1 Applying A&P to the Practice of Manual Therapy

Use this table to identify the study guide exercises and group activities that will help you explore or review each learning objective for the chapter.

No.	Learning Objective	Exercise	Study Group Activity (SGA)
1	Discuss the importance of the study of anatomy and physiology for manual therapy practitioners.		1
2	List and define the levels of complexity for body organization and provide an example of each.	1–3	2, 3
3	Define homeostasis and give a few examples of common homeostatic changes.	1, 3–6	2, 3
4	Explain the difference between the negative and positive feedback mechanisms used to maintain homeostasis.	1, 5	2, 3
5	Compare and contrast the benefits versus physiologic effects of manual therapy.	1, 7	2, 3
6	Distinguish between the structural and systemic effects of manual therapy.	1, 7	2, 3
7	Based on therapeutic intent, list and explain seven general manual therapy categories.	3, 8	2, 3
8	Name several examples of manual therapy techniques that fall into each of the seven categories.	8	2, 3
9	Identify the 11 body systems, including the primary components and general functions of each system.	9–11	2, 3

EXERCISE 1 • Key Terminology Crossword

Use this crossword to review and test your ability to define key terms from Chapter 1.

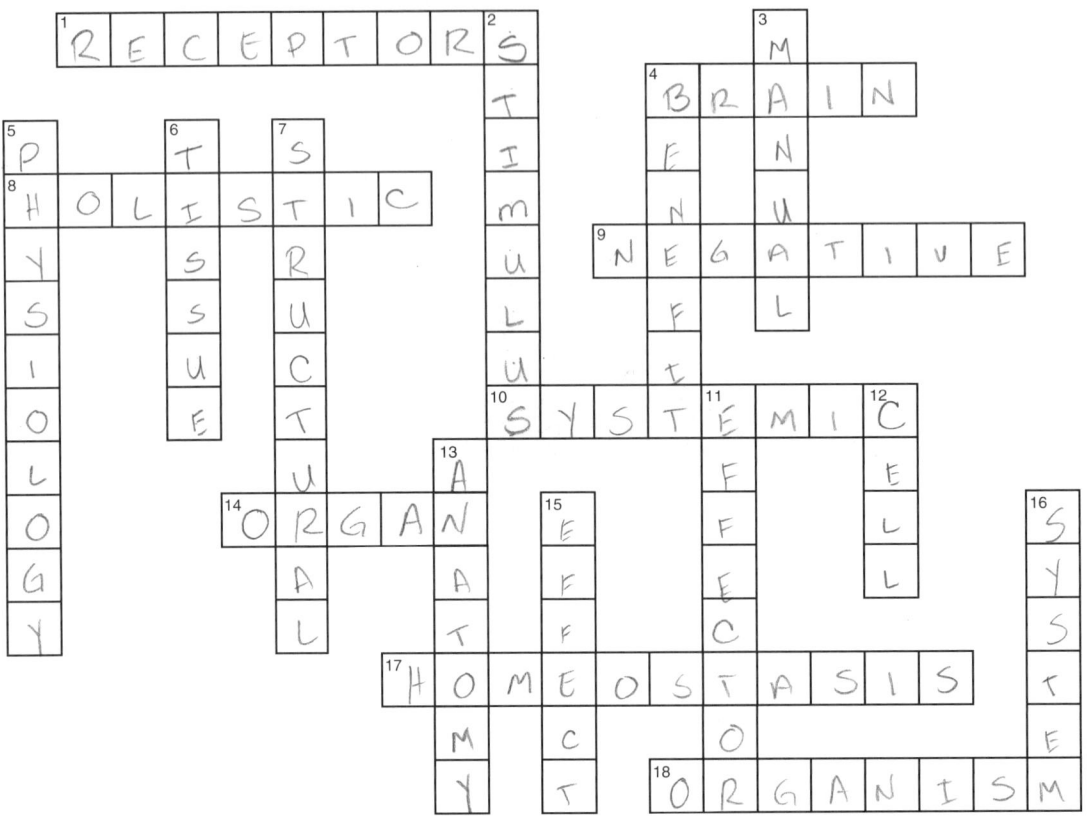

ACROSS

1. Sense organs sensitive to specific types of stimuli.
4. Can serve as the integration center in a feedback loop.
8. This health and wellness approach is guided by the principle that the physical body, cognitive processes (mind), and emotional or spiritual aspect are inseparable parts of a whole and integrated person.
9. The most common homeostatic feedback loop.
10. These regional or bodywide manual therapy effects are mediated by cellular, circulatory, and/or nervous system functions.
14. Group of tissues working together to accomplish specific tasks.
17. A level of internal stability or balance.
18. A living thing that functions as a whole.

DOWN

2. Any internal or external change in the environment.
3. Patterned and purposeful application of touch and/or movement with therapeutic intent.
4. A positive change in health or well-being caused by manual therapy regardless of the particular form utilized.
5. Study of the body's functional processes.
6. Group of like cells working together.
7. Manual therapy effects that create physical changes such as stretching or loosening.
11. Target cell, tissue or organ that responds to a specific stimulus.
12. Basic building block of the body.
13. The form and structure of an organism.
15. A specific and measurable change due to a particular manual therapy technique.
16. Group of organs working together to accomplish a specific set of tasks.

EXERCISE 2 • Levels of Organization

Color the diagram and fill in the appropriate labels for the five different levels of body organization. Provide a definition for each organizational level. If you need to refresh your memory, refer to Figure 1-1 in your text.

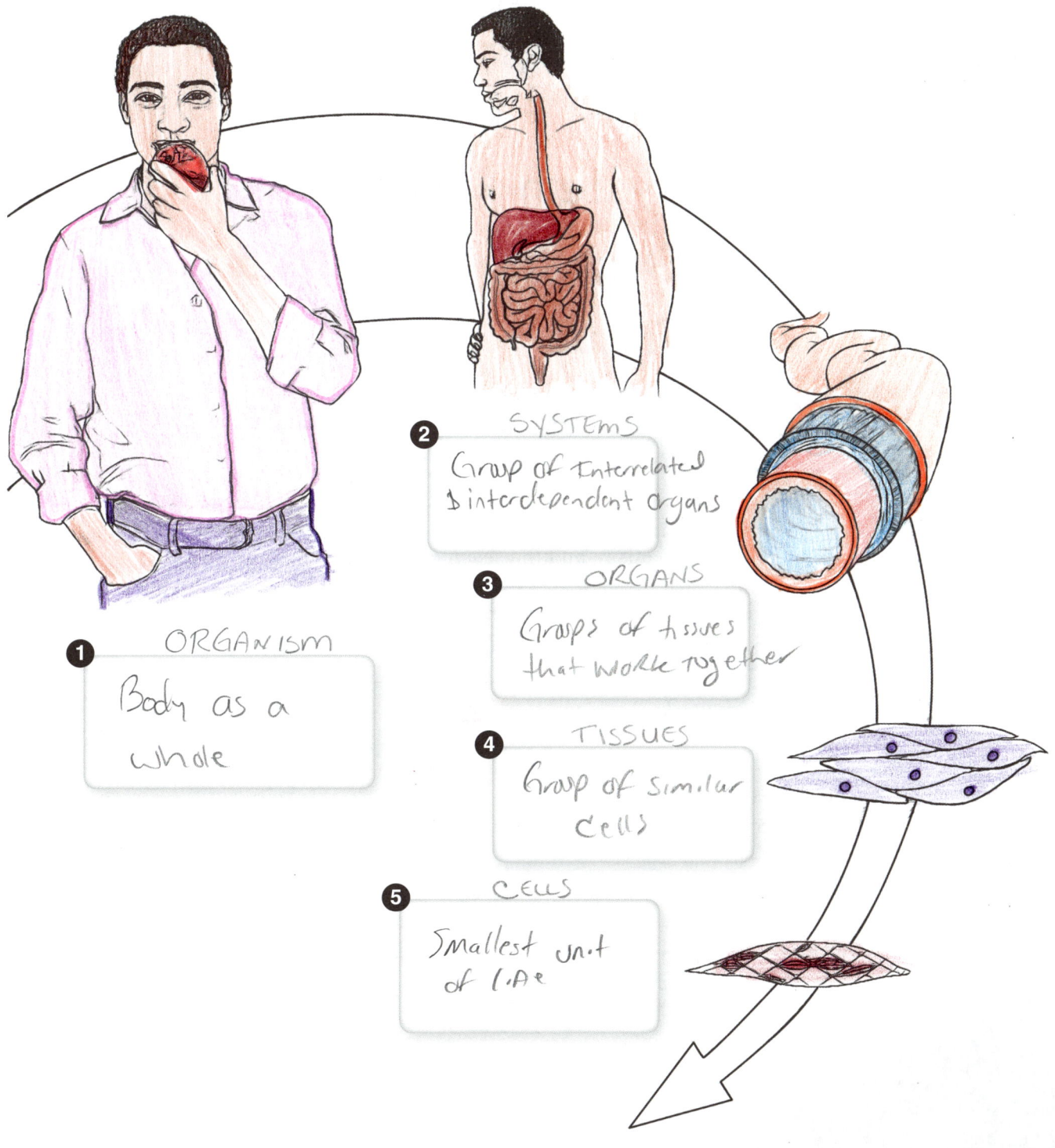

1. ORGANISM — Body as a whole
2. SYSTEMS — Group of interrelated & interdependent organs
3. ORGANS — Groups of tissues that work together
4. TISSUES — Group of similar cells
5. CELLS — Smallest unit of life

EXERCISE 3 • Mnemonics

Mnemonics are helpful memory cues for recalling lists of information. To create a mnemonic, identify the first letter of each word in the list you want to remember. Next, come up with a memorable saying by stringing together words that utilize the same first letters (silly or suggestive themes seem to work best). The following mnemonic is an example created for recalling the levels of body organization.

Body = Bodies
System = Sensing
Organ = Organized
Tissue = Touch
Cell = Chain-react

Use the spaces provided below to come up with mnemonics for the parts of a homeostatic feedback mechanism, and the seven categories of manual therapy.

Parts of a Homeostatic Mechanism
Stimulus—S So
Receptor—R Rebecka
IntegrationCenter—I Is
Effector—E Eating

Categories of Manual Therapy
Swedish—S So
Myofascial—M My
Neuromuscular—N Next
Lymphatic—L Lines
MovementTherapies—M May
Reflexive/Zone Therapies—R Repeat
EnergyTechniques—E EAchother

EXERCISE 4 • Homeostasis Flow Chart

Define the four components of a homeostatic feedback loop. Next color and complete the flow chart by placing each component in its correct position. Refer to Figure 1-2 in the text if you need to refresh your memory.

1. integration center (blue) _Nervous System or Endo Gland recieves input from Receptor_
2. stimulus (yellow) _Change in environment that disrupts homeostasis_
3. effector (red) _Responds_
4. receptor (green) _Senses Stimulus_

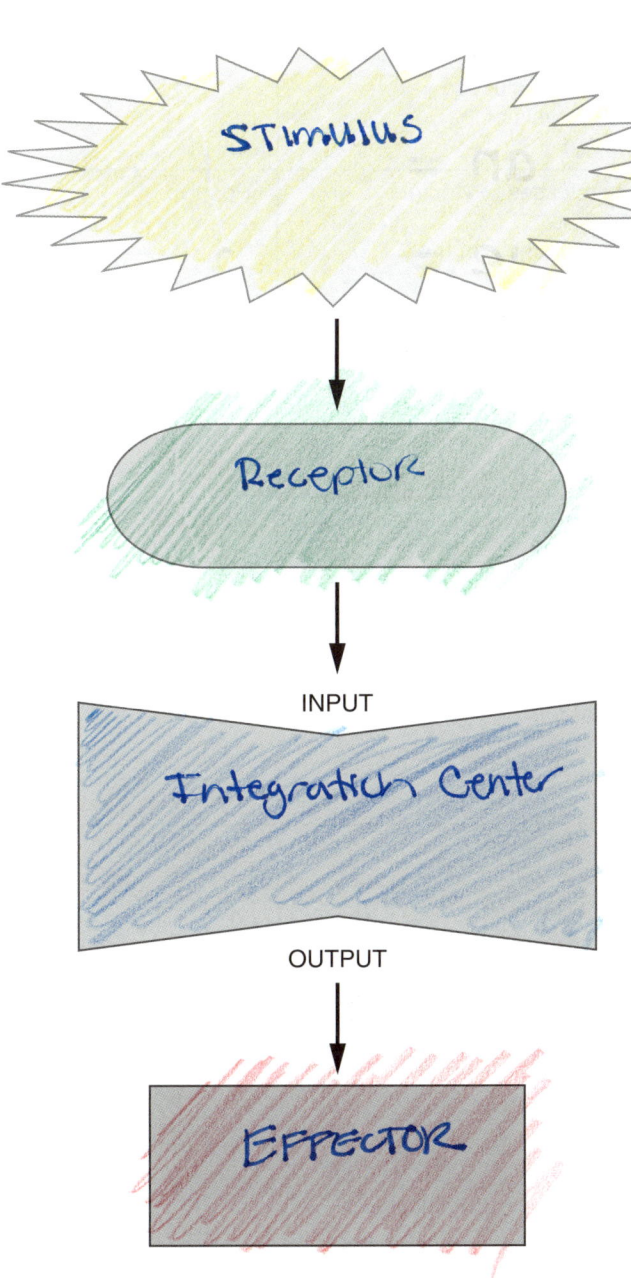

EXERCISE 5 • Charting Negative and Positive Feedback

Homeostatic mechanisms are either negative or positive feedback loops. In a negative feedback loop, the response of the effector 1. _Counteract or reverses_ the original stimulus, while in a positive feedback loop, the effector's response 2. _Reinforces/sustain_ the original stimulus. The chart below lists examples of homeostatic mechanisms and identifies each as either a negative or positive feedback loop. Fill in the missing information to complete the other examples.

Stimulus	Body's Homeostatic Response	Type of Feedback Loop
Increased levels of glucose in the blood	Pancreas releases insulin that allows body cells to increase their uptake and use of glucose that decreases the levels of glucose in the blood	Negative
Stretching of opening to the birth canal	Anterior pituitary releases oxytocin that increases uterine contractions and stretching of the birth canal by the baby	Positive
Drinking lots of water and increasing the fluid levels in the body	3. _Increased URINATION_	Negative
4. _↑ in HR & BP_	Decrease in heart rate to decrease blood pressure	Negative
Increased pH of the blood	Adjustments to decrease the pH of the blood	5. _Negative_
6. _Low level of Ca in Blood_	Parathyroid glands release parathyroid hormone that increases the breakdown of bone in order to increase the level of calcium in the blood	Negative

EXERCISE 6 • Linking Body, Mind, and Spirit

From a holistic perspective, the definition of homeostasis can be broadened to include the balance or dynamic equilibrium that exists between body, mind, and spirit. Explore this concept by writing down how the status of your body, mind, or spirit can affect the other aspects of this holistic balance. There are many correct answers for each graphic organizer. The answer key provides one example of each. Compare your answers with those of your classmates.

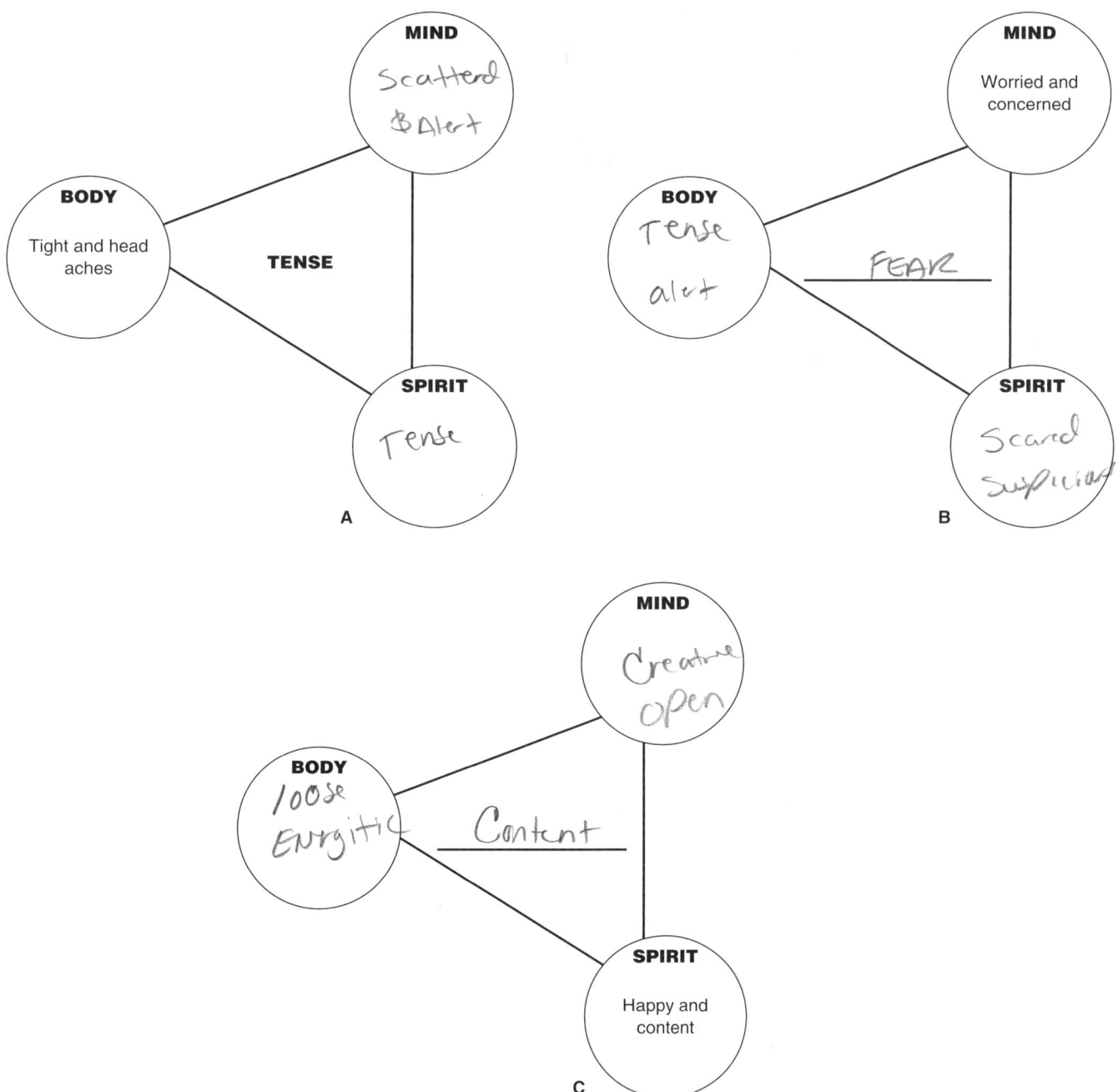

A.
- MIND: Scattered & Alert
- BODY: Tight and head aches
- SPIRIT: Tense
- (body-mind link): TENSE

B.
- MIND: Worried and concerned
- BODY: Tense, alert
- SPIRIT: Scared, suspicious
- (body-spirit link): FEAR

C.
- MIND: Creative, open
- BODY: loose, energitic
- SPIRIT: Happy and content
- (body-spirit link): Content

EXERCISE 7 • Benefits and Effects of Manual Therapy

Identify each of the following as either a benefit or physiologic effect of manual therapy by writing a **B** or **E** in the space provided.

1. __B__ Enhanced sense of well-being
2. __E__ Stretching muscles and connective tissue
3. __E__ Reduction of edema
4. __B__ Decreased anxiety/stress
5. __E__ Decreased pain
6. __B__ Improved mental focus
7. __B__ Improved sleep patterns
8. __E__ Loosening or broadening muscles and/or connective tissue
9. __E__ Unwinding muscles and connective tissue
10. __E__ Improved local venous flow

Identify each physiologic effect as either a structural or systemic effect by writing it in the appropriate column below.

STRUCTURAL EFFECT	SYSTEMIC EFFECT
2	3
8	5
9	10

Chapter 1 Applying A&P to the Practice of Manual Therapy

EXERCISE 8 • Manual Therapy Categories

Fill in the blanks in the table below. Refer to Table 1-1 in the text if you need to refresh your memory.

Category	Description	Primary Therapeutic Intention	Common Names
Swedish or Relaxation	1.	Relaxation Stress reduction Reconnecting and grounding	Relaxation massage Spa massage Stress reduction massage 2. 3.
Myofascial	Any technique focused on stretching, 4. _____, or 5. _____ fascia and other connective tissues Usually done without or with minimal amounts of lubricant	6. 7. 8. Improve local fluid flow	9. 10. 11. 12.
13.	Any technique that reduces resting muscle tension	Normalize muscle tension 14. 15. Improve range of motion (ROM)	Active Release Technique™ (ART™) Muscle Energy Technique® (MET) 16. 17. 18.
Lymphatic	Any system of light- to moderate-depth strokes based on anatomy and physiology of the lymphatic system	Stimulate edema uptake, 19. _____, and other lymphatic processes	Comprehensive Decongestive Therapy (CDT) 20. 21.
22.	Focused, patterned, conscious movement and/or positioning	23. 24. 25.	Alexander technique 26. 27. 28.
Reflexive/Zone Therapies	29.	Improve systemic and organ functions Decrease pain Enhance general well-being and energy flow	Acupressure Acupuncture Amma 30. 31.
32.	Touching/holding/stroking (with or without physical contact) of chakras, energy zones, or chi points	33. _____, 34. _____, or improve activity of energy (prana, Qi, ki, life force)	Aura techniques Ayurvedic Chakra balancing Touch for Health 35. 36.

EXERCISE 9 • Creating a Body Systems Table

Condensing information and organizing it in a table can make it easier to access and learn. Use the figures at the end of Chapter 1 and your own resources to create a quick reference for the systems of the body, their components, functions, and manual therapy connections. Some items have been filled in for you to get you started and the answer key offers possible responses.

Body System	Components	Functions	Manual Therapy Links
Integumentary	Skin & its glands Hair Nails Sensory receptors	1.	Therapeutic interface for touch therapies
Skeletal	2.	Structure Protects vital organs Levers for muscles Blood cell production Mineral storage	3.
Skeletal Muscular	4.	5.	Structural effects due to changes in muscles
Nervous	6.	Communication Coordination Control	7.
Endocrine	8.	Communication Coordination Control	9.
Cardiovascular	Blood Heart Blood vessels	10.	11.
Lymphatic	12.	13.	Specialty techniques boost fluid return and enhanced well-being improves immune function
Respiratory	Nose, sinuses, pharynx, larynx, trachea, bronchi, lungs	14.	15.
Digestive	16.	17.	Zone therapies target specific organs to improve function
Urinary	18.	Cleanses the blood Elimination of liquid wastes Regulation of pH, fluid, and electrolyte balances	Little direct effect except from zone therapies and lymphatic techniques
Reproductive	19.	Reproduction	20.

Chapter 1 Applying A&P to the Practice of Manual Therapy 11

EXERCISE 10 • Body Systems Anatomy Mind Map

Instead of a table, a mind map is an alternative way to organize information. Like a table, it condenses the information but organizes it spatially instead of linearly. Use the mind map below to identify the structural components of each body system. One system has been done for you to get you started and the answer key offers possible responses.

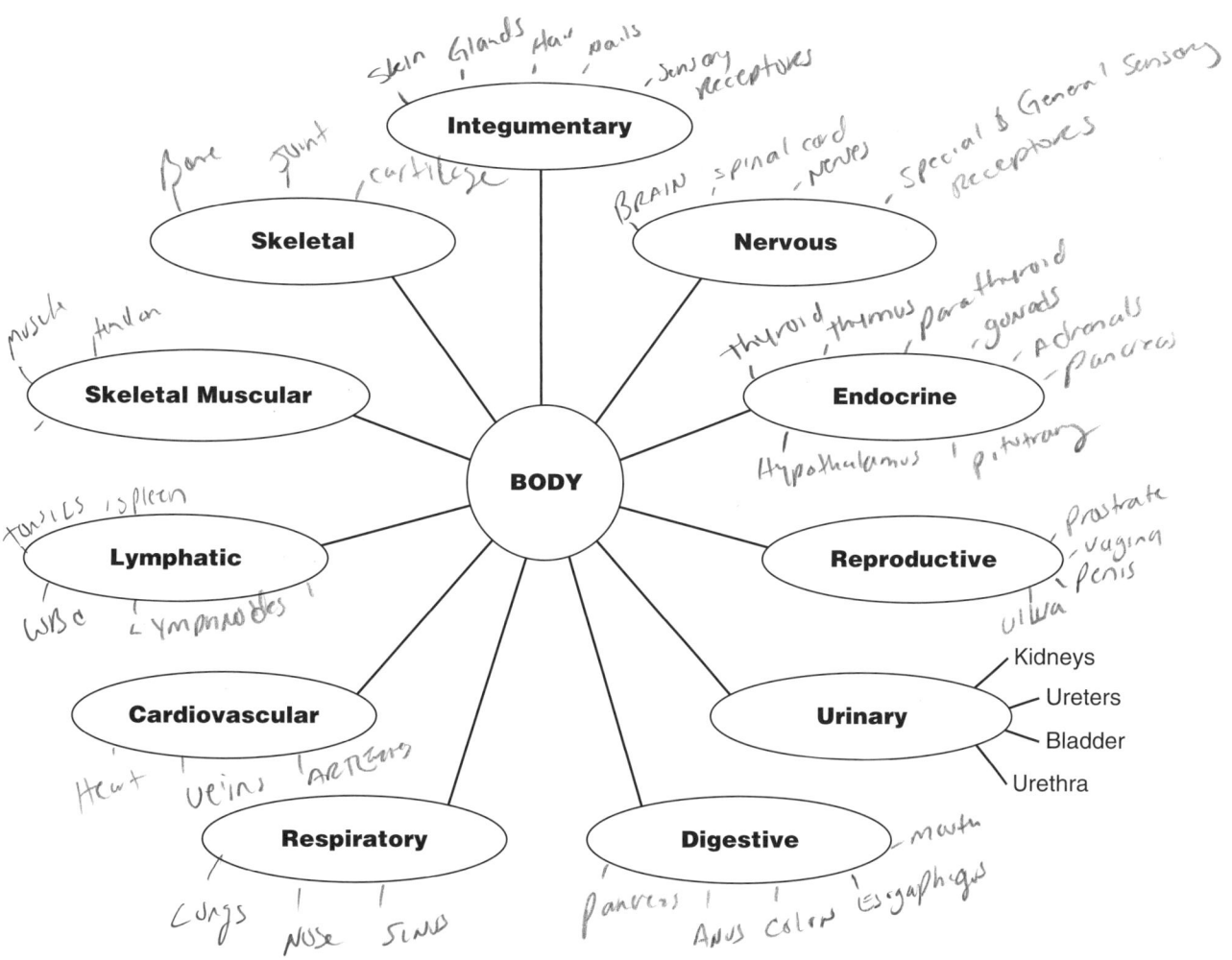

- Integumentary: skin, Glands, hair, nails
- Nervous: sensory receptors, BRAIN, spinal cord, nerves, Special & General Sensory receptors
- Skeletal: Bone, Joint, cartilage
- Endocrine: thyroid, thymus, parathyroid, gonads, Adrenals, Pancreas, Hypothalamus, pituitary
- Skeletal Muscular: muscle, tendon
- Reproductive: Prostate, vagina, Penis, uterus
- Lymphatic: tonsils, spleen, WBC, lymph nodes
- Urinary: Kidneys, Ureters, Bladder, Urethra
- Cardiovascular: Heart, veins, ARTEries
- Respiratory: Lungs, Nose, Sinus
- Digestive: mouth, pancreas, Anus, colon, Esophagus

EXERCISE 11 • Body Systems Physiology Mind Map

Use this mind map to note each system's functions. Again, one system is done for you to help get you started and the answer key offers possible responses. In addition, add colors to group systems together according to their common functions: covering; framework and movement; communication and control; circulation and body defense; metabolic processes and elimination; reproduction.

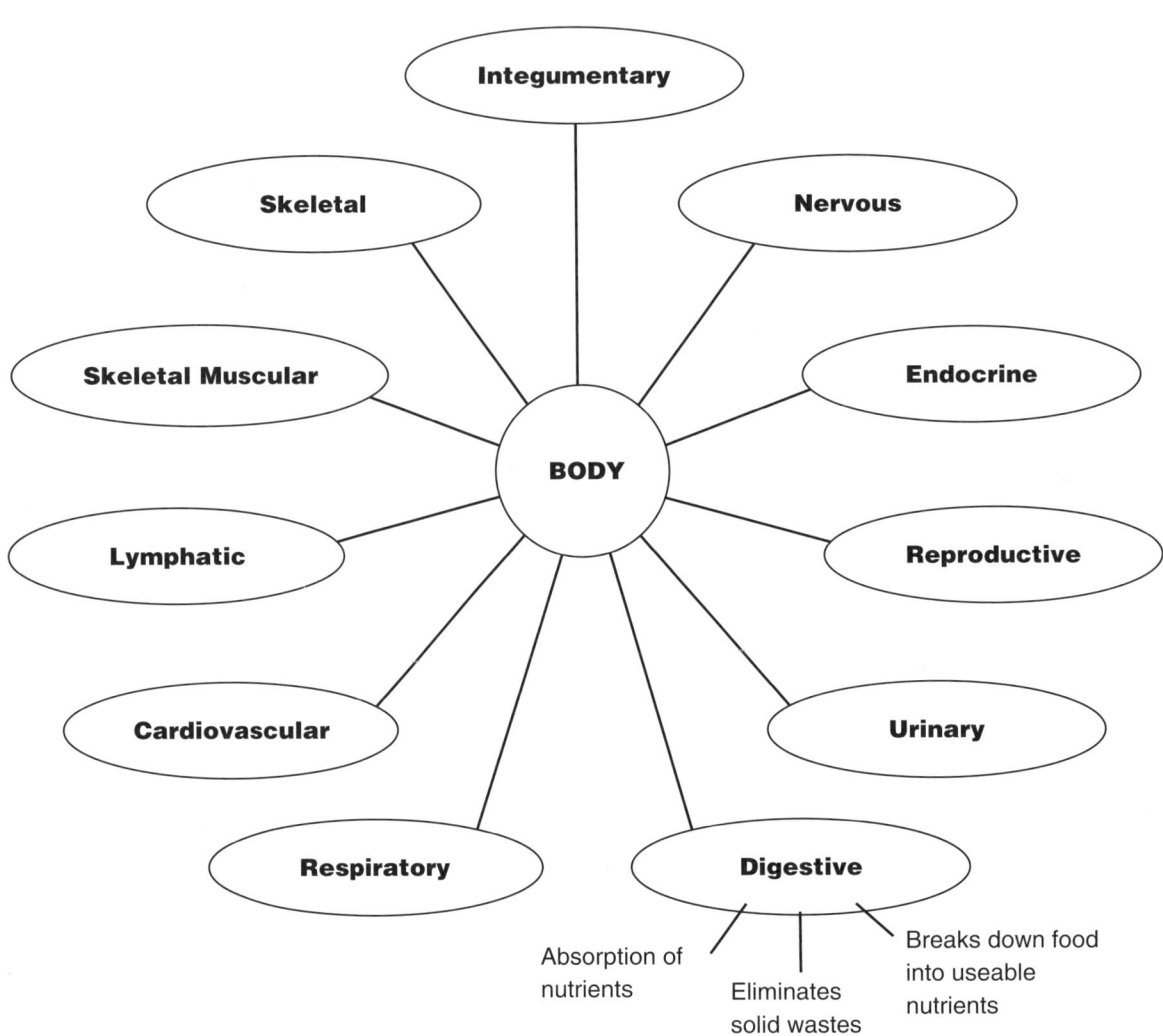

GROUP ACTIVITY 1 • Mind Mapping a Discussion

Mind maps can be helpful for tracking discussions especially during brainstorm or review sessions. Use this mind map to track ideas as you and your classmates discuss ways in which the study of anatomy and physiology is important for manual therapy practitioners. One example is provided to get you started. Feel free to add more bubbles as you come up with other ideas.

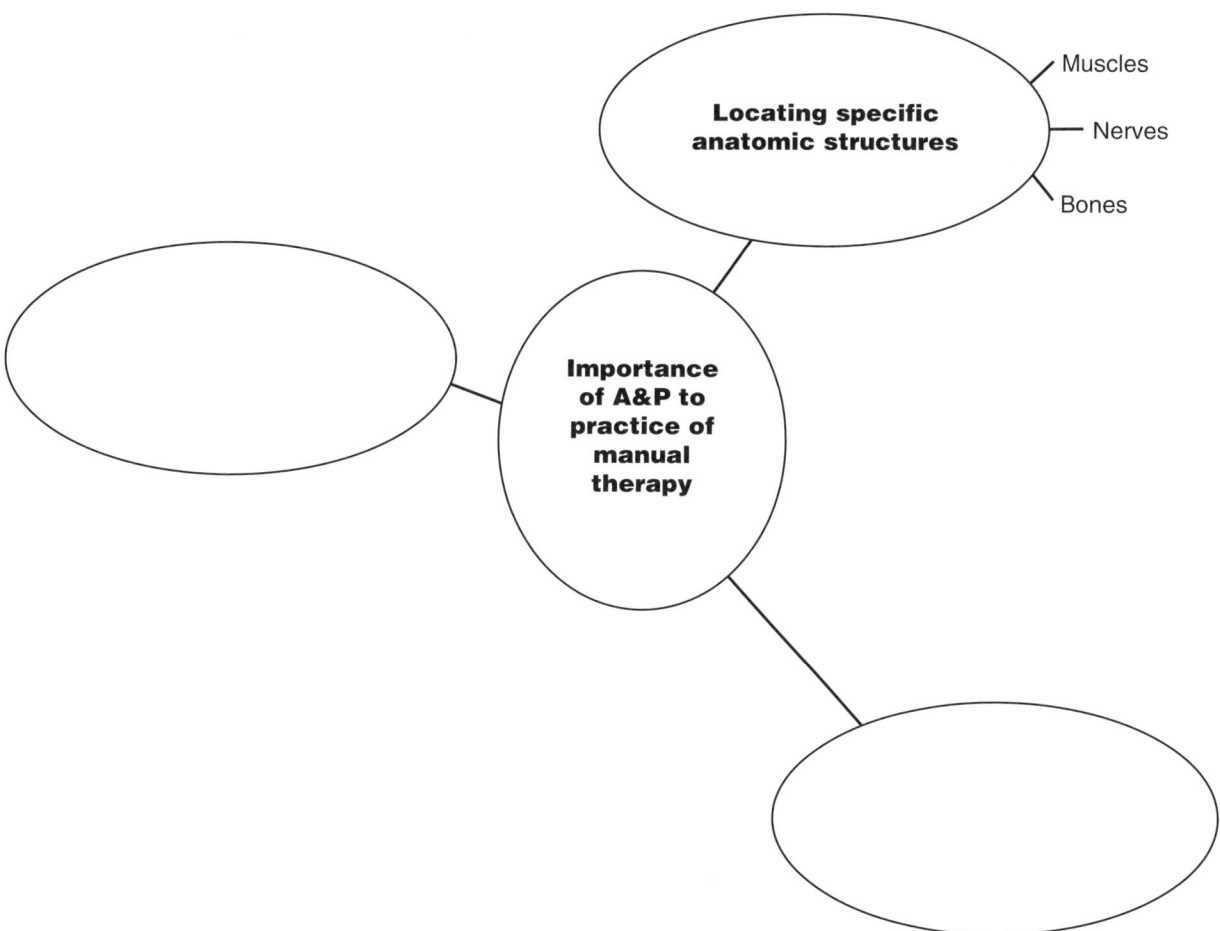

GROUP ACTIVITY 2 • Terminology or Mnemonic Charades

Charades, in which people "act out" the titles of books, movies, and other concepts, has long been a popular party game. Instead of using the standard book and movie titles, you can use charades to act out definitions for key terms or to share mnemonics with your study group. While playing a game may seem ridiculous and childish, the laughter and general silliness helps to ingrain the terms and/or mnemonics into everyone's memory making the game a fun and powerful study activity.

- Terminology—To review key terms, simply write the words on slips of paper and take turns acting out the definitions. Once the term is guessed, be sure everyone is familiar with the word and its definition before moving on to the next term.

- Mnemonics—This game of charades has many variations. It can be used to create and share mnemonics or to review mnemonics already created. To make new mnemonics, split into two teams. Assign each team a few lists of information for which they need to create a mnemonic. Once created, each team takes a turn acting out a mnemonic for the other team. Once they guess all the words in the mnemonic, there are two options: (1) review the list of information that the mnemonic was created to recall or (2) act out the list now that the team has the first letter of each item on the list. To use charades to review mnemonics, simply write the mnemonics on slips of paper like in regular charades and play the game as usual. When the clue is guessed, be sure everyone is clear what the mnemonic is used to recall.

GROUP ACTIVITY 3 • The Pyramid Game

This popular old game show format can be used as another way to help solidify your knowledge on any subject. In this game, a contestant has 1 minute (or whatever time period you choose) to correctly determine as many topic squares in the pyramid as possible. If they get all the topics of the pyramid correct, they earn 10,000 points. You can also assign "prizes" to the squares like cookies, chocolate, or doing a chore. There are three different roles to be played in the game:

- Contestant—a person in the group who is receiving clues and trying to determine the topic they describe
- Clue giver—a person that provides the clues to the contestant
- Timekeeper and judge—either one person or all other members of the study group

To set up a game, anyone except the contestant should create a game pyramid by writing a topic into each of the ten 1,000-point sections on the blank pyramid provided. For example, a game pyramid for this chapter might have body systems or types of manual therapy in each section. To play the game, the timekeeper starts the clock. With this clue, the clue giver looks at the first topic found in the bottom left section of the pyramid and provides one-word or short-phrase topic clues to the contestant. For example, clues for the respiratory system might be lungs, trachea, or breathing. The contestant must correctly guess the topic before the clue giver can move to the next block in that row (a new row always begins on the left side). Clue givers may not use any form of the topic's name in their clues. For example, you may not say *lymph nodes* as a clue for the lymphatic system, but you could say *nodes*, or *nodules*. If the judge determines a clue is improper, he or she "buzzes out" the clue giver, which causes the contestant to forfeit that square and its prize. The object of the game is for the contestant to determine every topic in the pyramid in the time period provided.

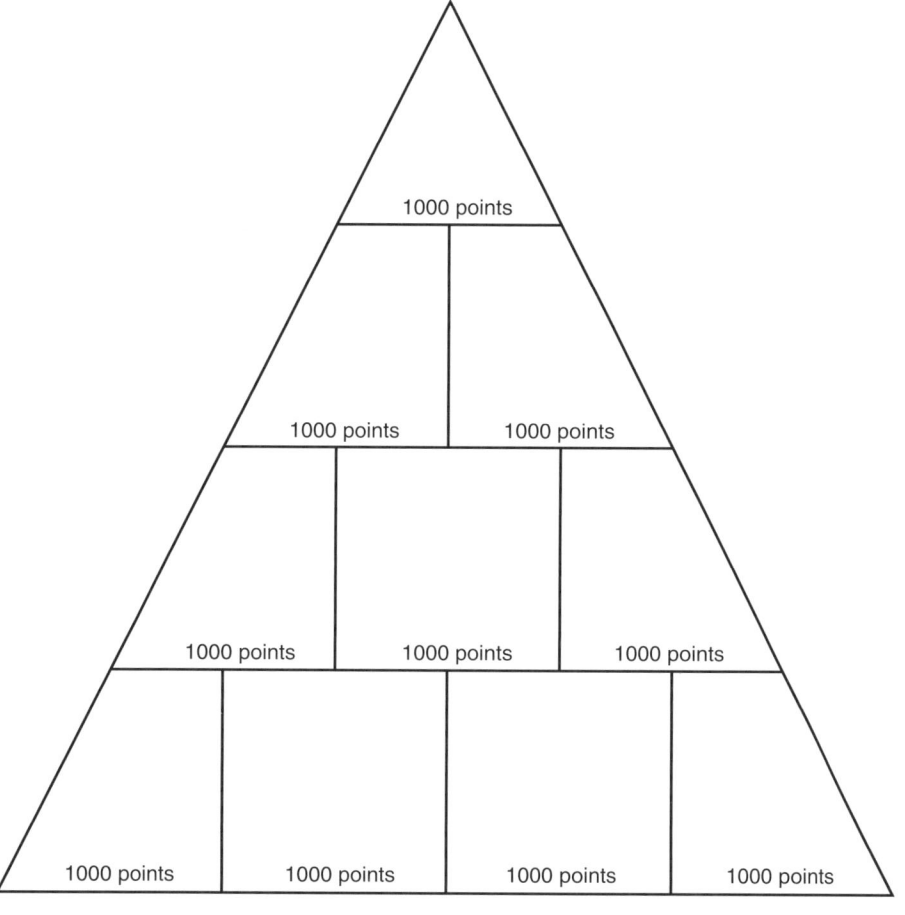

2 The Body and Its Terminology

Use this table to identify the study guide exercises and group activities that will help you explore or review each learning objective for this chapter.

No.	Learning Objective	Exercise	Study Group Activity
1	Describe and demonstrate anatomic position.	1	1, 2
2	Name and describe the three planes of the body.	1, 2, 11	1, 2
3	Demonstrate the use of proper terms for describing location and movement.	1, 3, 11	1, 2
4	List and define common medical prefixes, suffixes, and/or word roots.	1, 4, 11	1, 2
5	Use appropriate terminology to name and locate the primary body cavities and regions of the body.	1, 5–8, 11	1, 2, 3
6	List and define several common pathology terms.	1, 9, 11	1, 2
7	List four classes of disease and provide examples of each.	1, 10	1, 2

EXERCISE 1 • Flash Cards

Using index cards to create flash cards is a common study tool, especially for learning new terms and other straightforward declarative facts. For example, a flash card can have a new term on one side and its definition on the other, or a body system on one side and its components on the other. Flash cards help you study in two ways: (1) writing flash cards requires you to collect and organize new information and (2) the finished product is a portable study and review tool. The cards can be used while commuting via public transportation, waiting in line at the bank, or during a quick coffee break. You can use them to quiz study partners or organize them to help you keep track of which information you are sure of and what you need to continue to work on. Here are a few variations on flash cards:

- Color—Consider using different color cards or different color writing to categorize or organize flash cards. For example, in this chapter, you are learning terms for movement, location, body cavities, and body regions. Consider making each category of term a different color. This will help you determine which particular terms you need to focus your review and study on as well as which categories of terms are the most challenging for you.
- Diagrams and post-it notes—If you like to think in pictures instead of words, you may want to use blank body diagrams and post-it notes instead of flash cards. Print terms on post-its and simply stick the words to the appropriate body region on the blank diagram. If you need to learn verbal definitions, print up a chart that has all the definitions on it. Then use the same "sticky words," and match the correct term with the definition.
- Audio "flash cards"—If you spend long hours commuting in your car, reviewing information in an auditory manner with auditory flash cards could be a good option. To create these flash cards, you will need a tape recorder or a recording microphone for your iPod. Have a list of terms and definitions you want to review and make a recording that has pauses in it for you to repeat terms and/or define them. For example, you could record the word "gluteal" and then leave a space to repeat the term. Next record, "Gluteal means," and leave a pause of 5 to 10 seconds before saying, "Gluteal means buttocks." When you play the recording back, you will notice you have a space to repeat the term to help you practice the correct pronunciation as well as a space to define the term before the definition is given to you. This is similar to the way many people learn a foreign language.

EXERCISE 2 • Planes of the Body

Color and label each of the planes and cross sections of the body.

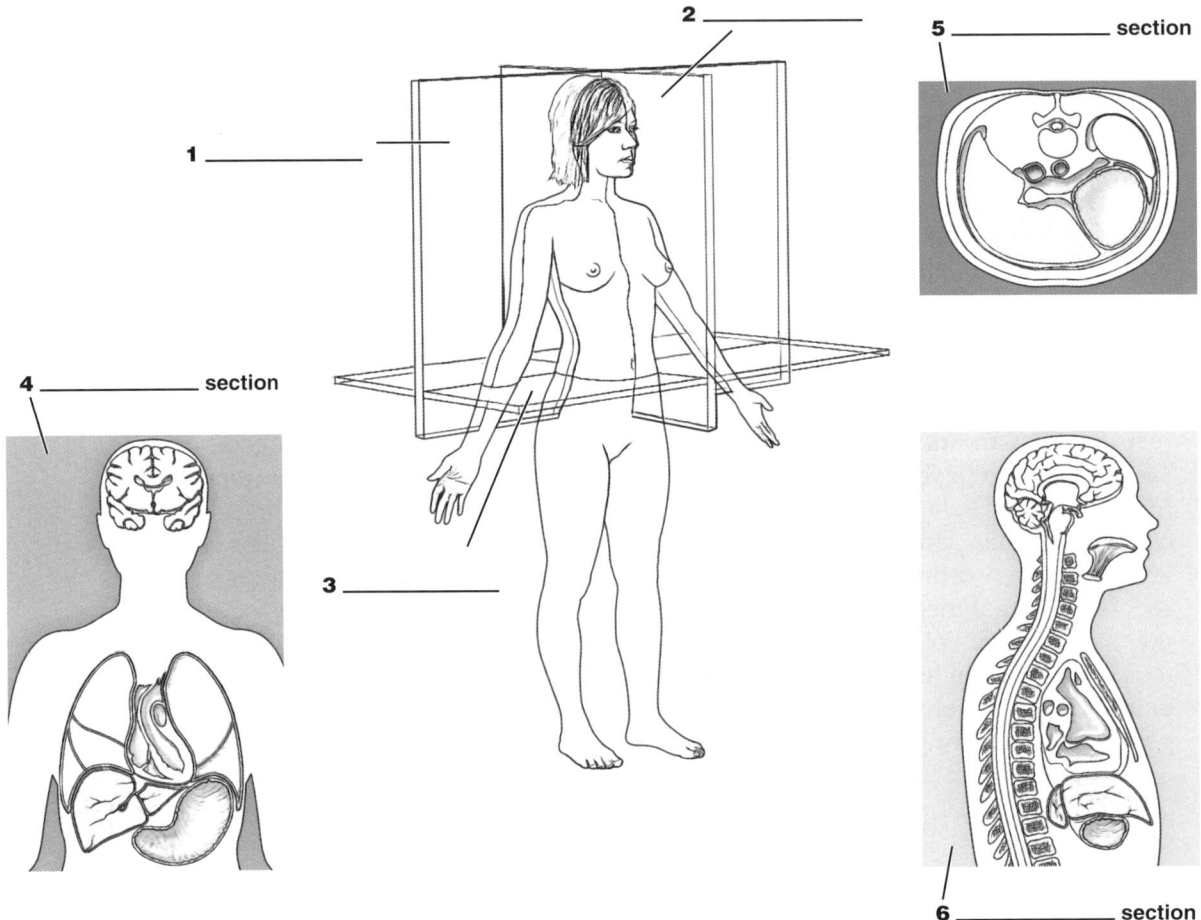

1. _____
2. _____
3. _____
4. _____ section
5. _____ section
6. _____ section

EXERCISE 3 • Location and Movement Terms Crossword

Use this crossword to review and test your ability to define the location and movement terms from Chapter 2.

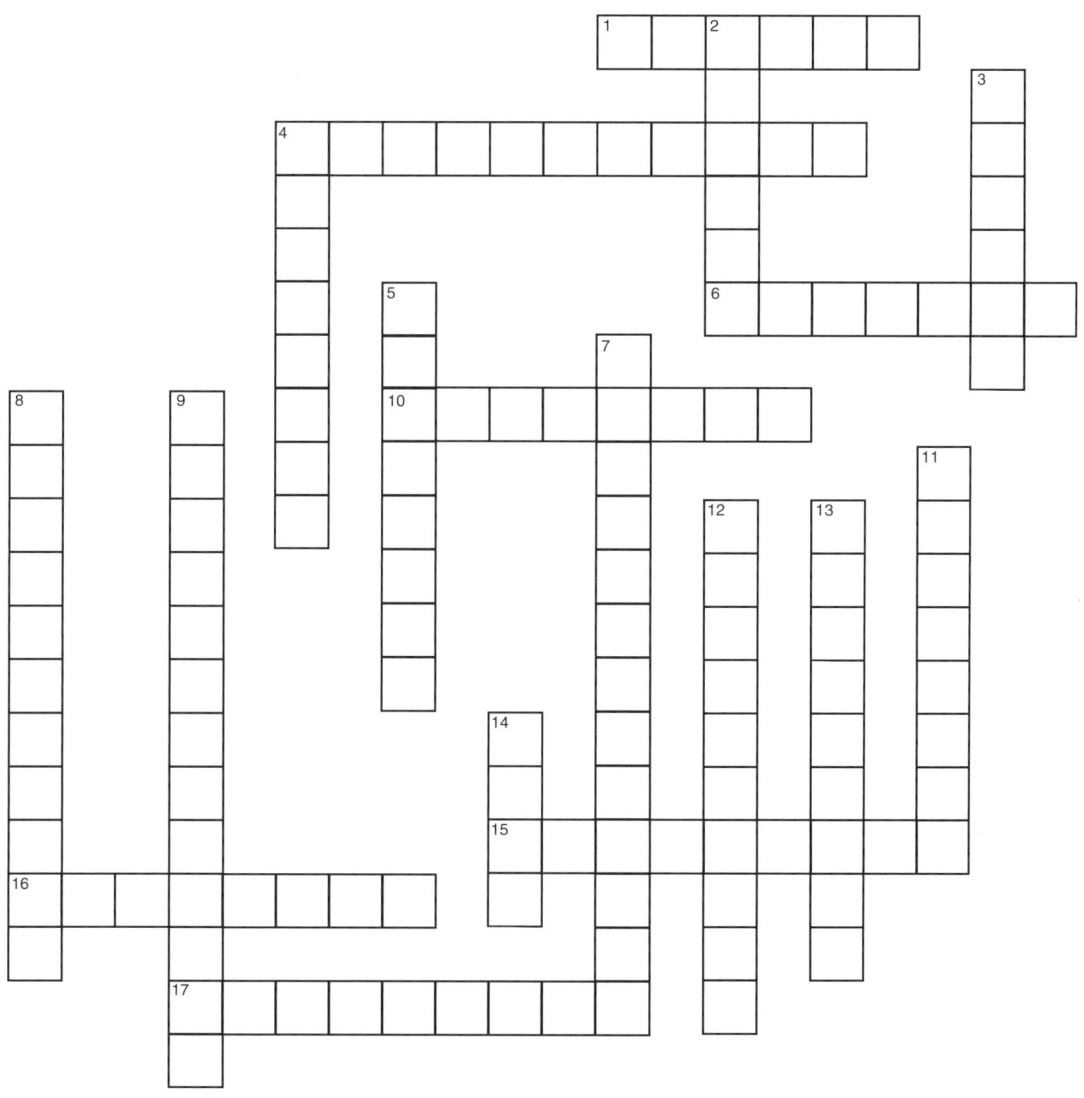

ACROSS

1. The sternum is _____ to the pectoral region.
4. On the same side of the median.
6. Farther from the mid-line.
10. Closer to the point of attachment.
15. Increasing the joint angle.
16. Front.
17. Moving away from the midline in the frontal plane.

DOWN

2. Another term for posterior.
3. The foot is _____ to the knee.
4. Below; caudal.
5. Another term for superior.
7. Multi-planar motion around a single point.
8. The scalp is _____ to the skull.
9. The eyes are _____ to one another.
11. Pivot around a single axis.
12. AB- or adduction in the transverse plane is referred to as _____.
13. The opposite of ABduction.
14. The bones are _____ to the skin.

EXERCISE 4 • Mix-and-Match Word Parts

Match the words in column A to their best definition from column B. Some of these words are made-up terms that you should be able to match by knowing the meaning of the prefix, suffix, and/or word root.

A:
_____ 1. Unicycle
_____ 2. Contradictions
_____ 3. Myositis
_____ 4. Interosseous membrane
_____ 5. Pseudonym
_____ 6. Tulipoma
_____ 7. Hemisphere
_____ 8. Malcontent
_____ 9. Retropatellar
_____ 10. Antechamber

B:
A. False name
B. One with poor socialization
C. One wheeled cycle
D. Opposing thoughts or ideas
E. Entry hall or room
F. Behind the knee cap
G. A membrane between two bones
H. Inflamed muscle tissue
I. Tumor on a cup-shaped flower
J. One half of a round object

Now that you get the idea, have some fun using the terms in Table 2-3 of the text to make up some of your own words and matching definitions.

Chapter 2 The Body and Its Terminology 21

EXERCISE 5 • Body Cavities Color and Label

Color both ventral cavities one color and the dorsal cavities another. Next, label each of the individual cavities. If you need to refresh your memory, refer to Figure 2-11 in your text.

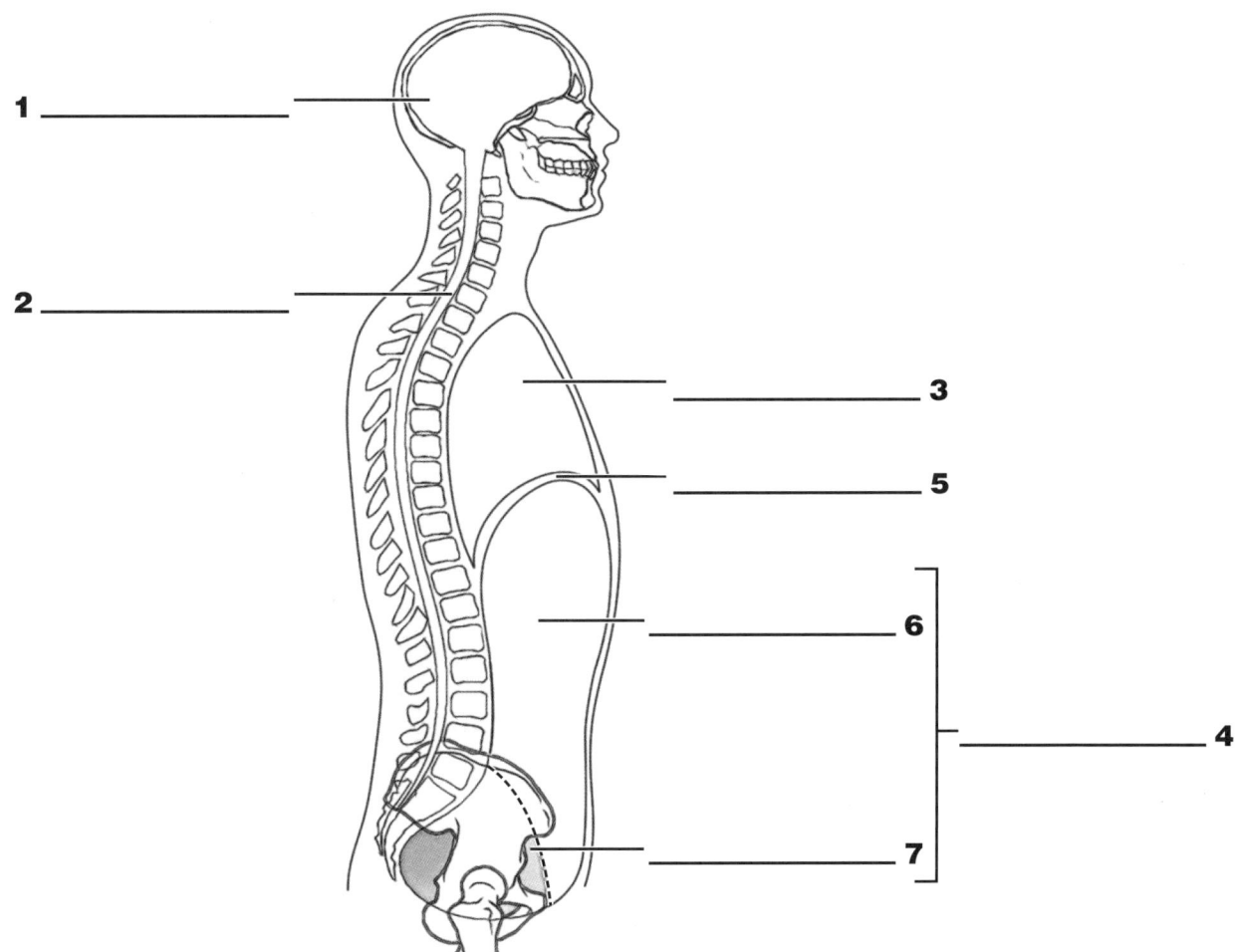

1 _____

2 _____

3 _____

5 _____

6 _____

4 _____

7 _____

EXERCISE 6 • Body Regions Matching

Match the name of the body region with the proper description.

_____1. Peroneal　　　　　A. Foot
_____2. Crural　　　　　　B. Head or cranium
_____3. Olecranal　　　　　C. Groin
_____4. Coxal　　　　　　D. Lower leg
_____5. Cephalic　　　　　E. Side of head
_____6. Thoracic　　　　　F. Back of hand
_____7. Pedal　　　　　　G. Posterior elbow
_____8. Sural　　　　　　H. Wrist
_____9. Temporal　　　　　I. Nose
_____10. Volar　　　　　　J. Lateral side of leg
_____11. Carpal　　　　　K. Lateral hip
_____12. Occipital　　　　L. Thigh; upper leg
_____13. Gluteals　　　　　M. Ribcage
_____14. Inguinal　　　　　N. Calf of leg
_____15. Lumbar　　　　　O. Armpit
_____16. Nasal　　　　　　P. Anterior upper chest
_____17. Femoral　　　　　Q. Posterior head
_____18. Axillary　　　　　R. Posterior knee
_____19. Pectoral　　　　　S. Low back
_____20. Popliteal　　　　　T. Buttocks

Chapter 2 The Body and Its Terminology 23

EXERCISE 7 • Body Regions Labeling

Label all of the body regions asked for on the diagram. If you need to refresh your memory, refer to Figures 2-8 through 2-10 in your text.

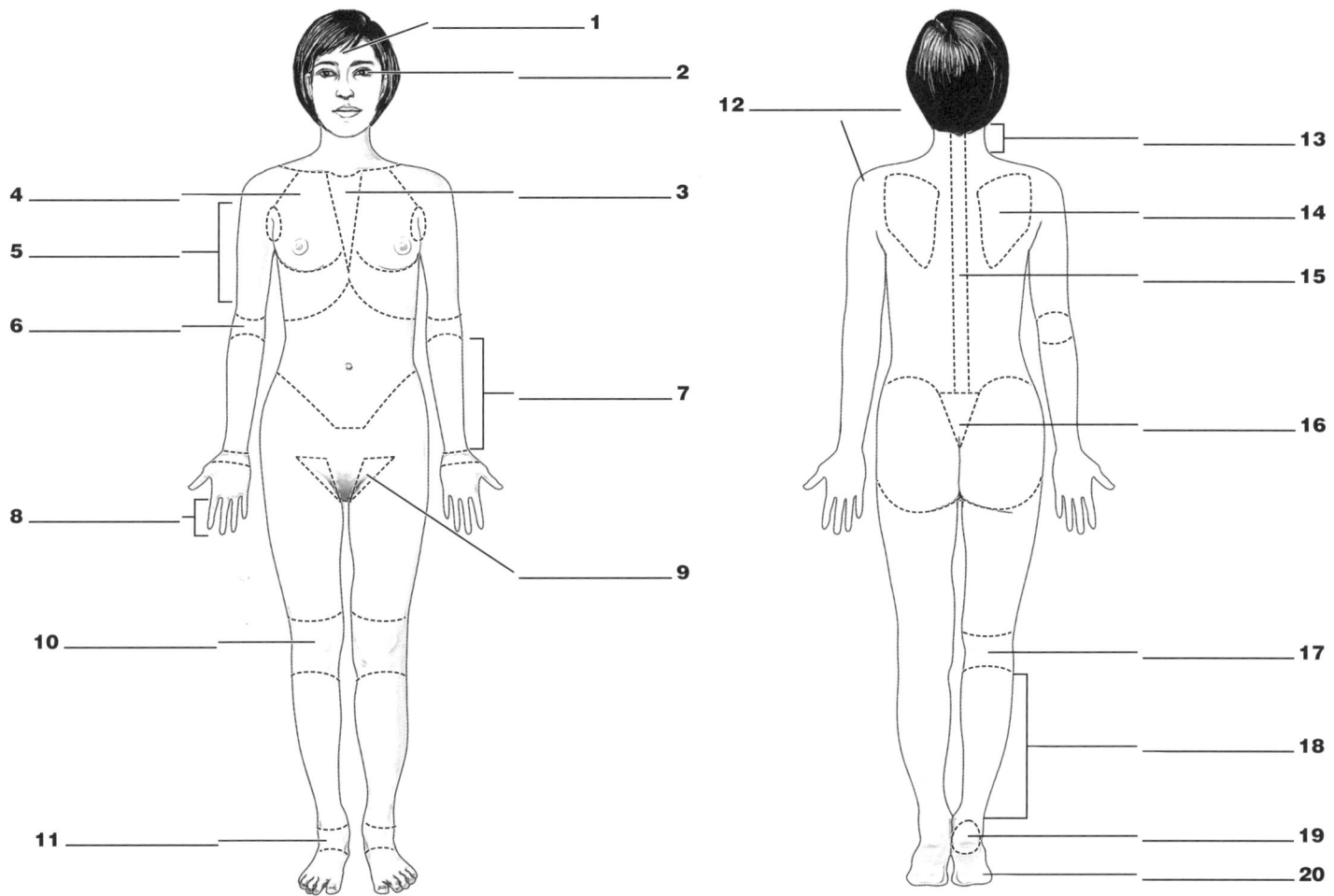

EXERCISE 8 • Abdominal Regions Labeling

Label all nine regions on the diagram. If you need to refresh your memory, refer to Figure 2-12B in your text.

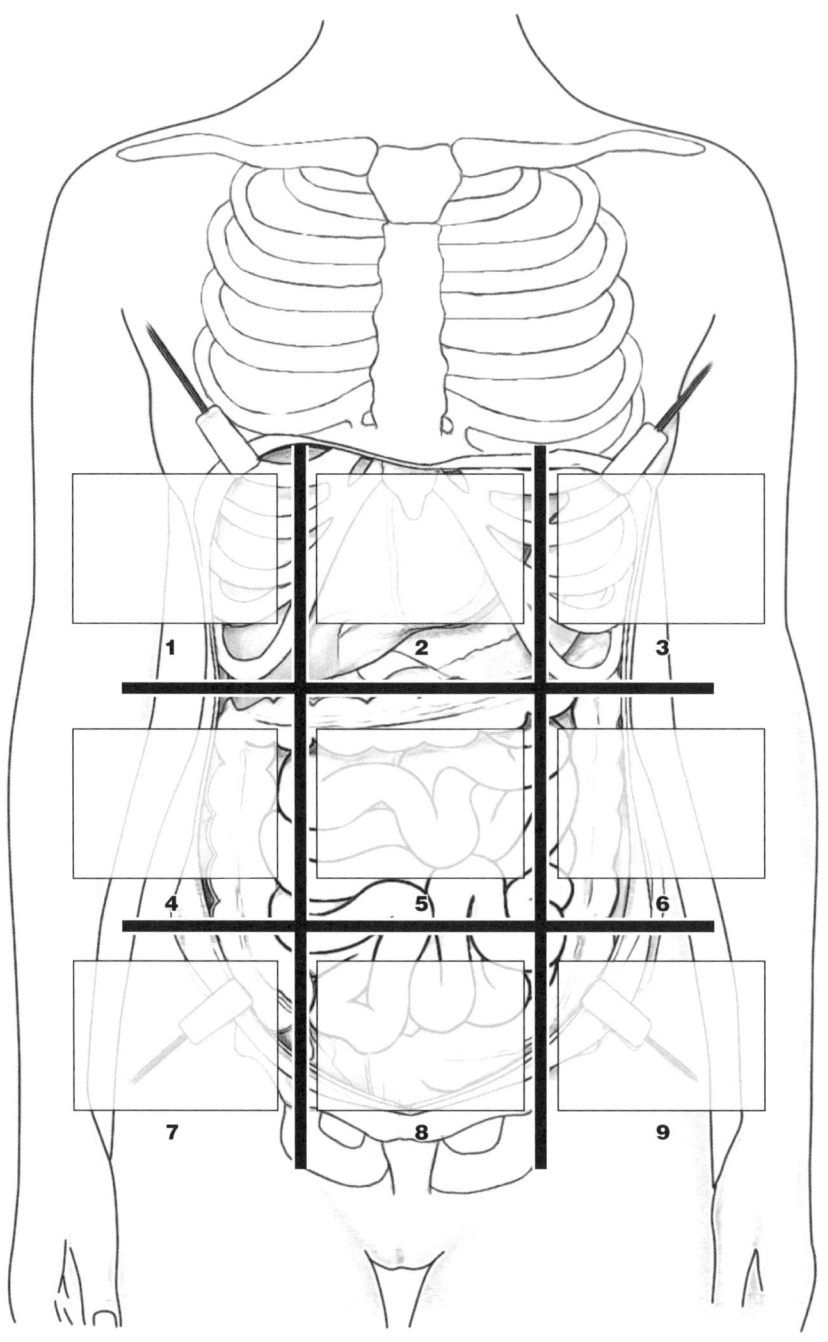

Chapter 2 The Body and Its Terminology

EXERCISE 9 • Pathology Terms Case Study

To review the pathology terms, answer the following questions using the case study below.

John Jones went to his doctor with a sore throat and headache. He explains that he has been feeling tired and generally run down for a few days, but yesterday he woke up with a severe sore throat that feels scratchy, swollen, and it hurts to swallow. He didn't sleep well last night and thinks he has a fever as well. The doctor's examination finds swollen lymph nodes in his neck, a fever of 102°, as well as red and pus-marked tonsils. He tells John that he has tonsillitis and that he needs to have his tonsils removed as soon as possible. The doctor believes John will recover completely within 2 or 3 days after surgery with a prescription of antibiotics.

1. What is the etiology?
   _____
   _____

2. What is the diagnosis?
   _____
   _____

3. What are the symptoms?
   _____
   _____

4. What are the signs?
   _____
   _____

5. What is the prognosis?
   _____
   _____

EXERCISE 10 • Classes of Disease Table

Fill in the spaces in the table below that lists the four major classifications of pathologies, their definition, and examples of each.

Disease Classification	Description	Example
Infectious	1.	2.
3.	4.	Lung cancer Mesothelioma Asbestosis
5.	Disease caused by particular genetic trait or flaw passed from one generation to the next	6.
Nutritional and Lifestyle	7.	8.

EXERCISE 11 • A&P Terminology Crossword

Use this crossword to review and test your ability to define a variety of terms from Chapter 2.

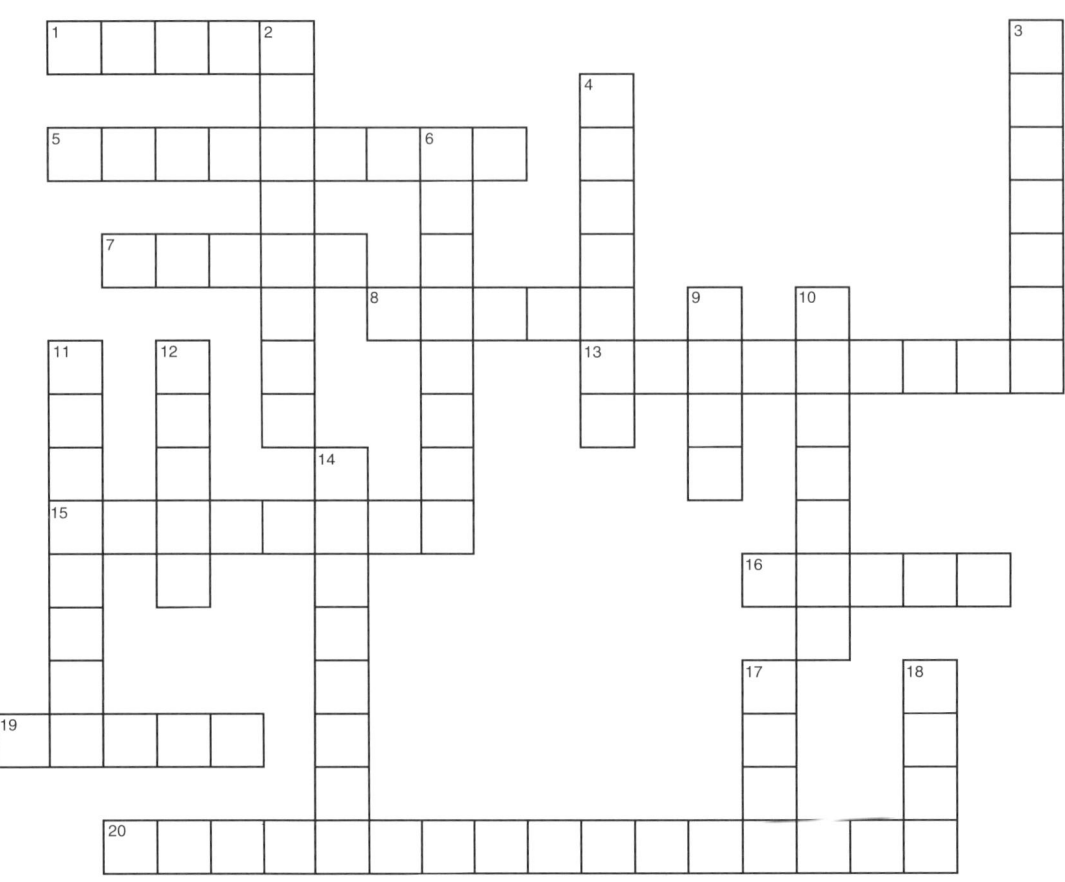

ACROSS

1. Sudden or rapid onset.
5. Posterior knee.
7. Tarsal.
8. The term arthritis means inflammation of a _____ (refer to your word parts).
13. Posterior elbow.
15. Neck region.
16. The prefix pseudo means _____.
19. A bone breaking cell could be called an osteo_____ (refer to your word parts).
20. A sign or symptom that could be made worse by a particular course of treatment.

DOWN

2. The cause of a disease.
3. Forehead.
4. A subjective indicator of disease.
6. Point of the shoulder.
9. To describe a layer around something else, the prefix _____ can be used.
10. Chronic diseases and conditions have a _____ or long-term onset.
11. Upper arm.
12. Fluid found within a cell can be called _____ cellular fluid (refer to your word parts).
14. Area of the shoulder blade.
17. Pedal.
18. A fever is a _____ of disease because it is measurable.

GROUP ACTIVITY 1 • Draw That Term!

This variation on the popular game Pictionary will allow two or more teams of players to review terminology in a new and fun way. If you actually have the game, you can play it as directed, except use your own terminology flash cards to provide the words for playing instead of the word cards provided with the actual Pictionary game. If you do not have a game board, use a point system to determine a winner. A turn starts when an illustrator draws a term from the pile of flash cards. The illustrator has 1 minute to try and illustrate the term for both teams. The team that guesses the term correctly receives a point. Choose another illustrator to draw a term from the pile and play again. The first team to 7 points wins.

GROUP ACTIVITY 2 • Concentration

The memory game Concentration can be used as a game for reviewing definitions and other flash card information. In this game, pairs of cards are placed face down and players take turns turning over cards and looking for matching pairs. If a player uncovers a match, he or she keeps the cards and gets another turn. If a player does not find a match, the next player takes his or her turn. To play this game, use your flash cards to create a set of cards with terms only and a set of cards with definitions only. Then place all the cards face down. A match is created when you locate both the term and its definition. This game challenges your memory to recall definitions as well as location of the cards. Also, it provides a more active learning experience than a pencil and paper matching exercise.

GROUP ACTIVITY 3 • Terminology Twister

This game can be played with three to six people.

- One caller
- Two to five players

Materials needed:

- One die
- Flash cards with body region terms. For decorum's sake, remove pectoral, pubic, genital, and inguinal regions from the pile.

Directions:

1. Determine which player will go first and the order of play.
2. The caller rolls the die to determine which hand the first player will be using for his or her turn. An odd number requires the player to use his or her right hand and an even number his or her left hand.
3. Next, the caller draws one card from the pile and announces the region on the card.
4. The first player places his or her hand as determined by step 2 on the announced body region of the second player and must maintain contact until directed to move that hand during another turn.
5. The caller repeats steps 2 and 3 for the second player who follows directions as outlined in step 4, and so forth for each player in the game.
6. Players can help each other with terminology.
7. The game ends when a player falls down or everybody decides to quit.

PRACTICE EXAM UNIT 1 • Chapters 1 & 2

1. What level of body organization does a group of like cells functioning together describe?

   A. Cells
   B. Tissues
   C. Organs
   D. Systems

2. The common qualities of all living organisms include functioning as a whole, use of nutrients, excretion of waste, reproduction, and a(n)

   A. requirement for oxygen and water to sustain life.
   B. skeletal or rigid framework.
   C. ability to move, grow, and adapt to their environment.
   D. ability to express and interpret emotions.

3. What is the anatomic term for the chest region of the body?

   A. Pectoral
   B. Thoracic
   C. Axillary
   D. Clavicular

4. According to the common medical terminology, the description of how things are put together is called and how they function is termed

   A. architecture and functionality.
   B. structure and action potential.
   C. anatomy and physiology.
   D. architecture and physiology.

5. What are the names of the two dorsal cavities of the body?

   A. Pelvic and thoracic
   B. Cranial and thoracic
   C. Vertebral and pelvic
   D. Cranial and spinal

6. Which of these is the best definition of homeostasis?

   A. The cooperative functions between body systems
   B. A range of physiologic balance, or dynamic state of equilibrium within the body
   C. The constant monitoring and regulation of all body responses
   D. The process of sensing and responding to changes in the external environment

7. Which of these physiologic effects is considered a structural effect?

   A. Relief of pain
   B. Increased circulation
   C. Loosening adhered connective tissue
   D. Improved sleep patterns

8. Reduced anxiety and an improved sense of overall health are examples of the _____ of manual therapy.

    A. systemic physiologic effects
    B. structural physiologic effects
    C. placebo effects
    D. benefits

9. The definition for all forms of reflexive or zone therapy is those that

    A. apply light or deep pressure to stimulate dermatomes, zones, or points of the body.
    B. gently slide over zones on the surface of the body to improve circulation of blood.
    C. employ Eastern forms of bodywork to stimulate emotional release and energy flow.
    D. apply deep and sustained pressure over defined energy points on the hands and feet.

10. Which cardinal plane divides the body into a right and left side?

    A. Coronal
    B. Horizontal
    C. Lateral
    D. Sagittal

11. Communication between and control of all other body systems are the functions of what body system?

    A. Skeletal
    B. Integumentary
    C. Circulatory
    D. Nervous

12. What is the anatomic term for the upper arm region of the body?

    A. Cubital
    B. Brachial
    C. Axillary
    D. Antecubital

13. What body plane divides the body into top and bottom?

    A. Sagittal
    B. Coronal
    C. Transverse
    D. Frontal

14. Hellerwork, Rolfing, and structural integration are all examples of what form of manual therapy?

    A. Swedish massage
    B. Deep tissue massage
    C. Neuromuscular
    D. Myofascial

15. What is the term for the organs, cells, or tissues that are signaled to change in order to maintain homeostasis?

    A. Effectors
    B. Integration centers
    C. Receptors
    D. Homeostatic organs

16. What anatomic term is used to describe the position of two structures on the same side of the sagittal plane?

    A. Contralateral
    B. Ipsilateral
    C. Unisagittal
    D. Homosagittal

17. Which body system helps regulate water and body temperature, serves as a large sensory organ, and provides a protective covering for the body?

    A. Sensory
    B. Integumentary
    C. Muscular
    D. Nervous

18. What is the term for movement away from the midline?

    A. Lateral rotation
    B. Horizontal flexion
    C. ABduction
    D. Adduction

19. Which of the two physiologic feedback mechanisms utilized to maintain homeostasis is most common?

    A. Negative
    B. Positive
    C. Neutral
    D. Autoregulation

20. What body system is responsible for returning proteins and 10% of capillary filtrate back into the bloodstream?

    A. Cardiovascular
    B. Digestive
    C. Respiratory
    D. Lymphatic

21. Which of the following forms of manual therapy techniques is best classified as a movement therapy?

    A. Active release
    B. Aston Patterning
    C. Swedish massage
    D. Trager

22. What is the simplest level of organization in the human body; the smallest unit capable of living on its own?

    A. Organ
    B. Cell
    C. Tissue
    D. Energy

23. What organ carries out key functions for both the digestive and endocrine systems?

    A. Spleen
    B. Liver
    C. Pancreas
    D. Kidneys

24. The location of the nose is best described as along the cardinal plane, and _____ to the eyes.

    A. transverse and lateral
    B. horizontal and superior
    C. sagittal and inferior
    D. anterior and medial

25. Using the nine-region method of dividing the abdominopelvic cavity, which of these is the best description of location for the pancreas?

    A. Left hypochondriac
    B. Epigastric
    C. Hypogastric
    D. Right hypochondriac

26. The four general classifications of diseases are environmental, hereditary, nutritional/lifestyle, and

    A. genetic.
    B. infectious.
    C. noncontagious.
    D. life threatening.

27. What medical term means the expected progression or outcome of a specific pathology?

    A. Diagnosis
    B. Sequela
    C. Etiology
    D. Prognosis

28. Which of these terms means that the specific cause of a disease or condition is unknown?

    A. Sequela
    B. Prognosis
    C. Idiopathic
    D. Etiology

29. What body region term describes the head?

    A. Cephalic
    B. Caudal
    C. Cervical
    D. Occipital

30. What word prefix means "related to or about the body?"

    A. humano-
    B. path- or patho
    C. myo-
    D. soma- or somato-

3 Chemistry, Cells, and Tissues

Use this table to identify the study guide exercises and group activities that will help you explore or review each learning objective for this chapter.

No.	Learning Objective	Exercise	Study Group Activity
1	Discuss the importance of understanding basic chemistry, structures, and functions of cells and tissues as they relate to the practice of manual therapy.		See Chapter 1—Activity 1
2	Name and explain the key inorganic and organic components of cells and tissues and explain the primary role of each.	1	1
3	Name the three structural components common to all cells and describe the general function of each.	2–4	1
4	Name and explain the function of the organelles in a cell.	2–4	1
5	Compare and contrast passive and active transport.	5	1
6	List and describe the different types of active and passive transport mechanisms.	5	1
7	Define, compare, and contrast cellular metabolism, anabolism, catabolism, cell division, and cell differentiation.	6	1
8	List the four categories of tissue found in the body, describe their distinguishing characteristics, and explain the general function and location of each.	7	1
9	Explain the different classifications of epithelial cells and tissues.	7	1
10	Name three types of muscle tissue and explain the distinguishing characteristics of each.	7	1
11	Name the two different types of nervous tissue and explain the function of each.	7	1
12	Name the common components of all types of connective tissue and list the different types of connective tissue and their common locations.	7	1

Chapter 3 Chemistry, Cells, and Tissues

EXERCISE 1 • Chemistry Crossword

Use this crossword to review and test your ability to define the chemistry terms and concepts from Chapter 3.

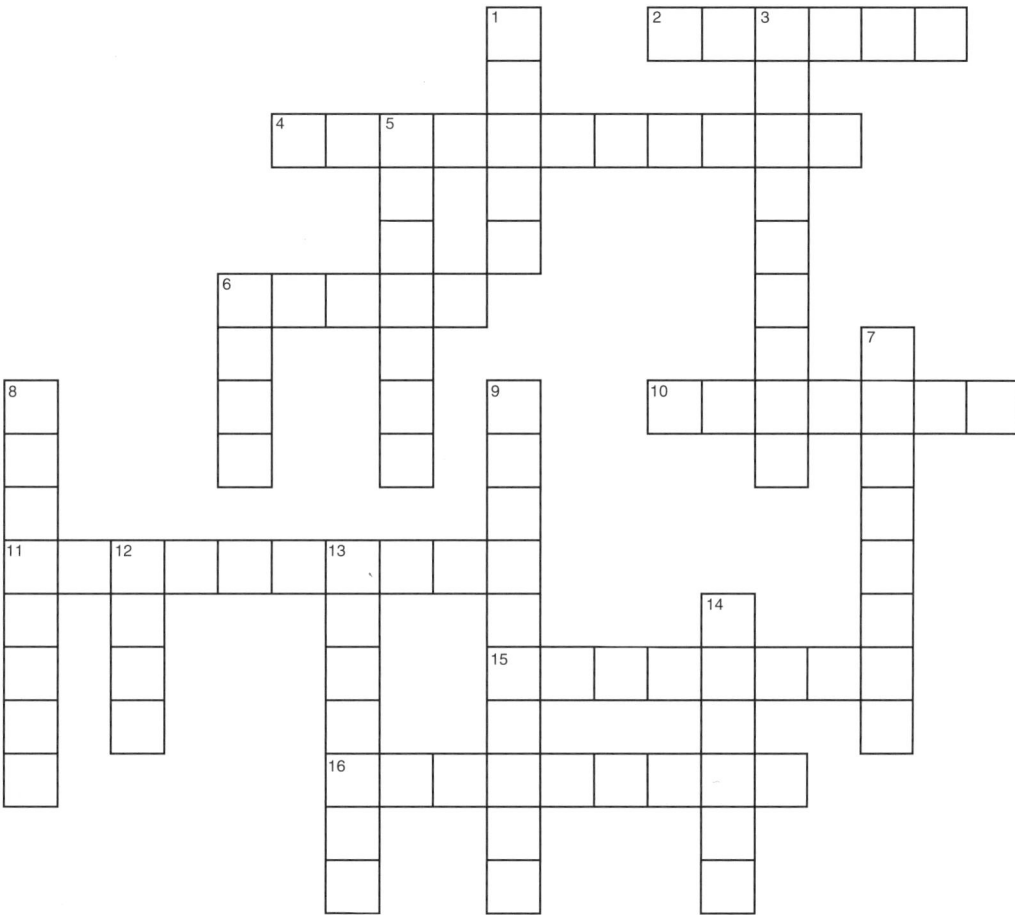

ACROSS

2 Fats.
4 Another name for an inorganic salt.
6 Small invisible units of energy that make up all elements.
10 A simple sugar; example of a carbohydrate.
11 Proteins are made of chains of 50–100 of these molecules.
15 As a free ion, _____ makes substances more acidic.
16 Compounds without carbon atoms.

DOWN

1 The compound comprised of 2 hydrogen atoms plus 1 oxygen atom.
3 Most abundant ion in intracellular fluid.
5 A molecule made from identical atoms.
6 A substance with a pH below 7.
7 A molecule made of two or more different atoms.
8 A synonym for basic.
9 Nucleic acids differ from proteins because they include these atoms.
12 Charged atoms or molecules.
13 This ion is important for muscle contraction, blood clotting, and bone structure.
14 Na^+.

EXERCISE 2 • Cellular Components Flow Chart

Place the terms into the flow chart to organize the information about cellular components.

centrosome
channel protein
cytoplasm
cytoskeleton
cytosol
DNA
effector proteins
endoplasmic reticulum
genes
genetic blueprint
Golgi apparatus
IMPs
linker protein
lysosomes
mitochondria
nuclear envelope
nucleolus
nucleus
organelles
organic compounds
phospholipid
plasma membrane
receptor proteins
ribosomes
transport protein
vesicle
water

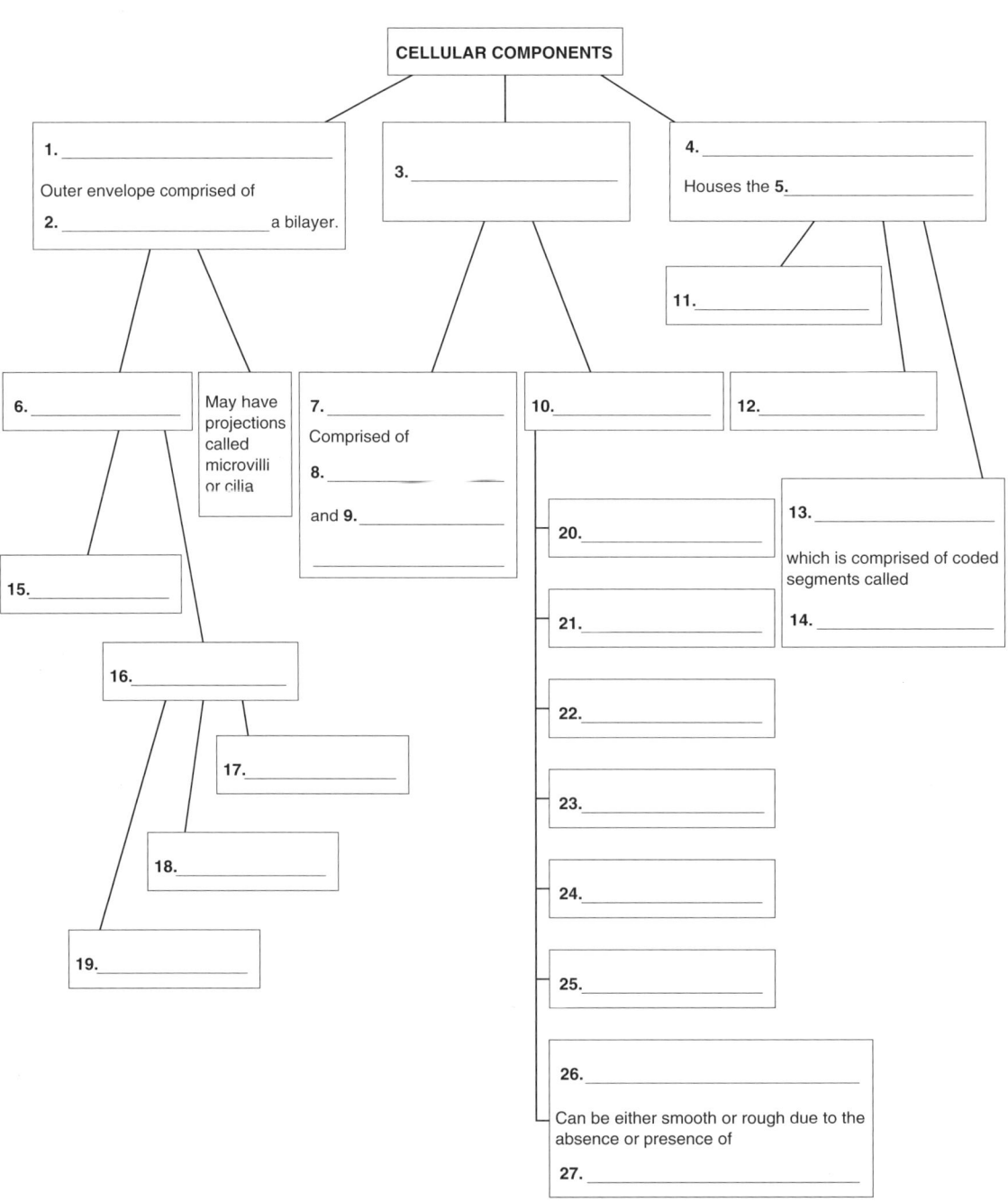

Chapter 3 Chemistry, Cells, and Tissues 37

EXERCISE 3 • Color and Label a Cell

Use this diagram to color and label the different components of the cell. If you need to refresh your memory, refer to Figure 3-4 in the text.

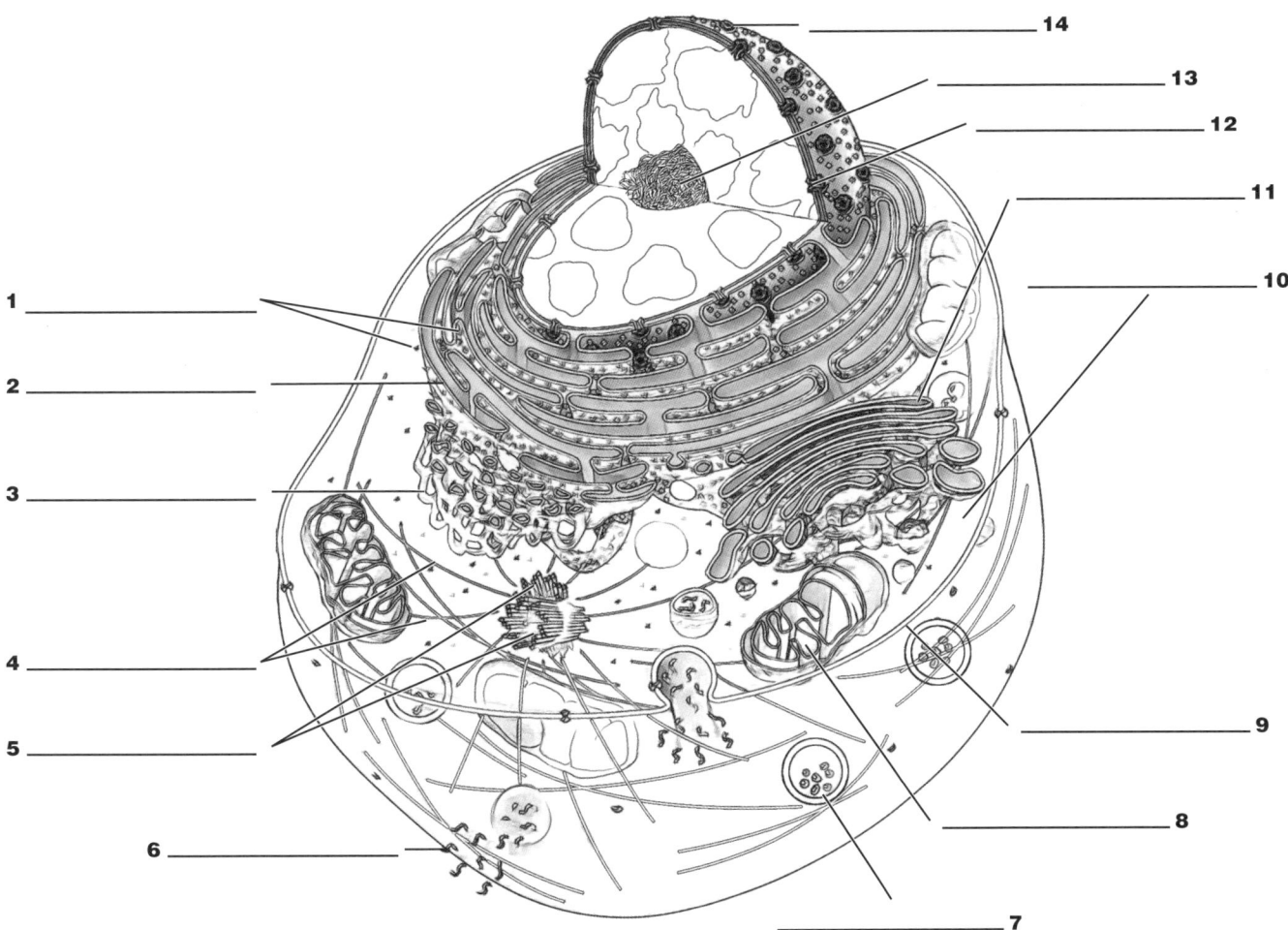

EXERCISE 4 • A Cell Analogy

Fill in the blanks for the following analogy for the cell.

A cell is like a city.

- The city limits resemble the **1.** _____ _____. This boundary surrounds the city and controls what comes in and what goes out.

- The town hall is the **2.** _____. It contains the Hall of Records that houses all the laws, building blueprints, and other records and is synonymous with the **3.** _____.

- The **4.** _____ are represented by the city's power plants that provide energy for the city.

- Because they provide protein, the numerous restaurants found within the city limits are **5.** _____.

- Delivery vehicles are **6.** _____ because they package items and deliver them to the city limits to be exported.

- The **7.** _____ of the cell are represented by the dump where food and trash are broken down.

- City roads resemble the **8.** _____ because they are transportation passageways. Some roads are **9.** _____ with lots of protein factories (restaurants, see #5), while others are **10.** _____.

Can you extend the analogy to include other components like IMPs, the centrosome, or the cytoskeleton?

EXERCISE 5 • Cellular Transport

Two-thirds of the total water in the human body can be found inside the cells; this fluid is known as **1.** _____ _____. The remaining one-third called **2.** _____ makes up the liquid component of blood, lymph, and the fluid that fills the small spaces between cells, called **3.** _____ _____. This fluid constantly circulates around the cells providing a dynamic medium from which nutrients are extracted and wastes released to support cellular activities. Movement of substances across the cell membrane can be divided into two general categories:

- **4.** _____ Transport—Mechanisms in which the cell does not expend energy because substances move according to either a concentration or pressure gradient.

- **5.** _____ Transport—Mechanisms that require the cell to use ATP because substances are being moved against the concentration gradient, engulfed, or secreted.

Which transport mechanisms are represented by the following diagrams?

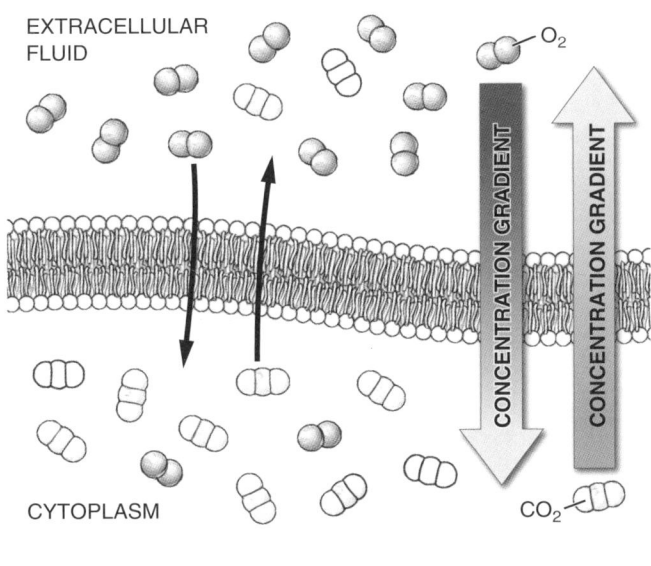

A _____

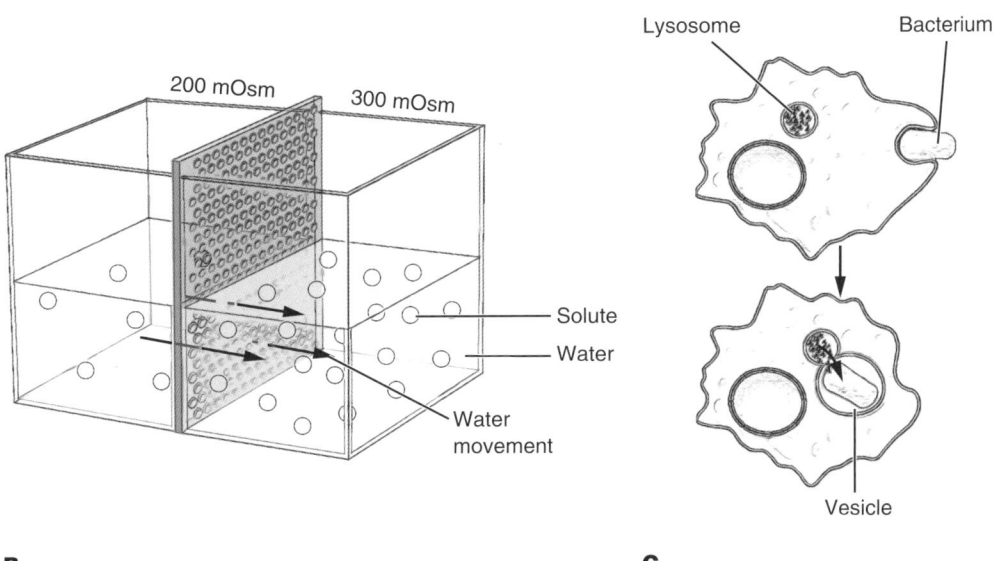

B _____   C _____

EXERCISE 6 • Cellular Processes Matching

Match the terms with their definition.

_____ 1. Metabolism   A. The storage form of glucose

_____ 2. Catabolism   B. The division of cytoplasm

_____ 3. Anabolism   C. A cell that can produce different types of cells

_____ 4. Protein synthesis   D. Chemical processes

_____ 5. Glycogen   E. Cell eating

_____ 6. Mitosis   F. A process of building up

_____ 7. Cytokinesis   G. Cellular reproductive process

_____ 8. Meiosis   H. Division of sex cells

_____ 9. Differentiation   I. A process of breaking down or apart

_____ 10. Stem cell   J. Secretion occurs through this process

_____ 11. Embryonic layer   K. A layer of cells that produces specific tissues

_____ 12. Filtration   L. Amino acid anabolism

_____ 13. Cell division   M. Passive transport with the pressure gradient

_____ 14. Phagocytosis   N. Nuclear division

_____ 15. Exocytosis   O. The process of cell specialization

EXERCISE 7 • Histology Concept Map

A concept map is an organizing tool. While similar to a mind map (Chapter 1, Exercises 10 and 11), a concept map goes further by asking you to show the relationship between linked items. Concept maps help you show and explain a hierarchy of information as you describe big ideas with supporting details. Look at the example below. Notice how it shows a flow of information from big ideas to smaller details. Each connecting line or stem is accompanied by a descriptive phrase or linking words that describe the connection represented by the stem.

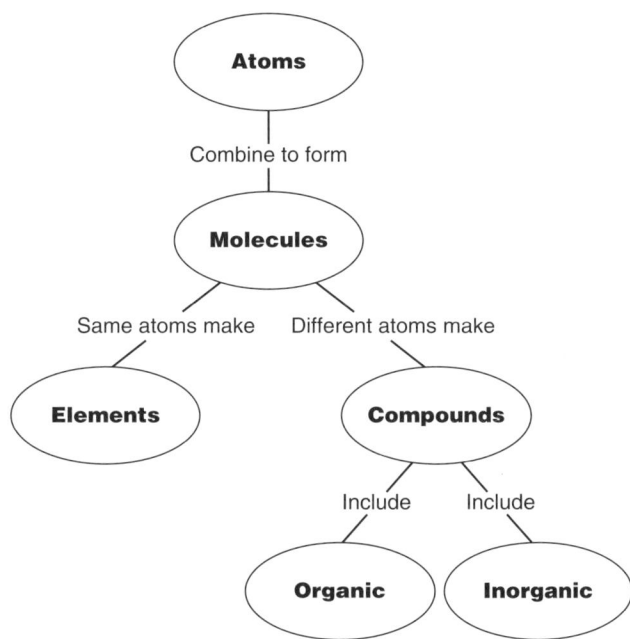

Using the terms and phrases provided, follow the directions to create your own histology concept map. You may want to refer to Tables 3-2 and 3-3 in your text to help with this activity.

Directions:

1. Pick out the largest or main concept(s) from the terms and phrases list provided.
2. Categorize the remaining terms and phrases according to your large concepts.
3. Rank the terms and phrases in each category listing them from most general to most specific. Cluster related ideas.
4. Arrange items in a downward flowing, branching structure and connect them with stems.
5. Add appropriate linking words to the stems to describe the connection represented.
6. Develop any cross linkages or connecting points you see now that your flow chart has been created.

Terms and phrases:

adipose
appearance and nervous system control
areolar
avascular
blood
bone
brain
cardiac
cartilage
cells
columnar
conductile
conducts electrical impulses
connective
covering organs
cuboidal
dense
disorganized
elastic
epithelium
fascia
fibers
fibrocartilage
fibrous
glial cells
ground substance
heart
hyaline
involuntary
ligament
lines, covers, protects, and secretes
lining body cavities
liquid
loose
lymph
muscle
nerves
nervous
neurons
nonconductile
nonstriated
organized
posture and movement
pseudostratified
reticular
shape and arrangement
simple
skeletal
skeletal muscles
skin
smooth or visceral
spinal cord
spongy
squamous
stratified
striated
supports, connects, protects, transports
supports, protects, and insulates neurons
tendon
types of tissues
voluntary
walls of internal organs and vessels

GROUP ACTIVITY 1 • Concept Mapping Together

The concept map activity described in Exercise 7 can be adapted in several ways to become a group activity. Here are some options:

- Work individually to create your concept maps. Then when finished, share and explain your creations to one another. This group activity will help expand everyone's thinking about the main topic as you see the various ways that people connect the same terms, phrases, and concepts.
- Create the concept map together. Again this will help expand everyone's thinking, but the comparison of connections comes through discussion as you work together to organize the terms and phrases into one concept map.
- Break your group into two or more teams. Each team produces a list of terms, phrases, or concepts that they would like to see organized into a concept map. Then exchange lists. Each team creates and presents a concept map for a list of terms and phrases provided by another team.

4 Body Membranes and the Integumentary System

Use this table to identify the study guide exercises and group activities that will help you explore or review each learning objective for this chapter.

No.	Learning Objective	Exercise	Study Group Activity
1	Discuss the importance of understanding the anatomy and physiology of the integumentary system as it relates to the practice of manual therapy.		See Chapter 1, Activity 1
2	Name the four types of membranes in the body and provide an example of each.	1, 2, 8	See Chapter 2, Activity 1
3	Describe the structure and list the general functions of each type of membrane.	1, 2, 8	
4	Name and explain the functions of the integumentary system, and describe the general structure and function of each layer of the skin.	1, 3, 4, 8	See Chapter 1, Activity 2
5	List the primary accessory organs of the skin and explain the function of each.	1, 4–6, 8	See Chapter 2, Activity 1
6	Name and explain the functions of hair, nails, and glands of the skin.	1, 5, 6, 8	
7	Name and explain the specific functions of cutaneous receptors, and describe their general location.	1, 5, 6, 8	
8	Discuss the links between the integumentary and nervous systems, and the importance of touch for neurological development and overall health.	8	See Chapter 1, Activity 1
9	List the four types of contagious skin conditions and provide an example of each.	1, 7, 8	See Chapter 2, Activity 1
10	List and describe the general signs and symptoms of several common noncontagious skin disorders and the ABCD warning signs of skin cancer.	1, 7, 8	See Chapter 2, Activity 1
11	Describe common integumentary system changes associated with aging and their implications for the practice of manual therapy.	8	See Chapter 1, Activity 1

EXERCISE 1 • Terminology Crossword

Use this crossword to review and test your ability to define the terms from Chapter 4.

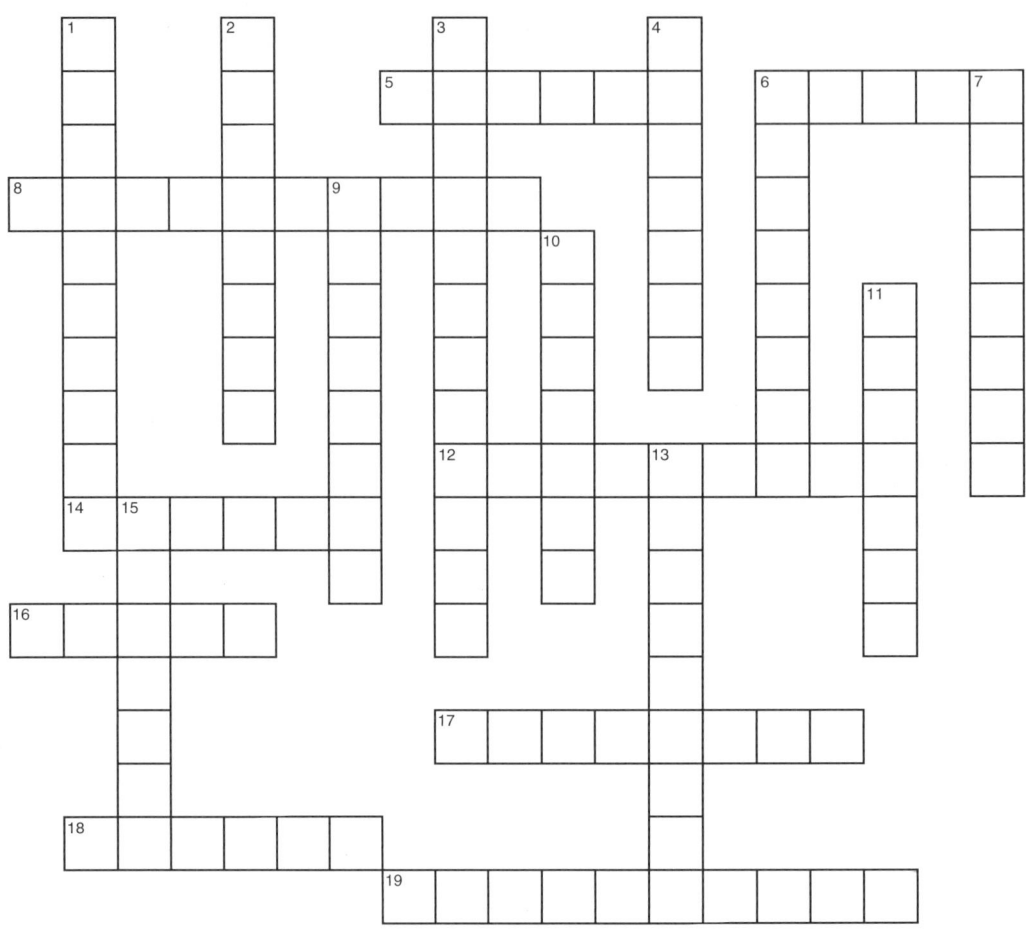

ACROSS

5. The arrector pili is a small _____ attached to the hair follicle.
6. The oil produced by the sebaceous glands of the skin.
8. A free nerve ending sensitive to chemicals released by tissue trauma; a "pain receptor".
12. The deeper region of the dermis.
14. Layers.
16. The thick and clear secretion produced by the membranes that line cavities with openings to the external environment.
17. The inner layer of a serous membrane.
18. The deeper connective tissue layer of the skin.
19. The ability to stretch.

DOWN

1. The superficial fascia; subcutaneous layer.
2. A specialized sweat gland found in the axilla and groin that becomes active at puberty.
3. All sweat glands are classified as _____ glands.
4. A brown skin pigment.
6. A connective tissue membrane that lines joint capsules.
7. The most serious type of skin cancer is malignant _____.
9. The outer layer of a serous membrane.
10. The tough water resistant substance found in many cells of the epidermis.
11. A common sweat gland.
13. The membrane that forms the skin together with the accessory organs.
15. This general sense includes the sensations of touch pressure, vibration itch and tickle.

EXERCISE 2 • Membranes Organizational Chart

Fill in the blanks of the organizational chart to visually organize the information about body membranes.

MEMBRANES

Definition = 1. Broad flat sheet of @ least 2 layers of tissue

Broadly classified as

2. Connective tissue

3. Epithelial

includes

5. Synovial Fluid
Structure: Joint capsules of synovial joints
Function: Protection, production of synovial fluid
Examples: Shoulder, elbow, hip, knee

5. Mucous
Structure: Lining cavities outside the environment
Function: Protection, production of mucus
Examples: Resp. Tract, GS Tract, urinary tract, vaginal tract

6. Serous
Structure: Peritoneum, pleura, pericardium
Function: Protection, production of serous fluid
Examples: Lines cavities in an enclosed environment

7. Cutaneus
Structure: Skin covers body
Function: Protection
Examples: Skin

EXERCISE 3 • Functional Mnemonic

In Chapter 1, Exercise 3 mnemonics were introduced as helpful memory cues for recalling lists of information. While this is true, learners must be careful to not confuse recall with understanding. Fill in the blanks below to come up with your own mnemonic for remembering the functions of the integumentary system. Additionally, explain each function of the skin to be sure you understand the function completely.

Protection—P _____
_____

Temperature regulation—T _____
_____

Excretion—E _____
_____

Absorption—A _____
_____

General sensory organ—G _____
_____

Synthesis of vitamin D—S _____
_____

Chapter 4 Body Membranes and the Integumentary System 47

EXERCISE 4 • Label and Color the Skin Diagram

Complete the diagram by labeling and coloring the structures of the skin.

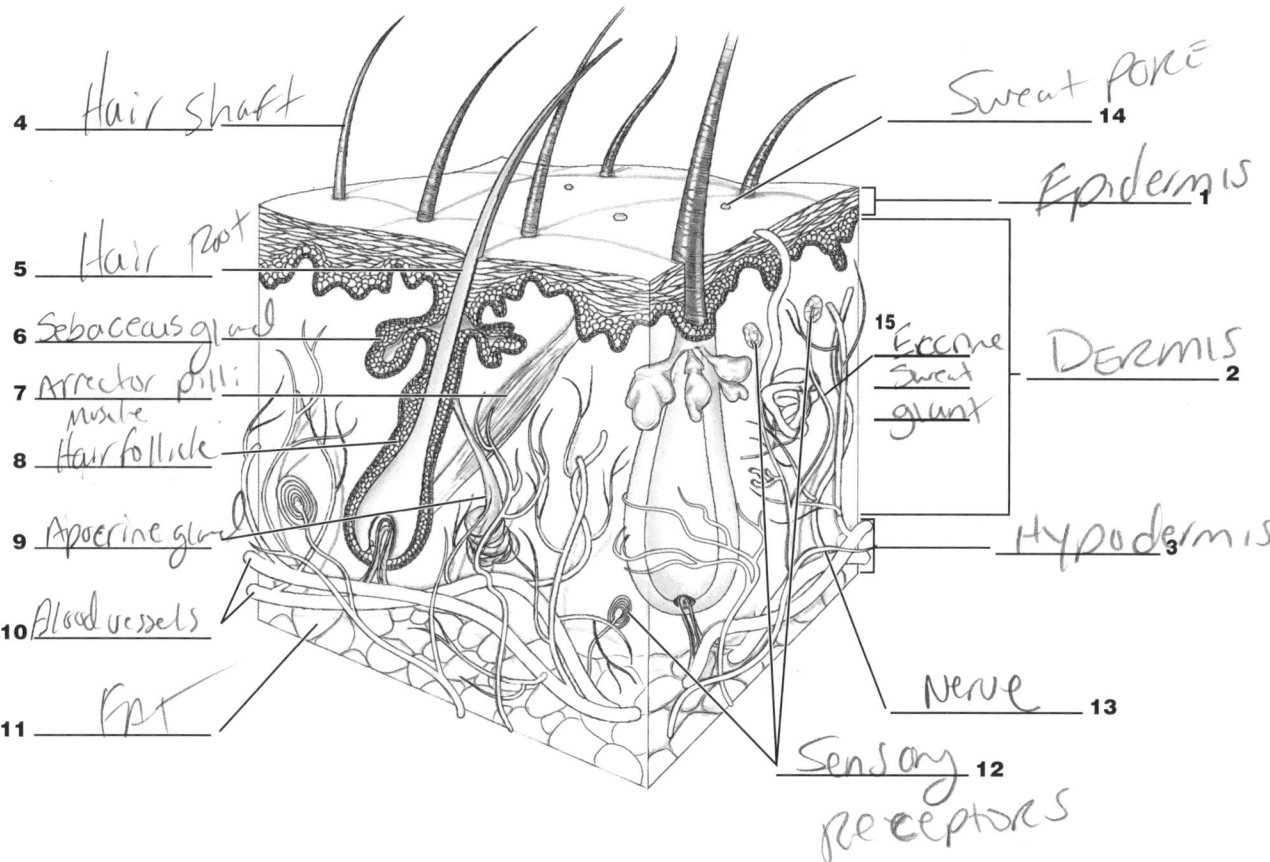

4. Hair shaft
5. Hair Root
6. Sebaceous gland
7. Arrector pilli muscle
8. Hair follicle
9. Apocrine gland
10. Blood vessels
11. Fat
12. Sensory receptors
13. Nerve
14. Sweat pore
15. Eccrine sweat gland
1. Epidermis
2. Dermis
3. Hypodermis

Study & Review Guide for Applied Anatomy and Physiology for Manual Therapists

EXERCISE 5 • Can You Picture It?

Because memories are often stored visually, it can be easier to recall images instead of remembering specific verbal explanations. Instead of structural diagrams and words, try drawing pictures or doodles that represent the functions of each of the following accessory organs of the skin.

Cutaneous receptors

Hair

Nails

Sebaceous gland

Sudoriferous gland

Chapter 4 Body Membranes and the Integumentary System

EXERCISE 6 • Matching Structures and Functions

Match the structures below with their specific functions.

___E___ 1. Hair follicle
___I___ 2. Fingernail
___D___ 3. Arrector pili
___L___ 4. Sebaceous gland
___C___ 5. Sudoriferous gland
___H___ 6. Eccrine gland
___M___ 7. Apocrine gland
___B___ 8. Nociceptor
___K___ 9. Merkel disc
___F___ 10. Meissner corpuscle
___N___ 11. Pacinian corpuscle
___G___ 12. Ruffini corpuscle
___J___ 13. Hair root plexus
___O___ 14. Sebum
___A___ 15. Epidermis

A. Protects the body from invading pathogens and the sun
B. Sensitive to chemicals released by tissue damage
C. Produces sweat
D. Contracts to raise hairs trapping air for insulation of skin
E. Tube that shapes hair shaft as it grows
F. Sensitive to vibration and light touch
G. Sensitive to deep touch, pressure, and tissue distortion
H. Excretes sweat for thermal and water regulation only
I. Protects fingers; helps us scratch and grasp small objects
J. Senses movement of hair shaft
K. Sensitive to light touch
L. Excretes oil
M. Excretes sweat with traces of lipids and pheromones
N. Sensitive to high-frequency vibrations and deep pressure
O. Lubricates and softens the outer surface of the skin

EXERCISE 7 • Pathology Mind Map

Fill in the mind map to visually organize the information on diseases of the skin. You may want to add items to your map such as specific examples, signs, or symptoms of some of the skin conditions.

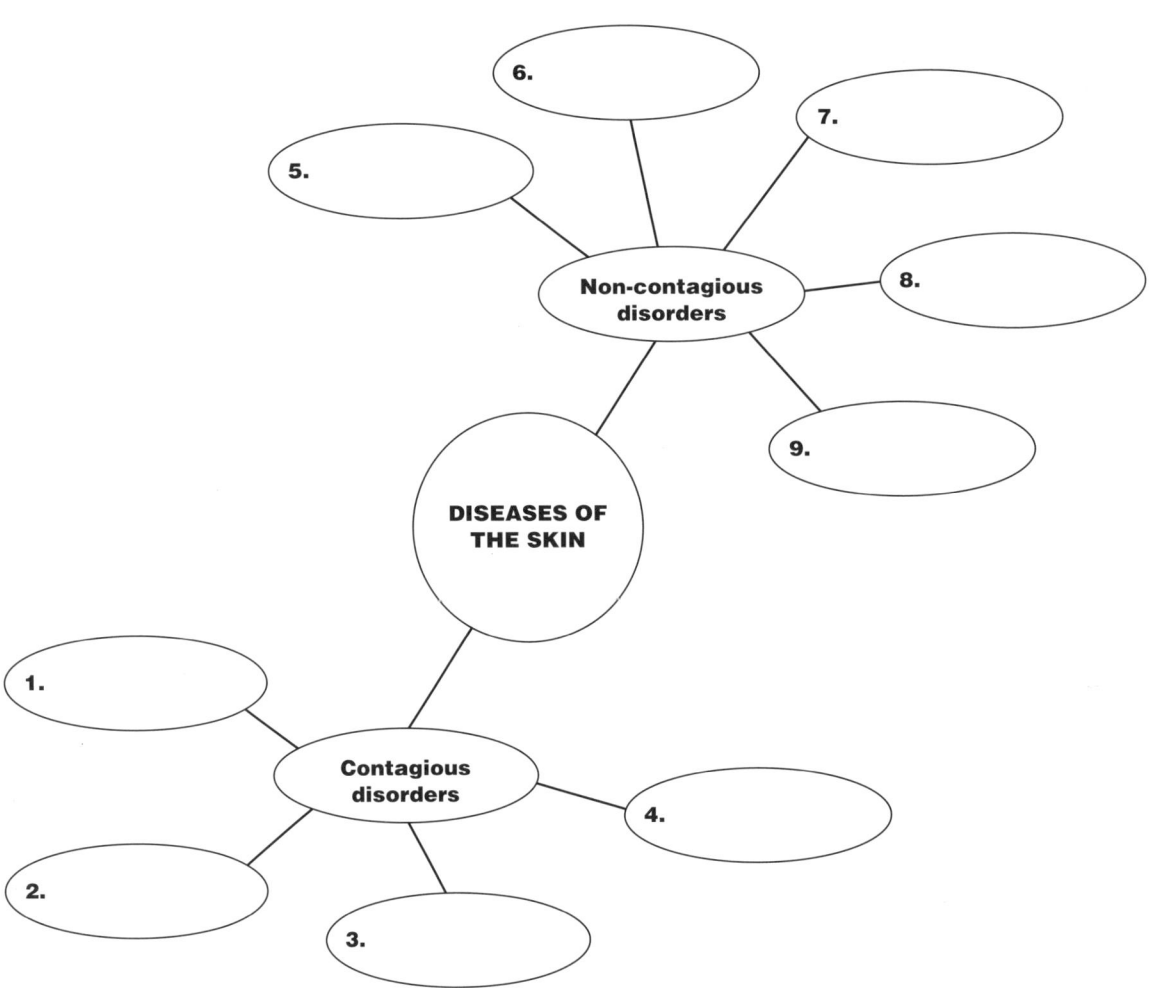

EXERCISE 8 • Pestilent Poetry

You may be more comfortable reading and writing poetry and song lyrics than science and medical terminology. Consider applying your talent to help you remember anatomy, physiology, or pathology terms and concepts. Write a Limerick about Boils or a Sonnet to Psoriasis. Perhaps write a song about the layers of the skin, a cutaneous receptors rap, or rework the functions of the integumentary system as lyrics to the theme song from a favorite TV show or movie. Use your imagination.

Here is an example from 18th century Scottish poet Robert Burns. It's a bit disgusting, but it creates a vivid image.

Ode to the Louse

Ye ugly, creepin, blastit wonner,
Detested, shunn'd by saunt an' sinner,
How daur ye set your fit upon her -
Sae fine a lady!
Gae somewhere else and seek your dinner
On some poor body.

PRACTICE EXAM UNIT 2 • Chapters 3 & 4

1. Atoms bind together to form microscopic particles called what?

    A. Cells
    B. Compounds
    C. Elements
    D. Electrolytes

2. Compounds that release hydroxide ions in water are called bases, and they are designated as such by having a pH value of

    A. acidic; under 7.
    B. base; over 7.
    C. base; under 7.
    D. acidic; over 7.

3. The three types of epithelial membranes in the body are cutaneous,

    A. serous, and synovial.
    B. mucous, and synovial.
    C. parietal, and visceral.
    D. serous, and mucous.

4. What type of compound always contains carbon molecules?

    A. Inorganic
    B. Alkaline
    C. Acidic
    D. Organic

5. Which type of membrane lines the respiratory and digestive tract?

    A. Serous
    B. Mucous
    C. Synovial
    D. Cutaneous

6. What is the name of the membrane that lines the thoracic cavity?

    A. Parietal pleura
    B. Visceral pleura
    C. Parietal peritoneum
    D. Visceral peritoneum

7. The three common structural components of almost all cells in the body are a nucleus, cytoplasm, and

    A. cellular receptors.
    B. plasma membrane.
    C. demiorgans.
    D. alkaline membrane.

8. Skin cells that produce pigment are called
   A. pigment cells.
   B. keratinocytes.
   C. melanocytes.
   D. fibrocytes.

9. Which layer of skin is made up of fat tissue?
   A. Epidermis
   B. Dermis
   C. Hypodermis
   D. Hyperdermis

10. Which cellular organelle has the responsibility of providing a pathway for substances to move throughout the cell?
    A. Endoplasmic reticulum
    B. Mitochondria
    C. Golgi apparatus
    D. Lysosomes

11. What cell structure allows the cell to read and respond to its environment?
    A. Nucleus
    B. Mitochondria
    C. Endoplasmic reticulum
    D. Integral membrane proteins

12. The functions of the integumentary system are protection, absorption and secretion, synthesis of vitamin D,
    A. providing emergency nutrition, and regulating pH.
    B. temperature regulation, and sensory organ.
    C. sensory map, and stimulation of emotions.
    D. temperature regulation, and synthesis of sebum.

13. Which layer of skin contains the blood vessels and sensory receptors?
    A. Epidermis
    B. Dermis
    C. Subcutaneous
    D. Hypodermis

14. What structure in the cell produces the energy molecule ATP?
    A. Mitochondria
    B. Endoplasmic reticulum
    C. Lysosome
    D. Centrosome

15. The process of making new protein is controlled and directed by which structure in a cell?
    A. Nucleic proteins inside the nucleus
    B. Golgi apparatus in the cytoplasm
    C. Effector proteins in the plasma membrane
    D. Lysosome organelles

16. How much of the total water in a human body is intracellular fluid inside the cells?

    A. One-half
    B. One-quarter
    C. One-third
    D. Two-thirds

17. What layer of skin is also considered to be the superficial fascia of the body?

    A. Subcutaneous
    B. Dermis
    C. Papillary layer of dermis
    D. Granular layer of the epidermis

18. Which passive transport mechanism for moving things across the cell membrane occurs when there is a concentration gradient?

    A. Filtration
    B. Diffusion
    C. Facilitated diffusion
    D. Pinocytosis

19. What is the term for the passive transport process where water moves from an area of higher to lower concentration?

    A. Hydrofiltration
    B. Facilitated diffusion
    C. Osmosis
    D. Oncotic motion

20. What is the function of keratin in skin?

    A. Adds pigment to the epidermis to protect it from sun
    B. Toughens the epidermis and makes it water-resistant
    C. Serves as a natural emollient for all layers of skin
    D. Stimulates the sudoriferous glands

21. What kind of pressure is created when fluids press against a barrier?

    A. Osmotic
    B. Oncotic
    C. Hyperhydrotic
    D. Hydrostatic

22. What type of cellular transportation is it when ATP is used to transport things up a concentration or pressure gradient?

    A. Diffusion
    B. Facilitated diffusion
    C. Active transport
    D. Osmosis

23. Which of the following is an example of anabolism?

    A. Protein synthesis
    B. Breaking fat into fatty acids
    C. Using ATP for energy
    D. Pinocytosis

24. What type of stem cells is only capable of producing blood, bone marrow, fat, bone, ligament, and muscle cells?

    A. Totipotent
    B. Pluripotent
    C. Multipotent
    D. Omnipotent

25. When the nucleus duplicates its DNA and then divides to form two identical nuclei with the same genetic blueprint, it is called _____.

    A. cytokinesis
    B. mitosis
    C. meiosis
    D. nucleic partitioning

26. What is the anatomic name for sweat glands?

    A. Keritinocytes
    B. Sebaceous
    C. Sudoriferous
    D. Extrariferous

27. What type of gland secretes a milking, slightly viscous fluid that contains pheromones?

    A. Sebaceous
    B. Eccrine
    C. Merocrine
    D. Apocrine

28. The four types of tissue in the body are epithelial, connective, muscle, and

    A. skeletal.
    B. liquid.
    C. nervous.
    D. blood.

29. Which of the four types of tissue is "avascular?"

    A. Connective
    B. Epithelial
    C. Muscular
    D. Skeletal

30. Which type of muscle tissue is described as striated and involuntary?

    A. Skeletal
    B. Visceral
    C. Cardiac
    D. Fibrous

31. What types of stimulus are the cutaneous receptors of the skin sensitive to?

    A. Touch, pressure, temperature, pain
    B. Pain, pressure, torsion, tearing
    C. Vibration, cold, movement, light
    D. Light, temperature, pain, chemicals

32. Pacinian and Ruffini corpuscles as well as the hair root plexus of skin are all examples of what type of cutaneous receptor?

    A. Nociceptors
    B. Temperature receptors
    C. Light tactile receptors
    D. Deep tactile receptors

33. What type of cells form nervous tissue that protects, insulates, and is nonconductile?

    A. Neurilemma
    B. Neurons
    C. Neuroglial
    D. Neuronocytes

34. The three kinds of cells present in high numbers in almost all kinds of connective tissue are fibroblasts, mast cells, and

    A. astrocytes.
    B. macrophages.
    C. blood cells.
    D. chondrocytes.

35. Of the three types of connective tissue fibers, which is described as extensible and resistant to stretch?

    A. Reticulin
    B. Elastin
    C. Collagen
    D. Fibrin

5 The Skeletal System

Use this table to identify the study guide exercises and group activities that will help you explore or review each learning objective for this chapter.

No.	Learning Objective	Exercise	Study Group Activity
1	Provide several examples of how knowledge of bone and joint structures is applied in manual therapy practices.		See Chapter 1, Activity 1
2	List and explain the primary functions of the skeletal system.	2	
3	Name the primary bones of the skeleton and identify them as axial or appendicular.	1, 3, 7	1
4	Name the two types of bone tissue and describe the key features of each.	5	1
5	Name and describe each of the four bone classifications according to their shape.	4	1
6	Identify the key parts of a long bone and describe the makeup and function of each.	5, 6	
7	Name the key bone landmarks of the body and locate them on a diagram.	1, 7	1
8	Name and define the three structural and functional categories of joints and provide examples for each.	10	1
9	Name the five common structures of all synovial joints and explain the general function of each.	8	1
10	List the six types of synovial joints and provide examples for each in the body.	9, 10	1, 2
11	List and demonstrate the movement capabilities of each type of synovial joint.	9, 10	1, 2
12	Describe common skeletal system changes associated with aging and their implications for the practice of manual therapy.		See Chapter 1, Activity 1

EXERCISE 1 • Bony Terms Crossword

Use this crossword to review and test your ability to define the bone and landmark terms from Chapter 5.

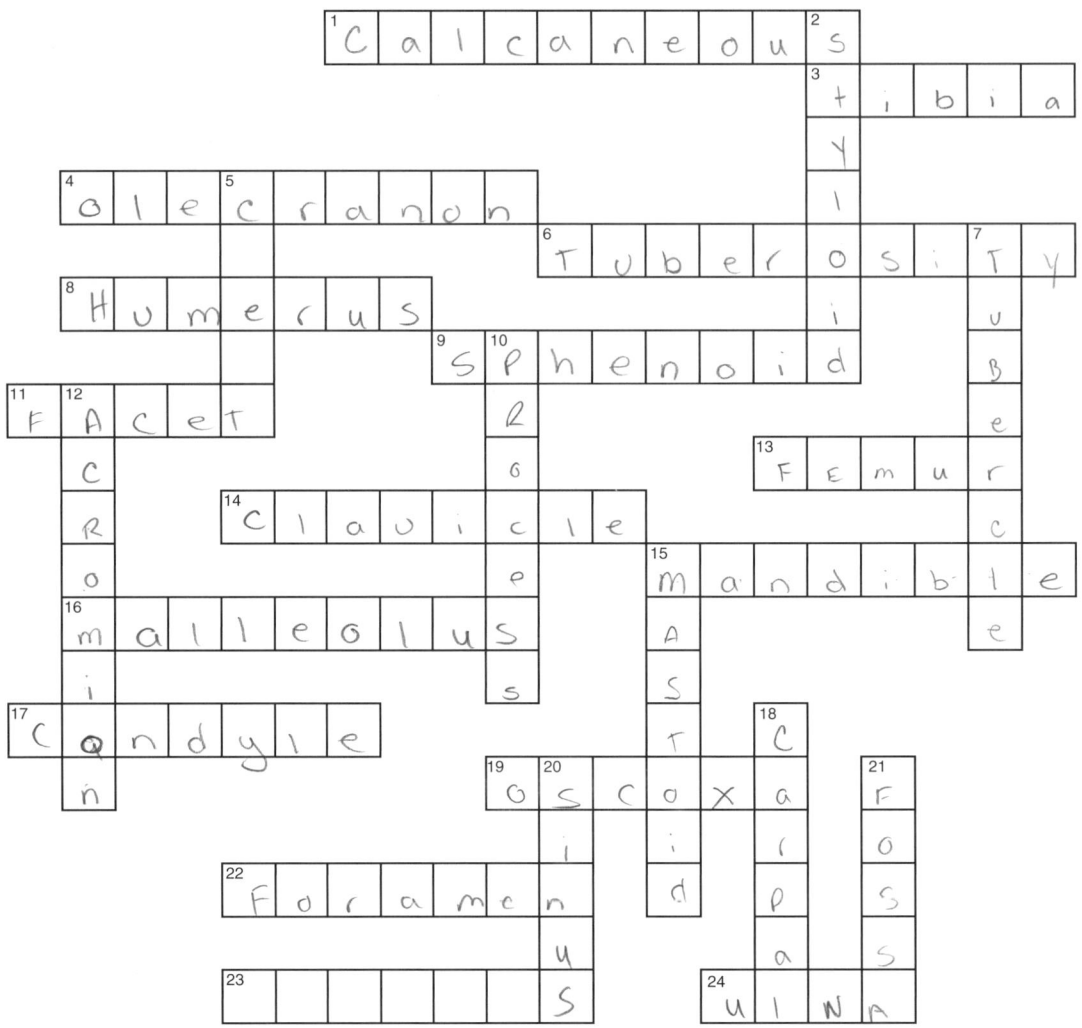

ACROSS

1. The heel bone.
3. Shin bone.
4. The point of the elbow; proximal posterior ulna.
6. A large bump such as the one on the tibia where the quadriceps attach.
8. Upper arm bone.
9. The butterfly shaped internal cranial bone.
11. A small flat articulating surface.
13. Thigh bone.
14. The collar bone.
15. Jaw bone.
16. A projection at the distal tibia or the fibula; "ankle bones".
17. A rounded projection at the end of the bone, often a point of articulation.
19. The fused ilium, ischium, and pubic bones; one side of the pelvis.
22. A hole in a bone for blood vessels or nerves.
23. The posterior process of a spinal vertebra.
24. Medial forearm bone.

DOWN

2. A needle-like process.
5. A sharp ridge.
7. A small bump such as the one on the humerus where the deltoid attaches.
10. A prominent projection.
12. Point of the shoulder; lateral projection of the scapula.
15. A process on the temporal bone just posterior to the ear.
18. A wrist bone.
20. A bone cavity.
21. A large saucer-shaped depression.

EXERCISE 2 • A Story of Functions

When you want to recall something specific, it is helpful to have a context for remembering. For example, when many of us want to remember the alphabet, we sing "The Alphabet Song," or when we want to recall the face of a loved one, we picture them doing something specific like laughing at a joke, playing ball, or doing the dishes. As learners, we can create context for important information by inserting facts into a story, drawing, poem, or song. Try writing a story or play where the characters are responsible for the functions of the skeletal system, or use the same information to write a poem or lyrics for a song.

Study & Review Guide for Applied Anatomy and Physiology for Manual Therapists

EXERCISE 3 • Label the Skeleton

Complete the anterior and posterior diagrams of the skeleton by coloring the axial and appendicular bones different colors. Write the name of each bone in the space provided.

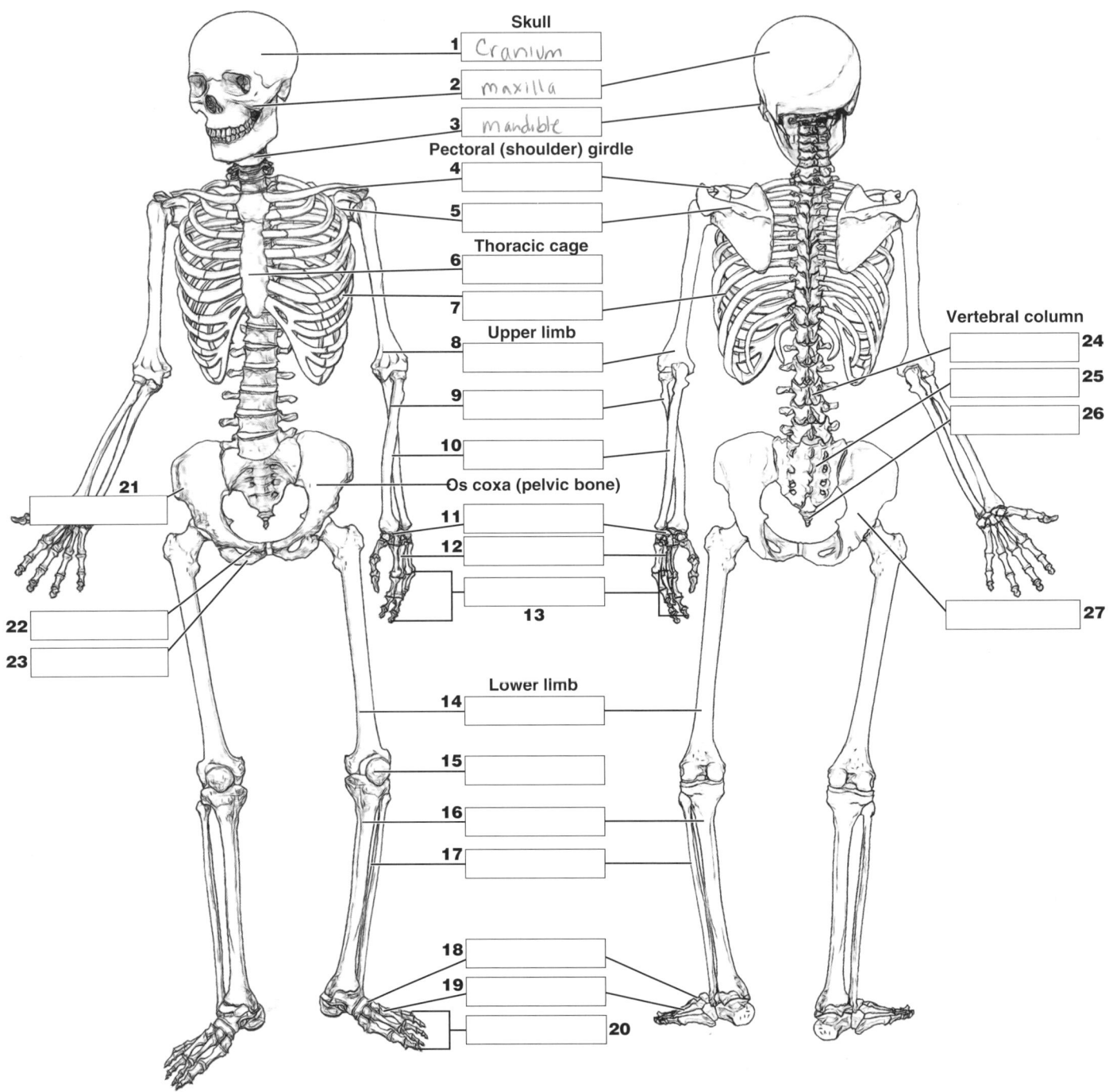

Skull
1. Cranium
2. maxilla
3. mandible

Pectoral (shoulder) girdle
4.
5.

Thoracic cage
6.
7.

Upper limb
8.
9.
10.

Os coxa (pelvic bone)
11.
12.
13.

Lower limb
14.
15.
16.
17.
18.
19.
20.

21.
22.
23.

Vertebral column
24.
25.
26.

27.

Chapter 5 The Skeletal System   61

EXERCISE 4 • Draw Me a Bone

Using the table below, list the four bone shapes in Sections 1 to 4. Then, in the space provided, draw a picture of each bone shape and list at least one example of each. Refer to Figure 5-3 in the textbook if you need to refresh your memory.

Shape	Picture	Examples
1.		
2.		
3.		
4.		

EXERCISE 5 • Parts of a Long Bone

Match the parts of a long bone with their description and/or function. Next, label each part on the diagram provided. If you need to refresh your memory, refer to Figure 5-4 in your textbook.

_____ 1. Epiphysis
_____ 2. Articular cartilage
_____ 3. Red bone marrow
_____ 4. Epiphyseal line
_____ 5. Spongy bone
_____ 6. Metaphysis
_____ 7. Diaphysis
_____ 8. Periosteum
_____ 9. Endosteum
_____ 10. Medullary cavity
_____ 11 Yellow bone marrow
_____ 12 Compact bone

A. Site of bone elongation; growth plate
B. Tough outer connective tissue covering
C. Bone end
D. Fatty tissue in medullary cavity
E. Region between epiphysis and diaphysis
F. Hematopoietic tissue
G. Comprises the shaft
H. Space in the middle of the shaft
I. Covers and protects bone ends; hyaline
J. Shaft of the long bone
K. Comprises the bone ends
L. Inner lining of the medullary cavity

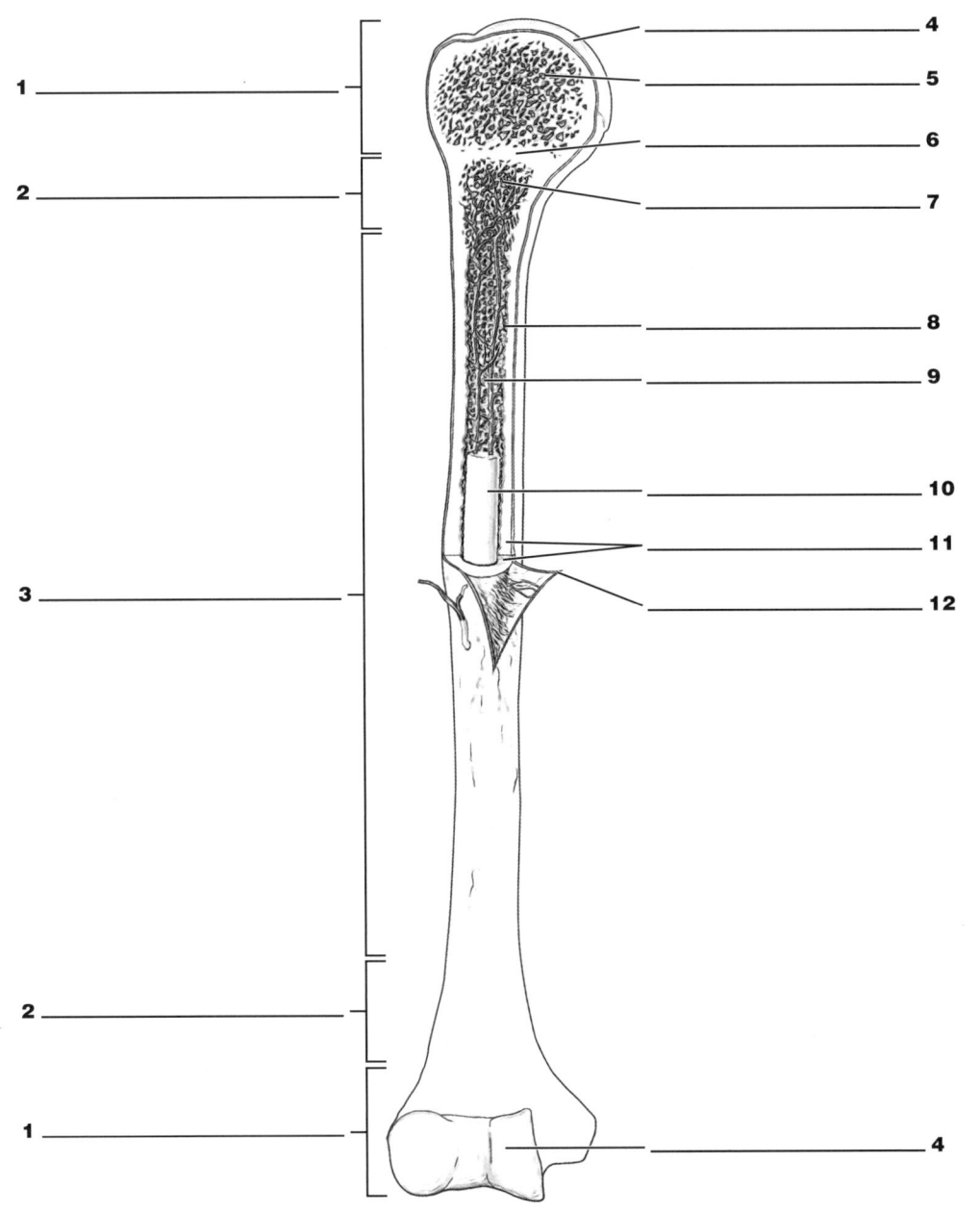

EXERCISE 6 • Build a Long Bone

Another way to learn the parts of a long bone is to build a model using some simple materials you can get at any home improvement store. To build this model of a long bone, you will need:

- A 6 to 12 in length of 1 in PVC piping
- Two caps to fit on the ends of your PVC pipe
- Silly putty
- Elastic food wrap
- Pink sponge pieces
- Yellow sponge pieces

The length of pipe represents the **1.**_____ or shaft of the bone. Therefore, the space inside is the **2.**_____ _____ that contains **3.**_____ _____ _____. This tissue is represented by the yellow sponge pieces that you can place inside the pipe. The PVC caps represent the ends of the bone or **4.**_____, where the **5.**_____ _____ _____ resides. Stuff the caps with red sponge pieces and attach them to the shaft. Use some silly putty to cover the very ends of the model to represent the **6.**_____ _____ that protects the bone ends from wear and tear during movement. Then wrap the entire length of the bone with elastic wrap to represent the **7.**_____, the connective tissue sheath that surrounds the bone.

EXERCISE 7 • Skeletal Landmarks Labeling

Match the bone or landmark with its label on the diagram.

_____ 1. Iliac crest

_____ 2. Lateral malleolus

_____ 3. Greater trochanter

_____ 4. Occipital bone

_____ 5. Olecranon process

_____ 6. Calcaneus

_____ 7. Patella

_____ 8. Inferior angle of scapula

_____ 9. Mastoid process

_____ 10. Acromion process

_____ 11. Mandible

_____ 12. Tibial tuberosity

_____ 13. Head of radius

_____ 14. Anterior superior iliac spine

_____ 15. Ischial tuberosity

_____ 16. Glenoid fossa

_____ 17. Spinous process

_____ 18. Lateral humeral epicondyle

_____ 19. Xiphoid process

_____ 20. Crest of tibia

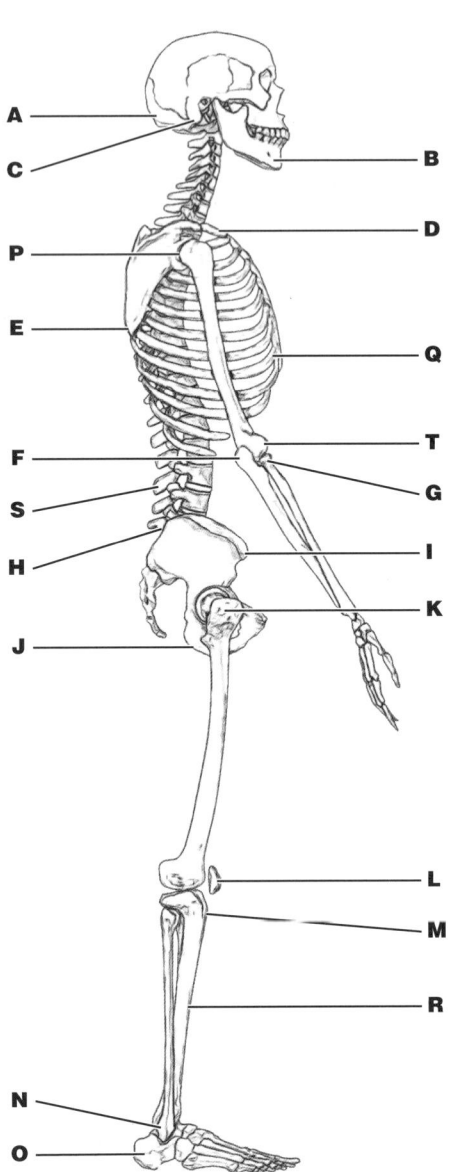

EXERCISE 8 • Color and Label a Synovial Joint

All synovial or diarthrotic joints share some common structural components. Color and label the sagittal section of the knee provided to review the structures of a synovial joint. If you need to refresh your memory, refer to Figure 5-24 in your textbook.

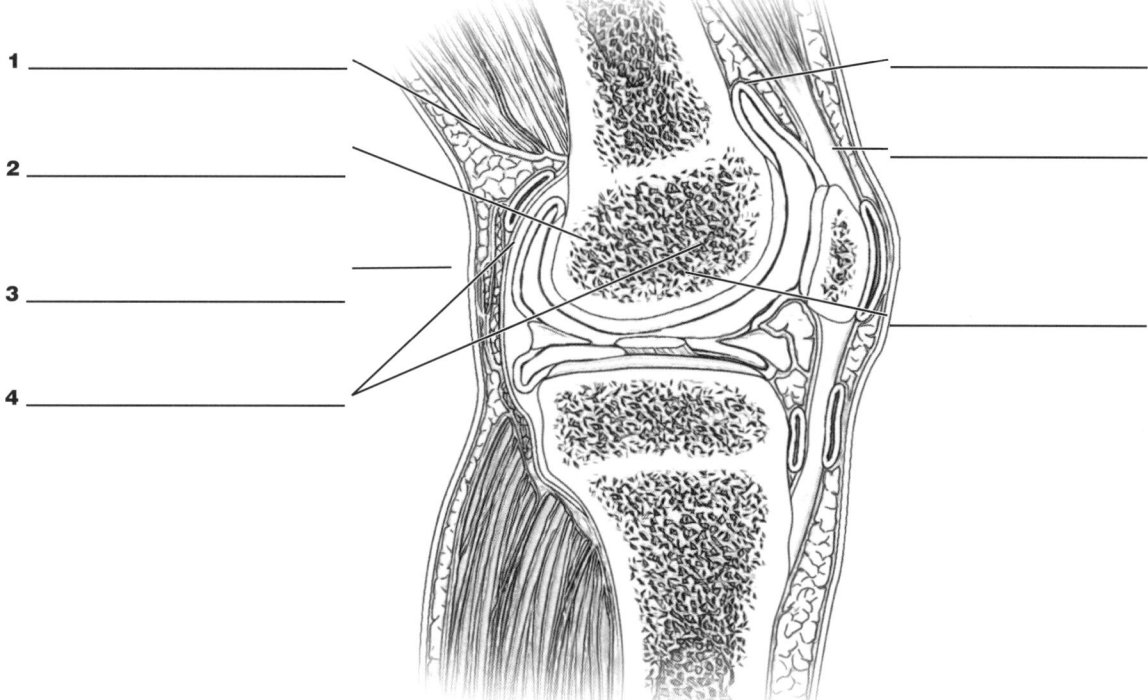

1 _____

2 _____

3 _____

4 _____

EXERCISE 9 • Diarthrotic Joint Movements

Complete the table below by identifying the type of joint and the movements allowed by each specific joint listed. The first one is done for you.

Specific Joint	Type	Movements
Atlanto - Occipital joint	Hinge	Flexion/extension
Atlantoaxial	1.	2.
Glenohumeral	3.	4.
Radioulnar	5.	6.
Humeroulnar	7.	8.
Radiocarpal	9.	10.
First carpometacarpal	11.	12.
Metacarpophalangeal	13.	14.
Interphalangeal	15.	16.
Iliofemoral	17.	18.
Femorotibial (knee)	19.	20.
Tibiotalar (ankle)	21.	22.
Talotarsal (subtalar)	23.	24.

EXERCISE 10 • Joint Crossword

Use this crossword to review and test your knowledge about joint classifications, names, and movements.

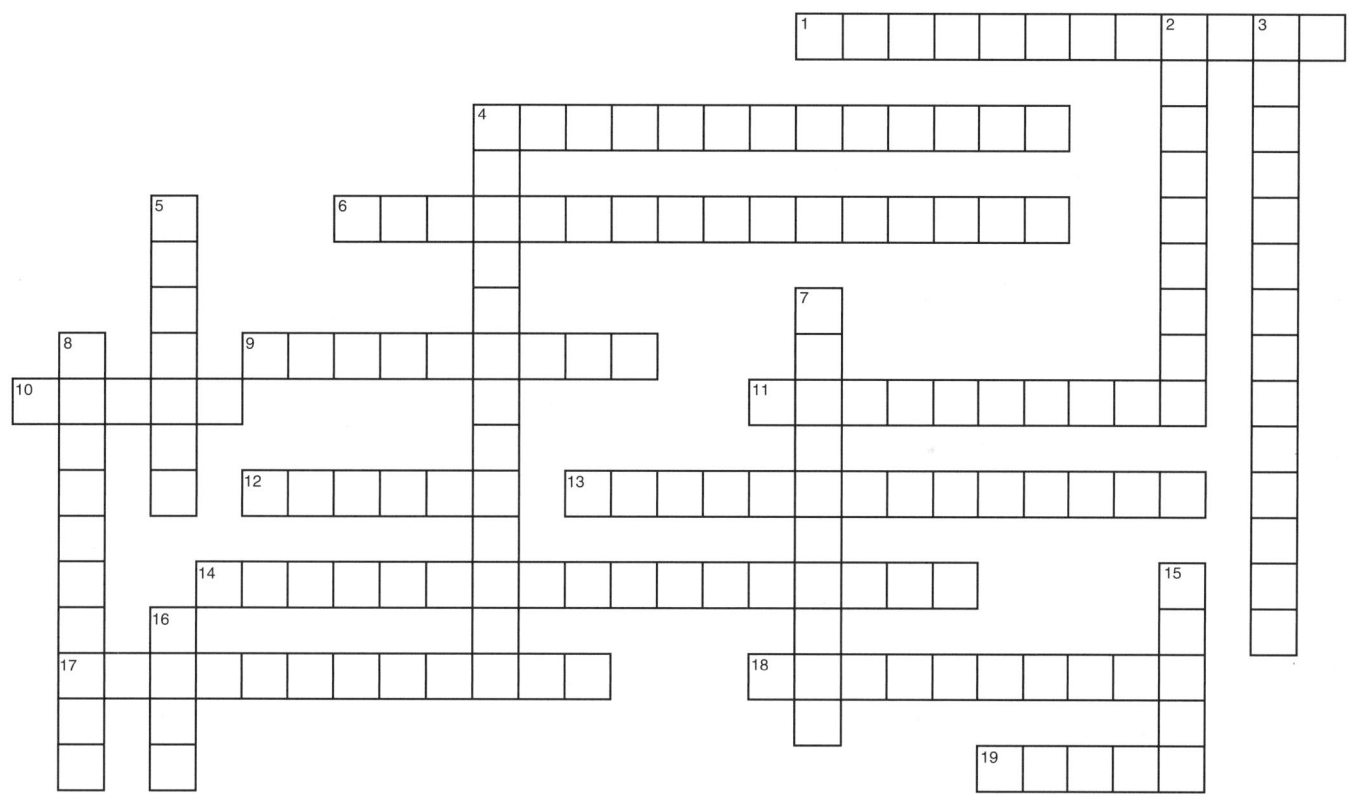

ACROSS

1. The shoulder joint.
4. Multiplanar movement about a single joint.
6. The joint between the manubrium and clavicle.
9. A synovial joint that allows movement in the frontal and sagittal planes.
10. A synovial joint that allows rotation only.
11. To draw a body part backward.
12. The joint category that includes the first carpometacarpal joint.
13. Rising up on the toes.
14. The TM in TMJ.
17. Immovable joint.
18. Turning the forearm so that the palm faces forward in anatomical position.
19. The tibiotalar joint.

DOWN

2. Upward movement.
3. Slightly movable joint.
4. The structural joint category that includes the pubic symphysis.
5. The structural joint category that includes the sutures of the skull.
7. The hip socket.
8. Synonymous with synovial joint.
15. A diarthrosis that allows flexion and extension only.
16. The tibiofemoral joint.

GROUP ACTIVITY 1 • Quiz Show

A game show format, based on the popular show "Jeopardy!" can be used to review the structures and function of any system in the body. Three or four "contestants" or two small teams play against each other, with one "emcee" managing the board and assigning points/money. In this game, the answers are revealed on the board, and contestants must then provide the proper question, by saying "what is..." at the beginning. For example, under a System Structures category, the answer for 11 points is "the lateral bone in the leg." The contestant wins the 100 points by saying, "What is the fibula?"

The game starts when the first contestant (decide who by age, shirt color, alphabetically, whatever) chooses a category and point value. The emcee reads the answer in that square to the contestants. The contestants must "buzz in" for the chance to provide the question. Whoever the emcee identifies as buzzing in first gets to provide the question they believe matches the clue. If they answer correctly, play continues with them choosing the category and dollar amount from the board for the next clue. If the contestant answers incorrectly, the other contestants may buzz in to provide their response. Again, play continues with the person who provides the correct response choosing the next clue to be read by the emcee. Consider setting a time limit for giving a response to a clue. You may also want to set a time limit for Level I or Level II,—say 10 minutes to complete the board or quit for the Final Level.

The final-level clue should be the most challenging. The emcee should choose this clue before the game begins. It could be something from a Pathology Alert, By The Way, or some extra detail your instructor added during lecture. The emcee provides the category description for the clue and each contestant secretly wagers any amount of his or her winnings he or she wants. Once the wagers have been secretly written down, the emcee reads the clue and each contestant writes down his or her response. Finally, each contestant reveals his or her response and wager. The wager amount is added to his or her winnings if the answer is correct or subtracted if it is wrong. The person with the highest total amount wins the game. Here are a sample game boards for the skeletal system.

LEVEL I

	'Dem Bones	Tissue? I Hardly Know You!	Joint Classification	Landmark Terminology	Specific Landmarks
100	This is the largest sesamoid bone in the body	This tissue is made up of osteons	The functional classification for joints with a fibrocartilage pad	The anatomic term for a hole or large opening in a bone	The round projection we sit on
200	Most of the bones in the appendages fall into this category	This tissue fills the medullary cavity	The structural classification for the joints between bones in the skull	A fossa is this type of landmark	The large projection off the temporal bone that can be palpated behind our ears
300	These two cranial bones form the superior portion of the skull	"Cancellous" is the anatomic name for this type of bone tissue	The radioulnar joint is an example of this type of synovial joint	A tubercle is a smaller version of this	The palpable proximal end of the fifth metatarsal
400	These three cube-shaped bones in the foot are anterior & lateral to the talus	These form the osseous bridges or lattice work throughout the spongy bone	This type of synovial joint is capable of all movements plus circumduction	A sharp line along the edge of a bone	The roughened ridge that runs the length of the posterior femur
500	This is the only moveable bone in the skull	The anatomic name for dense or hard bone	The anatomic name of the only saddle joint in the skeleton	The anatomic term for a small pit or depression	The posteriomedial bump on the proximal shaft of the femur

LEVEL II

	More Landmarks	Synovial Joint Structures	Special Movements	Common Names	What's Wrong?
200	The small groove in the proximal ulnar that receives the head of the radius	This forms as a sleeve around the bone ends that helps stabilize the joint	Turning the hand palm up	Glenohumeral joint	A decrease in bone density leading to brittle bones
400	The anterior thumb-like projection off the scapula	The inner lining of the joint capsule	Taking the arm away from the midline on the transverse plane	Tibiofemoral joint	Joint inflammation due to degeneration of the articular cartilage
600	The flat articular surface of the tibia	Fibrous connective tissue that attaches bone to bone	The scapular rotation involved in shrugging your shoulders	Humeroulnar joint	Joint inflammation due to degeneration of the synovial membrane
800	The anatomic terms for the distal projections of tibia and fibula; ankle bones	The smooth tough CT covering of the articular surfaces of bones	The motion that occurs when we stand on the outside of our feet	Coxal joint	Joint inflammation due to accumulation of uric acid crystals
1000	The needle-like projection just posterior to the mastoid process	Not present in all joints, this "synovial pillow" protects ligaments & tendons from sharp bone edges	The ankle motion of raising up on our toes	Talocrural joint	Abnormal lateral curvature of the spine

GROUP ACTIVITY 2 • Sculpting Statues

This game is an active way to practice movement and joint terminology. The object of the game is to sculpt or mold a person by providing verbal directions using the movement and joint terms. It can be played with three or more people.

- One model
- One "lump of clay"
- One or more sculptors

Directions:

1. The "lump of clay" is blindfolded.
2. The model strikes a pose that the sculptor(s) will attempt to sculpt.
3. Using technical terms, the sculptors provide directions to the blindfolded "lump of clay." For example, to get the clay to bend his or her elbow, the sculptors may direct the clay to, "Flex your humeroulnar joint."
4. The clay responds to each verbal direction to the best of his or her ability.
5. The game ends when the "lump of clay" resembles the model statue.

6 The Skeletal Muscle System

Use this table to identify the study guide exercises and group activities that will help you explore or review each learning objective for this chapter.

No.	Learning Objective	Exercise	Study Group Activity
1	Give several examples of how knowledge of the muscular system is applied in manual therapy practice.		See Chapter 1, Activity 1
2	List and describe the key characteristics and functions of skeletal muscle.	1	
3	Name and locate the major parts of a skeletal muscle.	2	1
4	Name and describe the distinguishing characteristics between fascia and tendons.	1, 3	1
5	Describe the microscopic arrangement of a skeletal muscle fiber.	4	1
6	Name the parts of a motor unit and explain the role of each in muscle contraction.	1, 5	1
7	Explain the key physiologic principles that govern the function of skeletal muscle, including sliding-filament mechanism, all-or-none response, threshold stimulus, and motor unit recruitment.	1, 5	1
8	List and explain the three major types of muscle contraction.	1	1
9	Explain the three primary mechanisms of producing energy for muscle contraction.	6, 7	
10	Explain muscle fatigue and oxygen debt.	1	
11	Name and describe the different types of fiber arrangements found in muscles of the body.	8, 11	
12	Name and describe the four major roles muscles play in creating and controlling movement of body parts.	9	1
13	Explain how muscles get their names.	10	
14	Describe the general location of the major muscles and the prime function(s) of each.	11–13	1–4
15	Describe common skeletal muscle system changes associated with exercise and aging and explain their implications for manual therapy practices.		See Chapter 1, Activity 1

EXERCISE 1 • Muscle Terminology Crossword

Use this crossword to review and test your knowledge of the general muscle anatomy and physiology terms from Chapter 6.

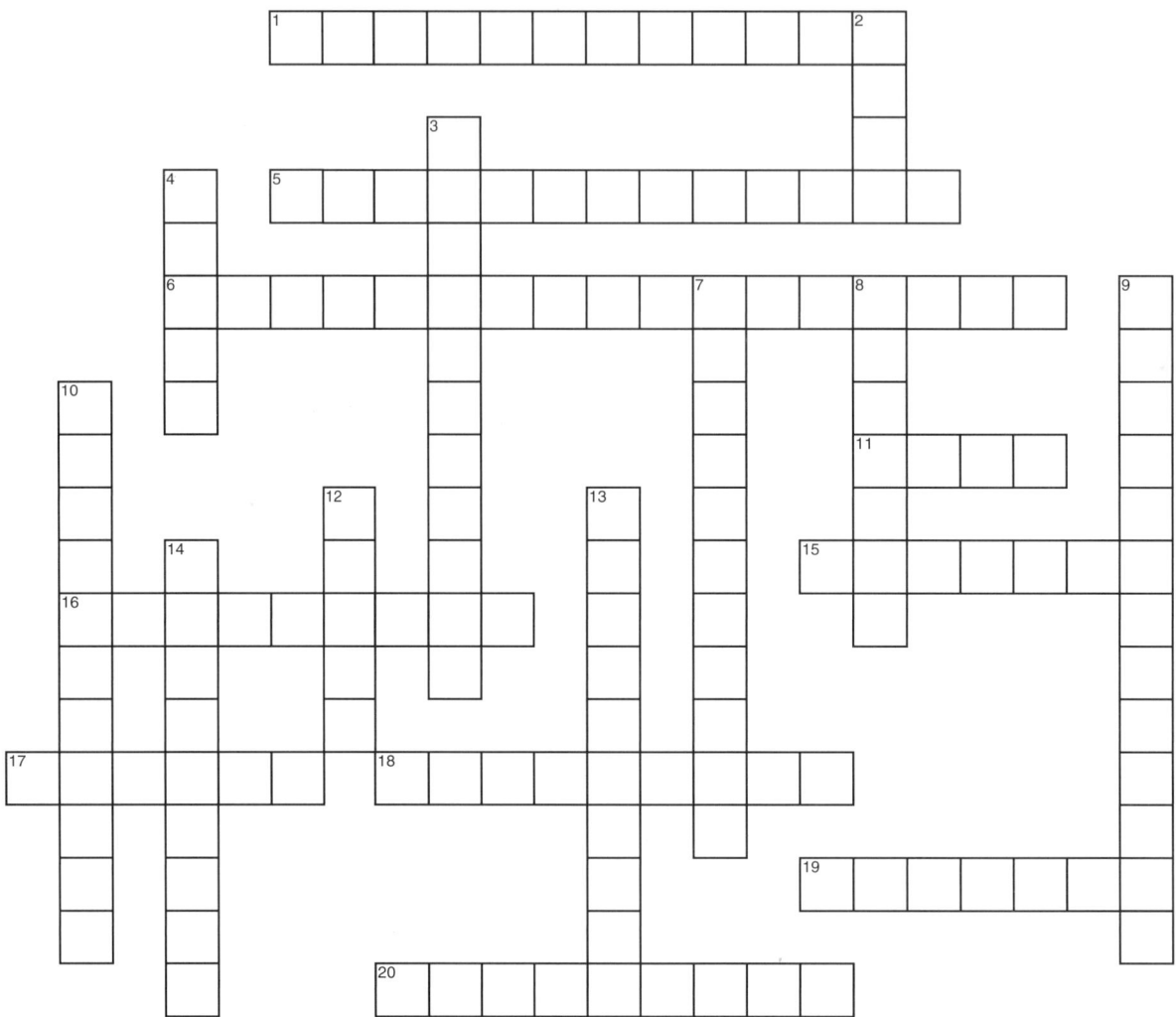

ACROSS

1. Type of fibrous connective tissue that makes up fascia.
5. The region of a muscle fiber that is highly sensitive to neurotransmitter.
6. Communicating chemicals released from a neuron.
11. The breakdown of ATP in muscle produces this byproduct which is why we shiver when we are cold.
15. The ability to rebound back to original shape and length.
16. Highly responsive to stimulation from the nervous system.
17. Muscles work together with ligaments and joint capsules to stabilize _____.
18. The minimum stimulus required to produce a response.
19. Inability to contract forcefully after prolonged activity.
20. A muscle contraction in which there is an increase in tension, but no change in length.

DOWN

2. The oxygen required by the body to metabolize lactic acid and replenish glycogen, creatine phosphate, and ATP stores after exercise.
3. Capable of forcefully shortening.
4. The type of contraction responsible for maintaining posture.
7. A nerve cell that stimulates multiple muscle fibers in a motor unit.
8. The organized fibrous connective tissue that makes up tendons is comprised of _____ packed collagen fibers.
9. Cork screw shaped protein that comprises collagen fibrils.
10. A broad flat sheet of organized connective tissue that attaches a muscle to bone.
12. An acute involuntary muscle contraction that lasts for several minutes; palpable as a knot.
13. The ability to lengthen.
14. An isotonic contraction in which the muscle produces tension while it is lengthening.

Chapter 6 The Skeletal Muscle System

EXERCISE 2 • Major Parts of a Skeletal Muscle

Color and label the diagram to identify the major parts of a skeletal muscle. Refer to Figure 6-1 in the textbook if you need to refresh your memory.

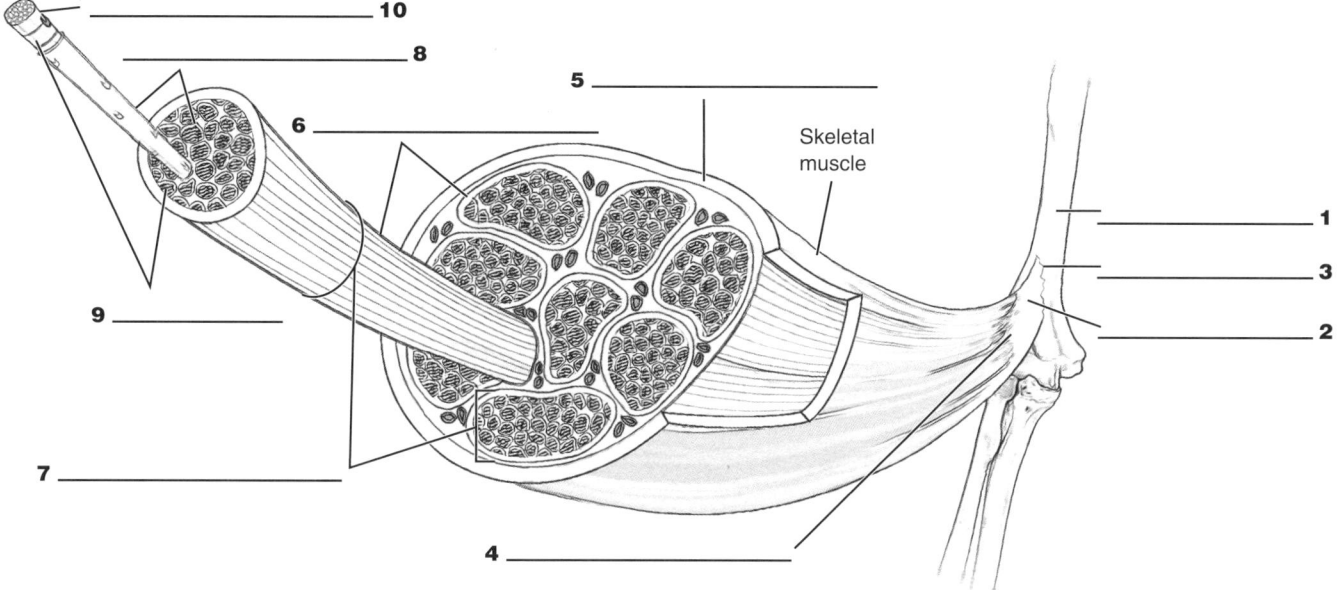

EXERCISE 3 • Comparing Fascia and Tendons

Venn diagrams are simple graphic organizers that provide a visual display of similar and different attributes between two items or sets of information. Each circle in the diagram represents one item or set of information. Where the circles overlap, record characteristics that are shared between the two items. Record the characteristics in which they differ in the other regions.

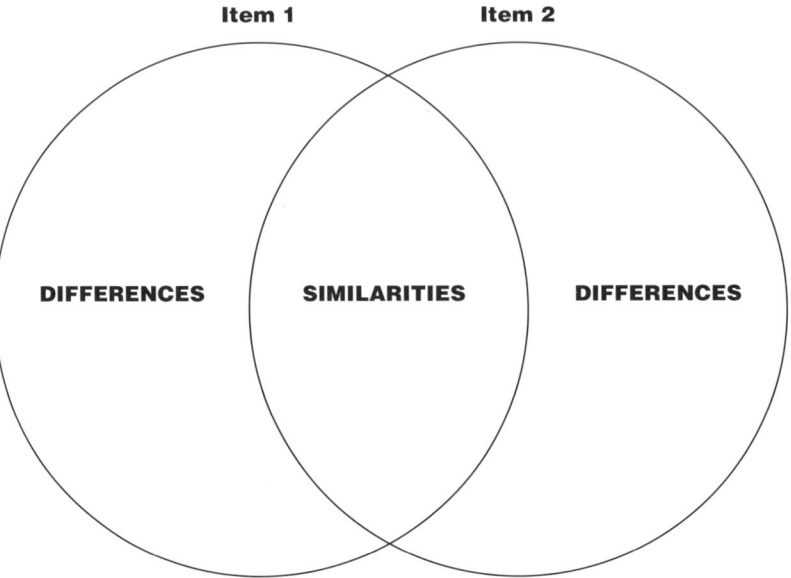

Use the Venn diagram below to compare and contrast the structural and functional characteristics of fascia and tendons. An example of one shared characteristic, that is, comprised of fibrous connective tissue, has been placed in the area of overlap to get you started.

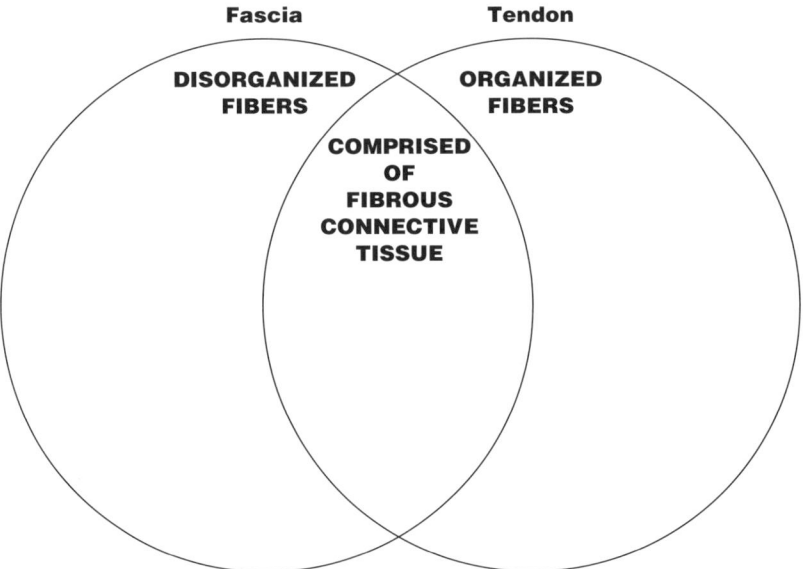

Chapter 6 The Skeletal Muscle System

EXERCISE 4 • Skeletal Muscle Fiber Organization

Match each organizational component with its definition or functional description. Then use the terms to label the diagram of a skeletal muscle fiber. Refer to Figure 6-2 in the textbook if you need to refresh your memory.

_____ 1. Muscle fiber
_____ 2. Myofibrils
_____ 3. Mitochondrion
_____ 4. Sarcoplasmic reticulum
_____ 5. Sarcolemma
_____ 6. Myofilaments
_____ 7. Myosin
_____ 8. Actin
_____ 9. Z line
_____ 10. A band
_____ 11. I band
_____ 12. Sarcomere

A. The ER of a muscle fiber
B. The thin myofilament
C. Light area of sarcomere; contains thin filaments only
D. Small cylindrical organelles that make up a fiber
E. Actin and myosin
F. A muscle cell
G. The functional unit of contraction
H. Dark area of a sarcomere created by thick filaments
I. The thick myofilament
J. Many of these produce ATP for the muscle cell
K. The plasma membrane of a muscle fiber
L. Boundary between two sarcomeres

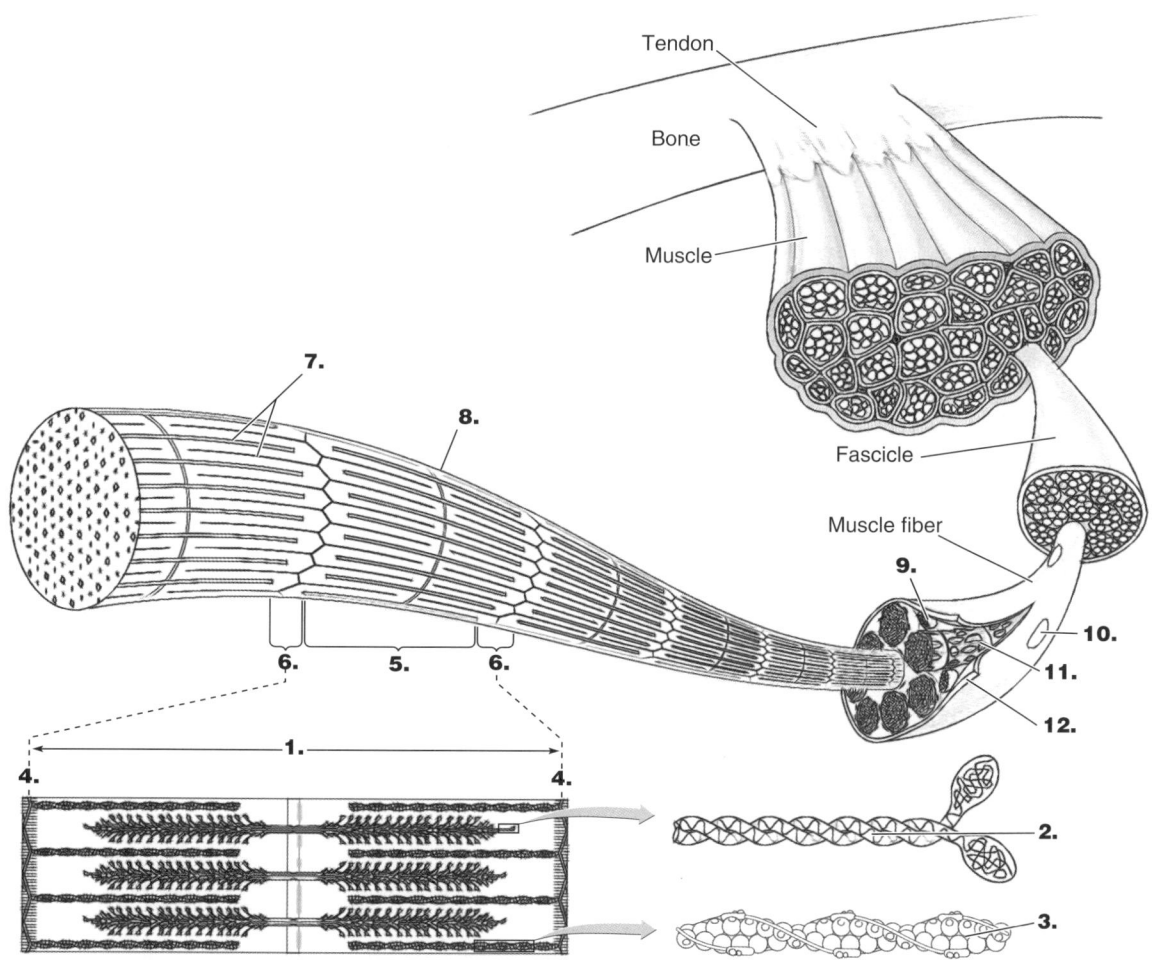

EXERCISE 5 • Skeletal Muscle Contraction

Fill in the blanks to describe the process of muscle contraction.

The physiology of muscle contraction is explained through a model called the **1.**_____. This model lays out the key physiologic events that create the shortening of the **2.**_____ when muscle cells are signaled to contract by the nervous system. The coordination between the nervous and muscular systems occurs through the functional structure called a **3.**_____, which is comprised of a **4.**_____ and the multiple muscle **5.**_____ it innervates. The structural interface between these structures is a microscopic space called the **6.**_____. A muscle contraction is initiated when **7.**_____ are released from the vesicles in the knobs of the **8.**_____ into this space or junction to stimulate the **9.**_____ of the muscle fibers.

A contraction only occurs when enough stimulation is delivered to the fibers. This minimum amount of stimulus is called a **10.**_____. A physiological principle known as the **11.**_____ applies to each individual motor unit. This principle states that if **12.**_____ is reached, **13.**_____ the muscle fibers in the motor unit will fully contract. If not, **14.**_____ of the fibers will contract. The nervous system regulates the force of muscle contraction by controlling the number of motor units stimulated within any given muscle. The regulation of a muscle's effort by increasing or decreasing the number of motor units stimulated is called **15.**_____ or **16.**_____.

When a muscle is stimulated to contract:

1. **17.**_____ ions stored in the **18.**_____ are released into the sarcoplasm.

2. The presence of these ions exposes binding sites on the **19.**_____.

3. The **20.**_____ bind to these exposed sites, forming cross bridges that **21.**_____.

4. ATP is used to detach the **22.**_____ so that they can flip forward to the next binding site. The net result is **23.**_____.

5. When the stimulus is removed, more energy is expended to pump **24.**_____ back into the **25.**_____, and chemical bridges can no longer form.

Chapter 6 The Skeletal Muscle System

EXERCISE 6 • Picturing Energy for Muscle Contraction

Color and label the diagrams to review the three methods of energy production for muscle contraction. If you need to refresh your memory, refer to Figures 6-7 and 6-8 in the text.

Direct Phosphorylation

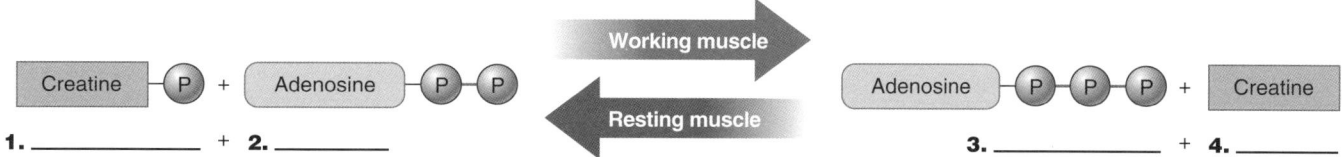

1. _____ + 2. _____   3. _____ + 4. _____

Glycolysis and Aerobic Cellular Metabolism

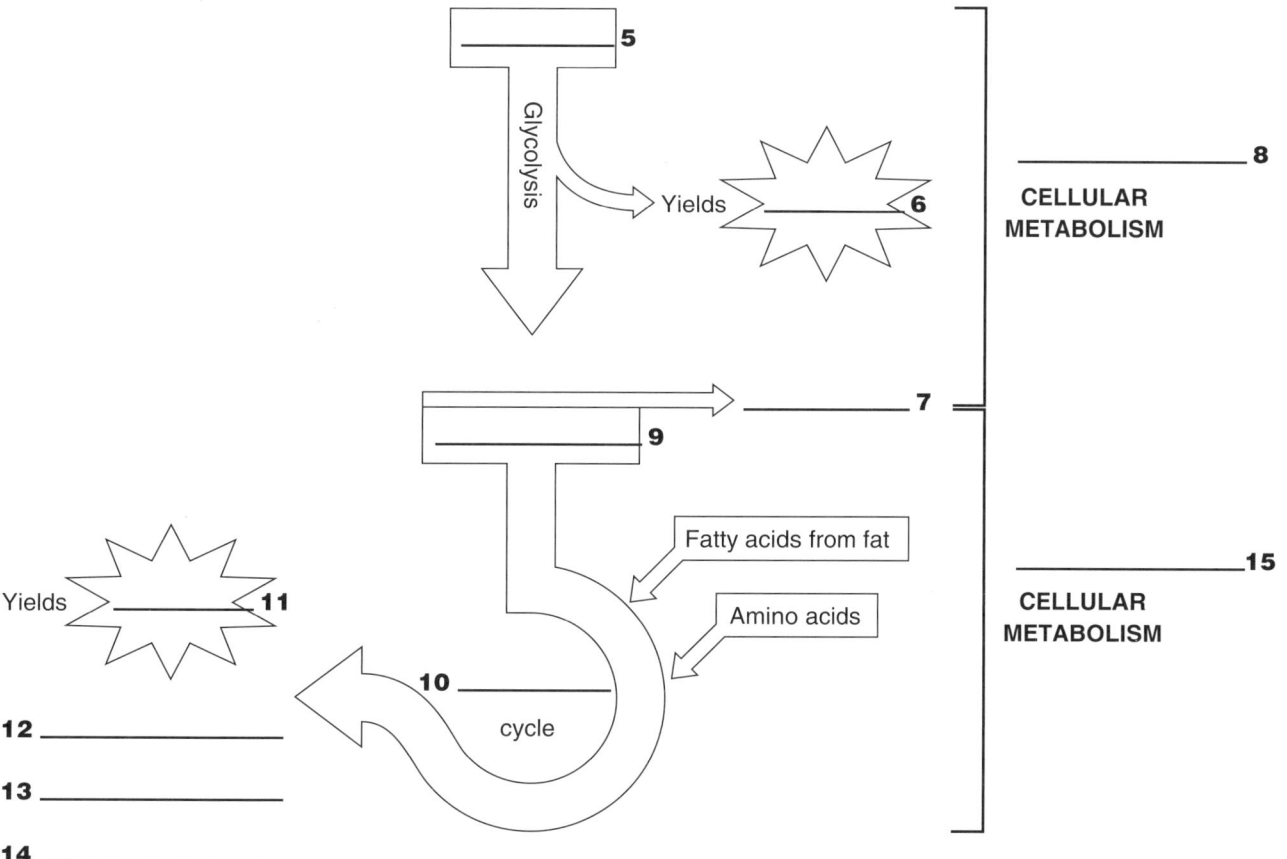

EXERCISE 7 • Organizing Methods of ATP Production

Use the table below to organize the key information about the three methods of ATP production for muscle contraction.

ENERGY FOR MUSCLE CONTRACTION

Method	Description	O_2 Needed?	By-Products
1.	Phosphate from creatine phosphate attaches to ADP to create ATP for short burst of activity	No, anaerobic process	2.
Glycolysis	3.	4.	ATP and pyruvic acid. Without oxygen, pyruvic acid converts to lactic acid
5.	6.	Yes, aerobic process	7.

EXERCISE 8 • Types of Fiber Arrangements

Muscles have a variety of fascicle or fiber arrangements that are an important part of their overall architecture. Complete the table on types of fiber arrangements by drawing a picture and providing at least one example of each. Refer to Figure 6-13 in the text if you need to refresh your memory.

FIBER ARRANGEMENTS

Arrangement		Picture	Example(s)
Parallel	Parallel		1.
	2.		Biceps brachii Biceps femoris
	3.		Orbicularis oris Orbicularis oculi
	Triangular		4.
Pennate	Unipennate		5.
	6.		Rectus femoris External obliques
	7.		Deltoid Triceps brachii

EXERCISE 9 • Muscle Assignments

Define the following muscle assignments:
- Agonist (prime mover)—_____
  _____
- Antagonist—_____
  _____
- Synergist—_____
  _____
- Stabilizer—_____
  _____

Next, complete the table by providing at least one agonist, antagonist, and synergist for each movement.

Movement		Prime Mover	Antagonist	Synergist
Knee	Extension	Rectus femoris	1.	2.
	Flexion	3.	4.	Semimembranosus Semitendinosus Gastrocnemius
Shoulder	Extension	5.	Pectoralis major Coracobrachialis	Teres major
	Flexion	6.	7.	8.
	Abduction	9.	10.	Supraspinatus
	Adduction	Pectoralis major	11.	12.
	Medial rotation	Subscapularis	13.	Pectoralis major Latissimus dorsi
	Lateral rotation	Infraspinatus	14.	15.

EXERCISE 10 • Naming Muscles

Use the mind map to show typical themes among muscle names. Provide as many examples as you can for each. An example has been provided to get you started.

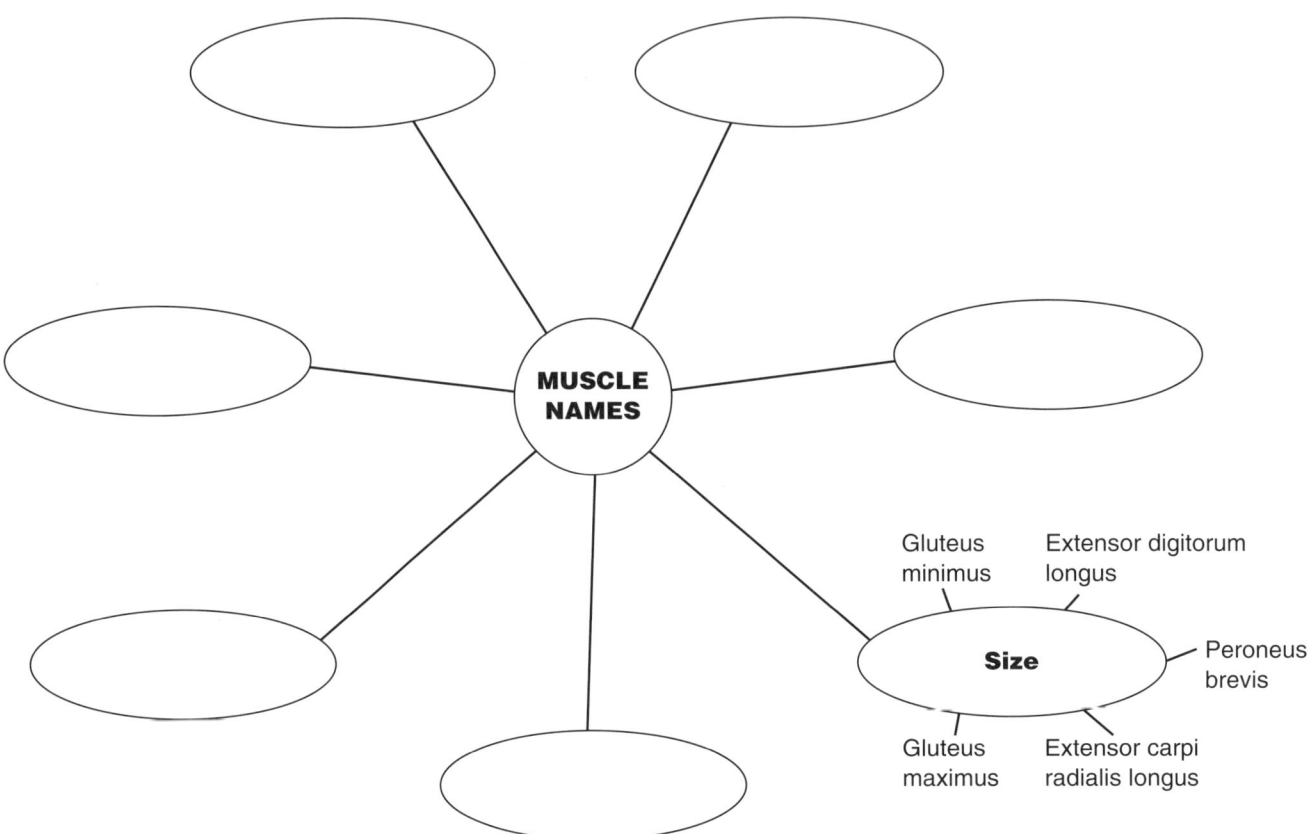

Chapter 6 The Skeletal Muscle System

EXERCISE 11 • Locating Major Muscles

Complete the diagrams by coloring and labeling the major muscles. If you wish to refresh your memory, refer to Figures 6-11 and 6-12 in the text. To find more specific muscle diagrams to label, go to the online resources available through the Point.

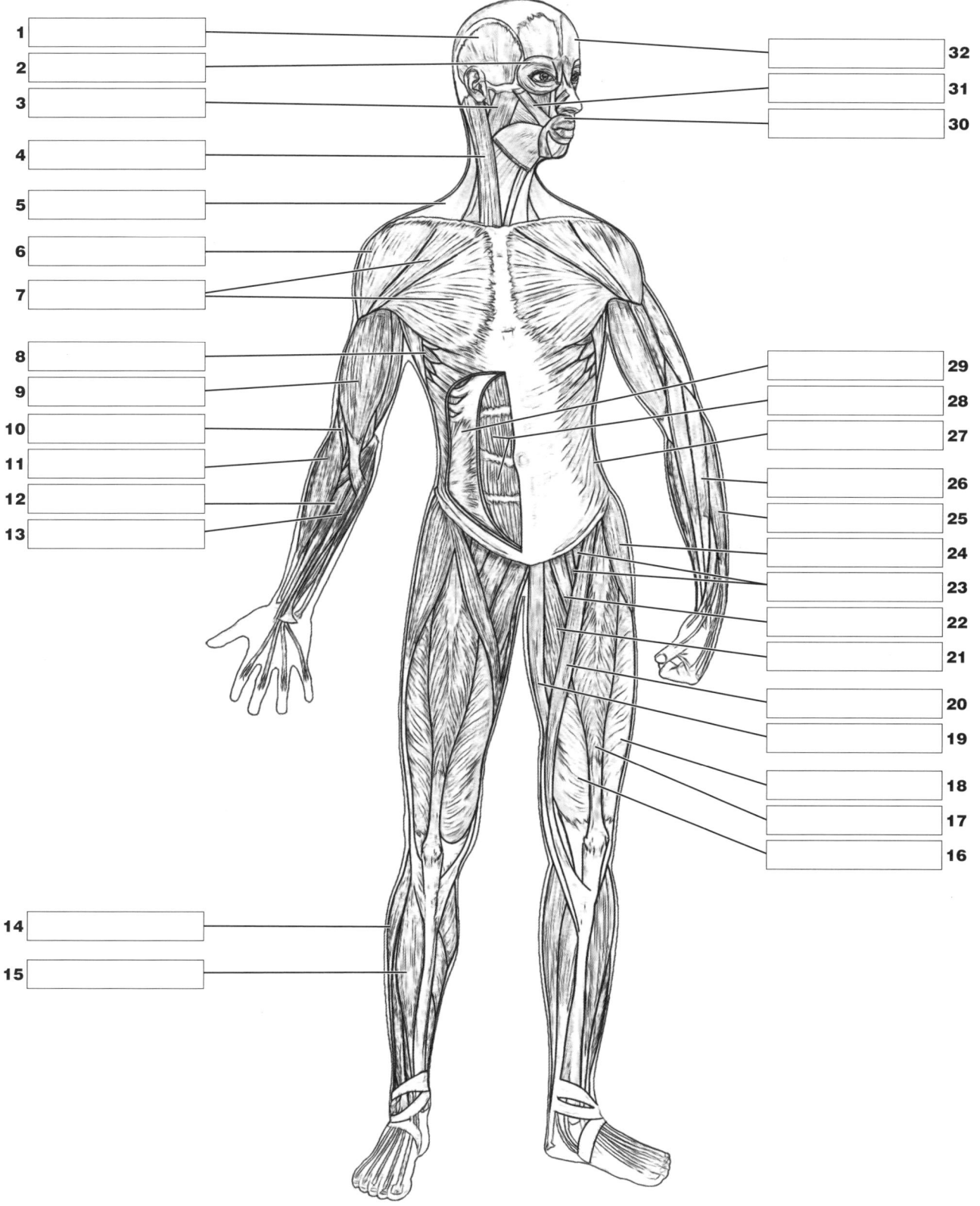

Anterior view

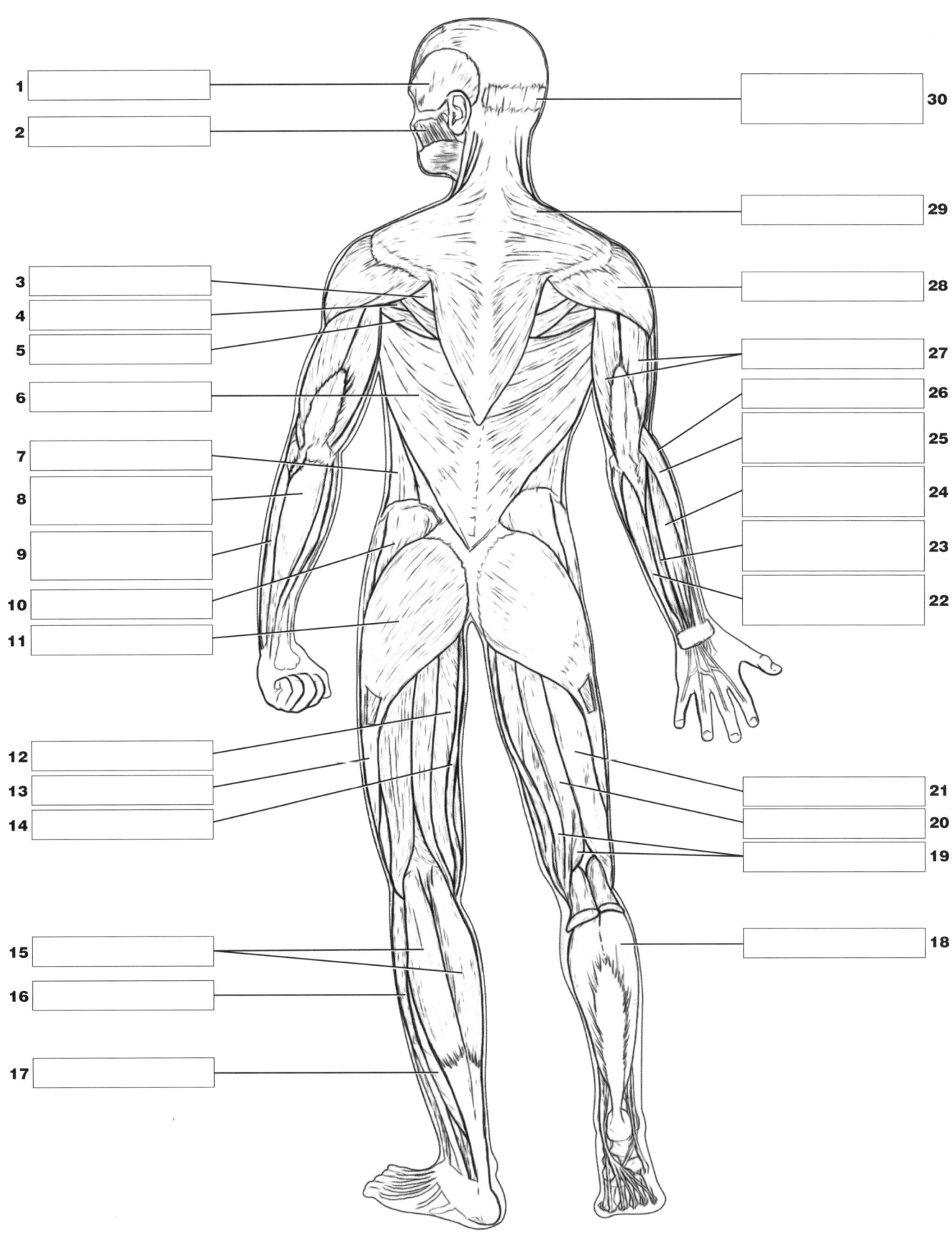

Posterior view

EXERCISE 12 • Building Muscles

It can help to use a model to learn origins and insertions and understand the actions of muscles. By molding clay or placing scarves, fabric cutouts, or therapeutic exercise bands on a skeleton, you can identify a muscle's specific location and see how it crosses joints to produce movement.

Use the recipe below to make large amounts of homemade play dough. Using a skeleton of any size, mold muscles from play dough onto the skeleton. Consider making several batches in different colors to layer muscles in the same region of the body. For example, to see how the three primary elbow flexors overlap one another in the elbow, make the brachialis one color, the biceps brachii another, and the brachioradialis a third.

Homemade Play Dough

Mix 2 1/2 cup flour, 1/2 cup salt, and 1 tablespoon alum thoroughly. Make a well in the middle of these dry ingredients and pour 3 tablespoon corn oil, 2 cup boiling water, and food coloring into the well. Stir well and then knead with hands until well mixed. Use flour on hands and kneading surface to keep the mixture from sticking. Continue to add flour to alleviate stickiness as necessary.

EXERCISE 13 • Memorizing Major Muscle Information

There are many ways to organize, review, and memorize the specific origins, insertions, and actions of the muscles. Many learners make or buy flash cards (for suggestions on how to make and use flash cards, see Chapter 2, Exercise 1), while others use mind maps or tables. For example, the two tables shown here organize the muscles by joint and list their actions before their origins and insertions. This organizational focus on function may be particularly helpful for kinesthetic learners who relate to action over origin and insertion. Notice that the primary functions are bolded, while secondary or assistive functions are in normal typeface. In addition, if you highlight each function with a different color, you will easily be able to identify all the muscles that contribute to a specific joint movement.

SCAPULOTHORACIC ARTICULATION

Muscle	Action(s)	Origin	Insertion
Trapezius 3 portions—upper, mid, lower	**Elevation** (upper) **Retraction** (mid) **Depression** (lower) Upward rotation of the scapula (upper; lower)	Occiput, nuchal ligament and spinous processes of C7–T12	Lateral one-third of clavicle, acromion process and full spine of the scapula
Levator scapulae	**Elevation** **Downward rotation** of the scapula	Transverse processes of C1–C4	Superior angle to the root of the scapular spine
Rhomboids	**Retraction** Downward rotation of the scapula	Spinous processes of C7–T5	Medial border of the scapula
Serratus anterior	**Protraction** **Upward rotation** of the scapula **Stabilization** of the scapula during shoulder movement	Anterolateral ribs 1–8	Vertebral border of the scapula
Pectoralis minor	**Protraction** **Depression** Downward rotation of the scapula	Anterior surface of ribs 3–5	Coracoid process
Subclavius	**Depression** of the clavicle **Stabilization** of the sternoclavicular joint	First rib	Inferior edge of the clavicle

Elevation: upper trap, levator scap; **Retraction:** mid trap, rhomboids; **Upward Rotation:** Upper and Lower trap, serratus.
Depression: L trap, pec minor, **Protraction:** serratus, pec minor; **Downward Rot:** levator, rhomboids, pec minor.

… Chapter 6 The Skeletal Muscle System 85

ELBOW (HUMEROULNAR) AND RADIOULNAR JOINTS

Muscle	Action(s)	Origin	Insertion
Biceps brachii	**Flexion** **Supination** Assists in shoulder flexion	Coracoid process and supraglenoid tubercle	Radial tuberosity
Brachialis	Flexion	Anterior distal half of the humerus	Coronoid process and ulnar tuberosity
Brachioradialis	Flexion	Lateral supracondylar ridge of the humerus	Styloid process of the radius
Triceps Brachii	Extension Assists in shoulder extension	Infraglenoid tubercle, proximal posterior and distal shaft of the humerus	Olecranon process
Anconeus	Extension	Lateral epicondyle of the humerus	
Pronator Teres	Pronation	Medial epicondyle of the humerus	Mid lateral shaft of the radius
Pronator Quadratus	Pronation	Distal anterior ulna	Distal anterior radius
Supinator	Supination	Lateral epicondyle of the humerus and posterior proximal ulna	Proximal lateral shaft of the radius

Humeroulnar joint motions: Flexion—biceps brachii, brachialis, brachioradialis; **Extension**—triceps brachii, anconeus.
Radioulnar joint motions: Supination—biceps brachii, supinator; **Pronation**—pronator teres, pronator quadratus.

GROUP ACTIVITY 1 • Quiz Show

The game show format can be used to review the structures and function of any system in the body. To review the directions for adopting this game for home play, see Chapter 5, Group Activity 1. Here are sample boards for the muscular system.

LEVEL I

	Functions and Junctions	Let's Get Connected	Under the Microscope	Movement Roles	Prime Functions
100	This function is how we get around	The type of fibrous connective tissue that makes up fascia	It is the plasma membrane of a muscle fiber	It is the muscle that contributes the most to a specific movement	It is the most superficial prime mover for elbow flexion
200	This function keeps us upright	A cord of organized fibrous connective tissue that attaches muscle to bone	It is the ER of a muscle fiber	These muscles assist the prime mover(s)	This is the prime function of the flexor carpi radialis
300	This by-product of contraction is important during winter	The connective tissue covering a muscle fascicle	It is the thick myofilament	Muscles in this role act as a brake to control the motion	Both the gastrocnemius and the soleus are prime movers for this action
400	The junction where skeletal muscle turns into fibrous connective tissue	The corkscrew-shaped protein molecules that make up collagen	It is the zigzagged border between two sarcomeres	The subclavius and subscapularis play this role during shoulder flexion and extension	The prime functions for this muscle are shoulder Abduction, flexion, and extension
500	The anatomic name for the junction between skeletal muscles and bone	A flat sheet of connective tissue that attaches muscle to bone	It is the dark area of the sarcomere	The type of contraction used by an antagonist	This trunk muscle serves as a prime mover in both hip and trunk flexion

LEVEL II

	Not All Contractions Are the Same	Origins	Insertions	Muscle Groups	I Am What I Do
200	This contraction generates force but no movement	Originates from the sternum and clavicle	The common tendon that inserts the gastroc and soleus to the calcaneus	This is number of hip adductors	It is a prime mover in dorsiflexion and inversion
400	This contraction generates both force and a change in length	The origin of the coracobrachialis	The common insertion of the quadriceps	The muscles on the posterior thigh responsible for knee flexion	I assist with knee flexion and have the prime function of hip adduction
600	This is an involuntary contraction of short duration	The common origin of the hamstring muscles	The fascial band formed by the gluteus maximus and TFL for insertion on the tibia	The most superficial group of the paraspinals	It is the strong medial rotator of the rotator cuff group
800	These contractions help us maintain our posture	The common origin of the wrist extensors	The insertion of the supraspinatus	The deepest abdominal muscle of the anterior abdominal wall	I extend the knee but also assist in flexing the hip
1000	Low-grade tension generated through tonic contractions	The medial humeral epicondyle	The insertion of the triceps brachii	The transversospinales group	I am an abdominal muscle that rotates the trunk to the opposite side

GROUP ACTIVITY 2 • Sculpting Statues

This game is an active way to practice movement and muscle knowledge. To play, first review the directions from Chapter 5, Group Activity 2. This time when you play, extend the information used for sculpting by adding muscle information. For example, instead of simply saying, "Flex your elbow," you could direct the lump of clay to, "Concentrically contract the biceps brachii of your right arm." Have fun using your new knowledge.

GROUP ACTIVITY 3 • Assessing End Feel

Review the information on passive range of motions and assessing end feels. In partners or groups of three, perform a P-ROM assessment for each movement in the following joints and note whether the end feel is soft, firm, or hard by checking the appropriate box. Since each person in your group may have different end feels for the same joint, assess each group member. Discuss your findings with each other and your instructor.

Joint	Movement	Soft	Firm	Hard
Elbow	Flexion			
	Extension			
Hip	Flexion			
	Extension			
	Abduction			
	Adduction			
Knee	Flexion			
	Extension			
Ankle	Dorsiflexion			
	Plantarflexion			
	Inversion			
	Eversion			

GROUP ACTIVITY 4 • Drawing Muscles

Many manual therapists use their knowledge of musculoskeletal anatomy everyday when working with their clients. For many learners, it is challenging to translate information that they have only seen presented as words in muscle tables and in two-dimensional drawings into the three dimensions of the body. One way to bridge this learning gap is use washable markers to draw muscles onto a willing partner. This can help you visualize the muscles' positions in relationship to one another and on a real live body.

PRACTICE EXAM UNIT 3 • Chapters 5 & 6

1. Which muscle attachment is generally on the nonmoving bone during motion?
   A. Distal
   B. Insertion
   C. Origin
   D. Lateral

2. Which of the following is an accurate description of the characteristics of skeletal muscle?
   A. Smooth and involuntary
   B. Striated and voluntary
   C. Striated and involuntary
   D. Smooth and voluntary

3. Functions of the skeletal system include protection of vital organs, providing a structural framework for the body and levers for movement, plus
   A. production of blood cells.
   B. storage of energy.
   C. vitamin D synthesis.
   D. generation of movement.

4. What type of bone tissue makes up the shaft of a long bone?
   A. Spongy
   B. Cancellous
   C. Cortical
   D. Fibrous

5. Which of these bones is classified as a cuboid or square bone?
   A. Scapula
   B. Vertebra
   C. Skull
   D. Calcaneous

6. Blood cell production occurs in what part of bones?
   A. Yellow bone marrow
   B. Red bone marrow
   C. Medullary tissue
   D. Dense bone

7. The functions of the muscular system are to maintain posture, create movement, and
   A. store energy.
   B. synthesize ATP.
   C. regulate temperature.
   D. generate heat.

8. A skeletal muscle fiber, or muscle cell, is made up of smaller fibers called
    A. Myofibers.
    B. Myofibrils.
    C. Myofilaments.
    D. Fibrous myocytes.

9. What is the anatomic name for the ends of a long bone?
    A. Epiphysis
    B. Diaphysis
    C. Medullary
    D. Epichondria

10. What is the function of a tendon?
    A. Stabilizing joints
    B. Increasing the force of contraction
    C. Connects muscles to bone
    D. Connects bone to bone

11. What is the bone landmark term for a rounded articular surface of a bone?
    A. Epicondyle
    B. Tubercle
    C. Condyle
    D. Articular protuberance

12. What portion of a muscle fiber is the actual contractile unit?
    A. Myofiber
    B. Sarcomere
    C. Sarcoplasmic reticulum
    D. Myofibrils

13. What fascial layer surrounds each skeletal muscle fiber?
    A. Epimysium
    B. Endomysium
    C. Perimysium
    D. Fibromysium

14. What is the function of articular cartilage?
    A. Cushions bone ends and stabilizes the joint
    B. Feeds the end of the bone
    C. Production of red blood cells
    D. Synthesizes synovial fluid

15. What is the anatomic name of the lateral projection off the spine of the scapula?
    A. Coracoid process
    B. Lateral angle
    C. Acromion process
    D. Scapular process

16. The mastoid process is a bone projection on which bone?

    A. Mastoid
    B. Occipital
    C. Scapula
    D. Temporal

17. What is the function of retinaculi in the muscular system?

    A. Separating the muscle groups in the thigh
    B. Attaching abdominal muscles to the ribcage
    C. Tension straps that hold tendons in place
    D. Serve as the central tendon of the diaphragm

18. When ligaments are stretched or torn, the injury is classified as what?

    A. Torsion trauma
    B. Strain
    C. Sprain
    D. Hematoma

19. What is the name for the narrow ridge that runs along the posterior femur?

    A. Femoral ridge
    B. Linea aspera
    C. Crest of the femur
    D. Linea femoralis

20. The myofilament bonding of a muscle contraction can only occur in the presence of what element?

    A. Calcium
    B. Potassium
    C. Sodium
    D. Oxygen

21. When threshold stimulus is applied to a motor unit, what happens?

    A. Some of the fibers in the unit contract fully.
    B. All fibers in the unit contract fully.
    C. All of the fibers in the unit partially contract.
    D. Minimal numbers of fibers in the unit contract strongly.

22. Fibrous joints that allow minimal or no movement are classified as

    A. diarthrosis.
    B. synovial.
    C. amphiarthrosis.
    D. synarthrotic.

23. Which of these joints is an amphiarthrosis?

    A. Pubis symphsis
    B. Sutures of the skull
    C. Sternoclavicular
    D. Facet joints between vertebrae

24. What types of synovial joint is the radial ulnar joint?
    A. Gliding
    B. Ball and socket
    C. Condyloid
    D. Pivot

25. The five common features of all diarthrotic joints are ligaments, synovial membrane, joint capsule, joint space, and
    A. bursa.
    B. hyaline cartilage.
    C. fibrocartilage.
    D. disorganized connective tissue.

26. Which muscle physiology reflex increases or decreases the number of motor units engaged according to the effort required for a movement?
    A. Sliding filament
    B. Muscle recruitment
    C. Graded response
    D. Myo-magnification

27. Which method of energy production for muscle contraction uses ATP stored in the skeletal muscle and produces only enough energy for a short-term effort?
    A. Glycolytic conversion
    B. ATP glycolysis
    C. Direct phosphorylation
    D. Anaerobic glycolysis

28. What type of joint allows flexion, extension, ABduction, and adduction only?
    A. Pivot
    B. Hinge
    C. Gliding
    D. Condyloid

29. The only saddle joints in the body are the articulation between what bones?
    A. Proximal and distal phalanges of the thumb
    B. First metacarpal and carpal
    C. Proximal row of carpals and radius
    D. Occipital bone and the first cervical vertebra

30. Which of these bones is part of the axial skeleton?
    A. Clavicle
    B. Scapula
    C. Sacrum
    D. Ilium

31. Which method of energy production generates the highest amount of ATP?
    A. Direct phosphorylation
    B. Anaerobic glycolysis
    C. Anaerobic metabolism
    D. Aerobic cellular metabolism

32. What type of muscle contraction increases muscle tension but does not result in movement?

   A. Isotonic
   B. Isometric
   C. Tonic
   D. Eccentric

33. What change occurs in the muscle during a concentric contraction?

   A. The muscle shortens.
   B. All motor units in the muscle are recruited.
   C. The muscle lengthens.
   D. Tension is decreased.

34. What is the name for the movement of turning the hand palm down?

   A. Supination
   B. Pronation
   C. Protraction
   D. Palmar rotation

35. How many thoracic vertebrae are there in the spinal column?

   A. 5
   B. 7
   C. 10
   D. 12

7 The Nervous System

Use this table to identify the study guide exercises and group activities that will help you explore or review each learning objective for this chapter.

No.	Learning Objective	Exercise	Study Group Activity
1	Discuss the importance of understanding the anatomy and physiology of the nervous system as it relates to the practice of manual therapy.		See Chapter 1, Activity 1
2	List and explain the primary functions of the nervous system, the two major divisions, and the key structural components of each.	2	2
3	Name and describe the key structural components of a neuron and the different types of neurons based on structure and function.	3	2
4	Name the different types of neuroglia plus the location and function of each.	4	2
5	Describe the general structure of a nerve and explain the difference between cranial and spinal nerves.	5	2
6	List the four cranial nerves that manual therapists need to know and explain why.	1	2
7	Name the four major nerve plexuses and the body regions they innervate.	1	2
8	List and explain the key events of nerve impulse conduction and synaptic transmission.	6	2
9	Explain the structure and function of a reflex arc.	7	
10	List six categories of sensory receptors, explain the sensitivity of each, and give an example of their location.	8	2
11	Explain the location, structure, and functions of the meninges and cerebrospinal fluid.	1, 9	2
12	Name the key structural features and regions of the spinal cord and explain the general functions of each.	10, 11, 14	1, 2
13	Name the key structural features and regions of the brain and explain the general functions of each.	2, 12, 13, 14	2
14	Compare and contrast the key structural features of somatic and autonomic motor pathways of the peripheral nervous system.	14, 15	2
15	Name, compare, and contrast the structural features and functions of the two motor divisions of the autonomic nervous system.	14, 16	2
16	Discuss the effects of aging on the nervous system		See Chapter 1, Activity 1

EXERCISE 1 • Nervous System Crossword

Use this crossword to review and test your knowledge of some of the nervous system's structures and functions.

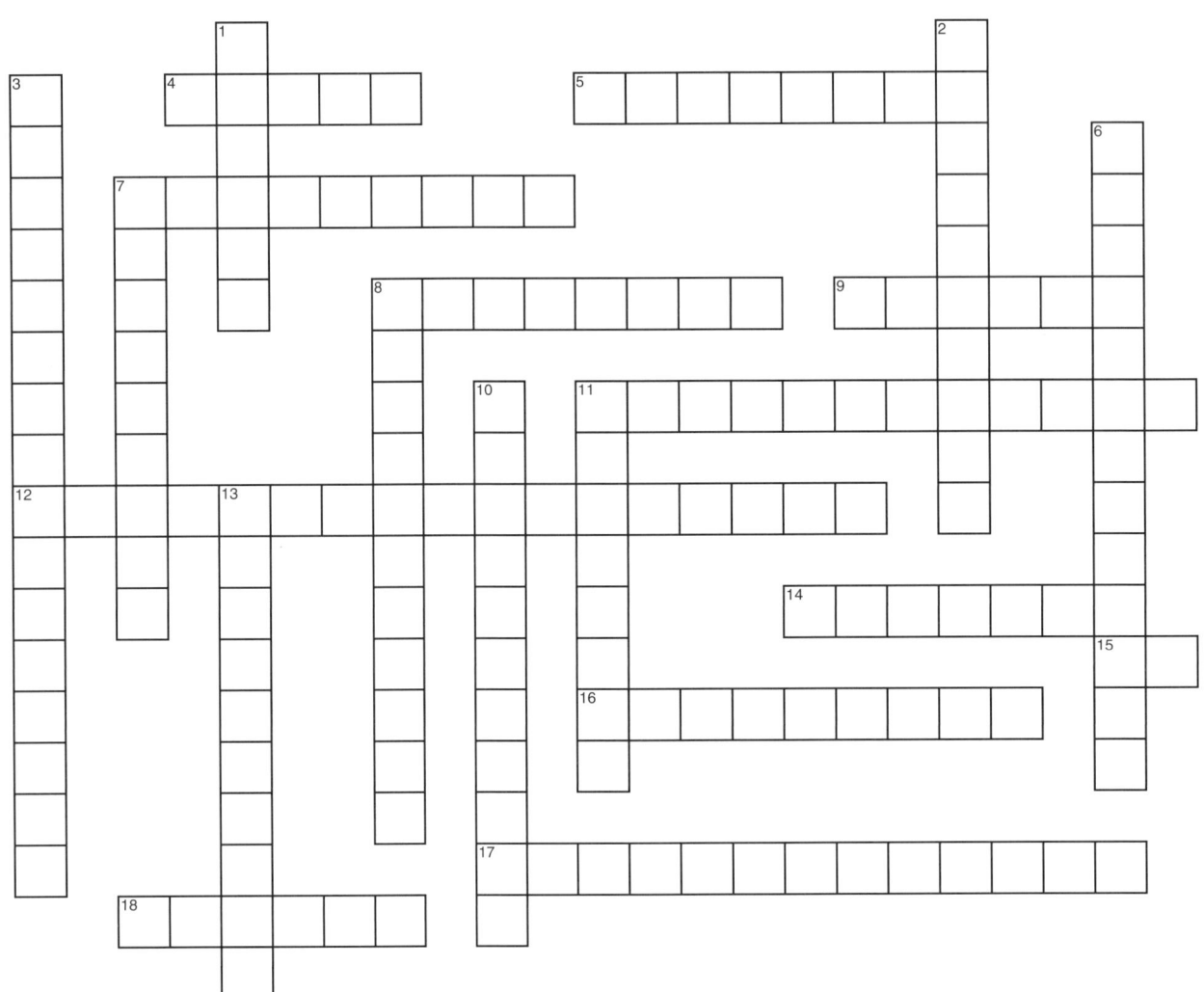

ACROSS

4 Cranial nerve that innervates the diaphragm and viscera.
5 Meningeal layer that supports the large blood vessels on the surface of the brain and spinal cord.
7 Tough outermost meningeal layer.
8 Nerve plexus that innervates the head and neck.
9 Nerve plexus that consists of L1 through L4 spinal nerves.
11 Specific gray matter motor regions of the cerebrum.
12 Boundary that protects brain from pathogens present in blood.
14 Muscle(s) innervated by a specific spinal nerve and cord segment.
15 The number for the accessory cranial nerve.
16 Meningeal layer where cerebral spinal fluid circulates.
17 Colorless fluid that cushions and nourishes the structures of the CNS.
18 Cranial nerve affected by Bell's palsy.

DOWN

1 Nerve plexus whose branches include the sciatic nerve.
2 Cranial nerve V.
3 The brain stem region that contains the respiratory rhythmicity and cardiovascular centers.
6 Specialized capillaries lined with ependymal neuroglia that produce CSF.
7 Area of skin innervated by sensory fibers from a specific spinal nerve and cord segment.
8 Horse's tail of the spinal cord.
10 A neural circuit in which several neurons synapse on a single neuron.
11 Nerve plexus whose branches include the axillary, radial, and ulnar nerves.
13 A neural circuit in which one neuron synapses with several neurons.

EXERCISE 2 • Functional Organization of the Nervous System

Under the umbrella of the nervous system, there are two major divisions. Fill in all of the components of the system below starting with the two major divisions. Then use blue to color the divisions and structures responsible for sensory functions, green for integrative functions, and red for motor functions. If you need to refresh your memory, refer to Figures 7-1 and 7-28 in your textbook.

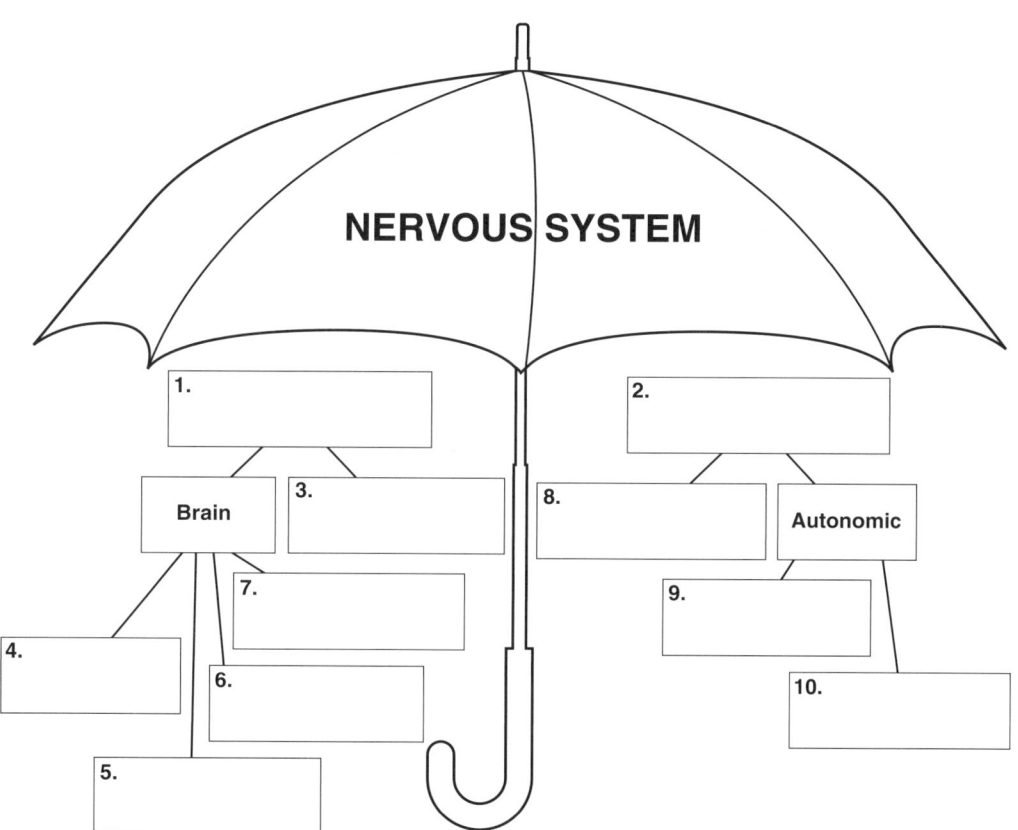

EXERCISE 3 • Neuroglia Mind Map

Complete the mind map by filling in the names and functions of the six types of neuroglia. Color the neuroglia found in the CNS green and those found in the PNS purple.

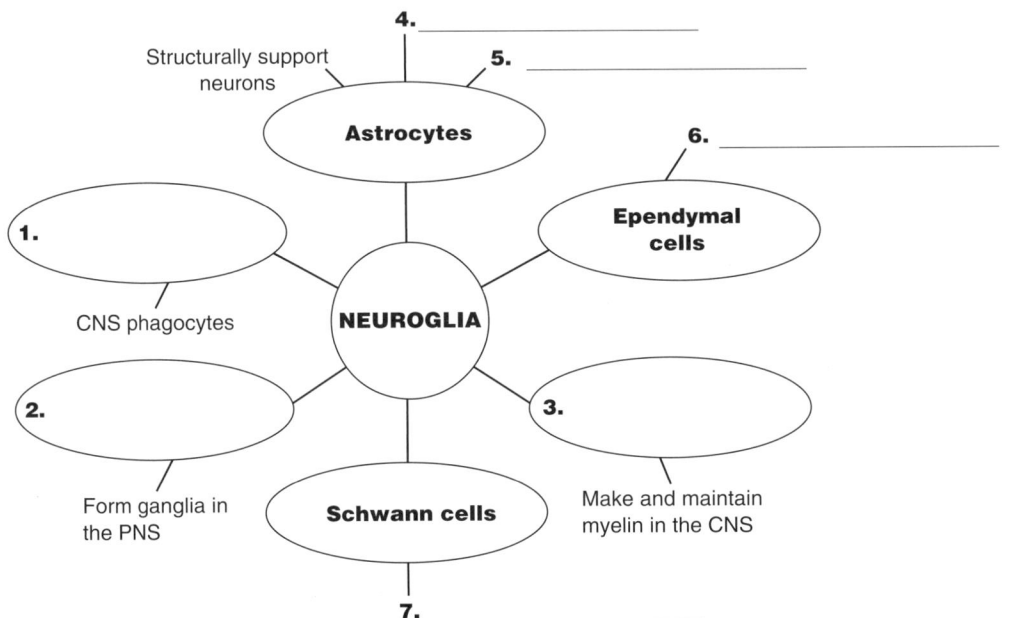

EXERCISE 4 • Neurons: Matching Parts

Color and label the diagram of a neuron. The terms in the matching exercise may provide you clues, or if you need to refresh your memory, refer to Figure 7-2 in your textbook. Complete the matching exercise by placing the letter of the answer that best matches the term provided in the diagram.

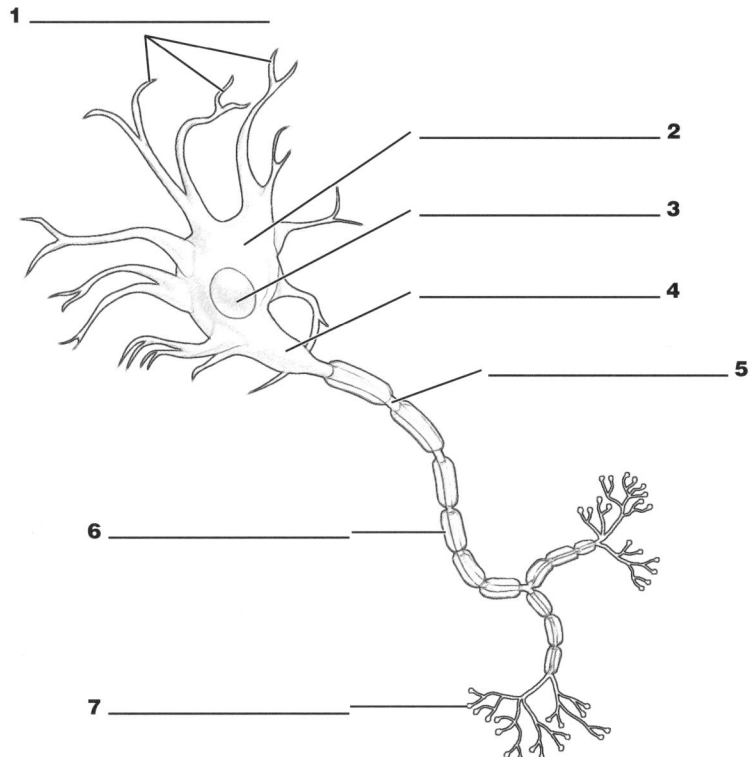

Matching:

_____ 1. Axon
_____ 2. Axon hillock
_____ 3. Axon terminal
_____ 4. Myelin
_____ 5. Cell body
_____ 6. Dendrites
_____ 7. Nucleus
_____ 8. Sensory neuron
_____ 9. Interneuron
_____ 10. Motor neuron
_____ 11. Unipolar
_____ 12. Bipolar
_____ 13. Multipolar
_____ 14. Neurilemma
_____ 15. Synaptic bulb

A. Location of the synaptic bulbs
B. Carries impulses to the CNS
C. Carries impulses to effectors
D. Transmits impulse away from the cell body
E. Transmit impulse toward the cell body
F. Plasma membrane of a Schwann cell
G. Location of the neuron's nucleus
H. Many dendrites and one axon
I. Contains vesicles with neurotransmitter
J. Region where an action potential is generated
K. Cell body between one dendrite and one axon
L. Location of DNA
M. One fiber with a cell body off to one side
N. Insulating sheath of fat
O. Found only in the CNS

EXERCISE 5 • Structure of a Nerve

A nerve is a bundle of axons with its connective tissue coverings and blood vessels outside the CNS. There are _____ pairs of _____ nerves exiting the underside of the brain, and _____ pairs of _____ nerves that relate to the segments of the spinal cord. Color and label the parts of a nerve on the diagram below. If you need to refresh your memory, refer to Figure 7-5 in your textbook.

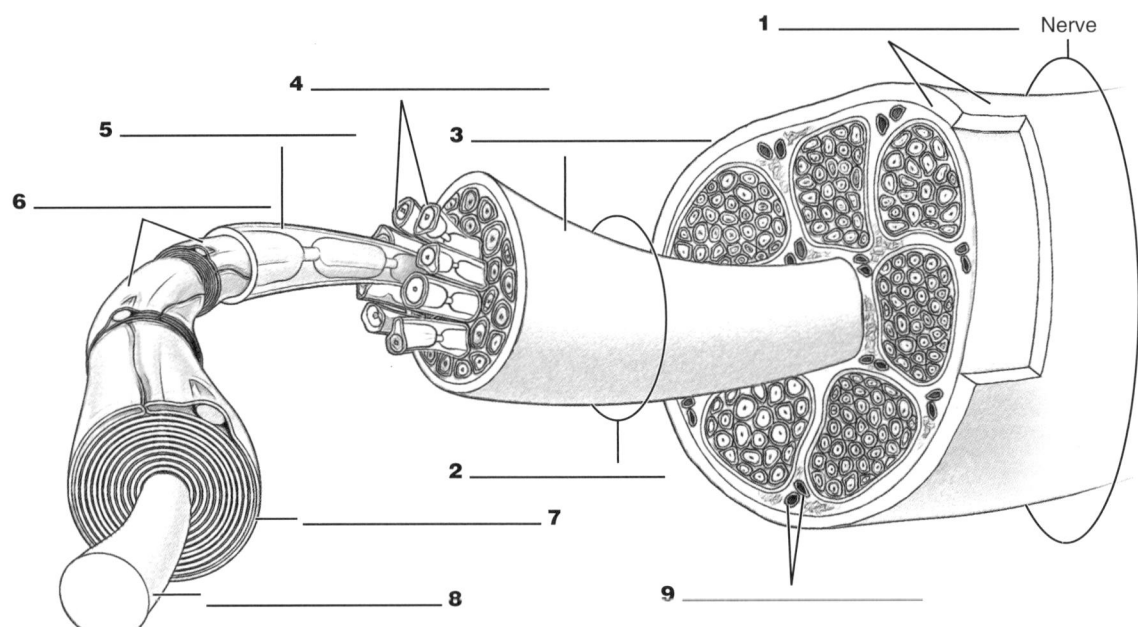

EXERCISE 6 • A Story of Impulse Conduction

Taking the steps of a physiologic process and turning them into a story can help with understanding and recall. The following provides one example of how a story about the key steps of nerve impulse conduction and synaptic transmission might begin. Have fun completing this story or write a different story altogether.

Once upon a time, a traveler named "Impulse" entered the tiny hamlet of Neurolandia and traveled down the main street named Neuron Avenue. Because of his rather gloomy and negative attitude, Impulse created change wherever he walked...

EXERCISE 7 • Diagram a Reflex Arc

Reflexes are automatic and involuntary responses that require little interpretation by the integrating center. A reflex arc is a simple neuronal pathway that provides a predictable 1. _____ _____ for a specific 2. _____ _____.

3. _____ _____ reflexes are managed by two-neuron reflex arcs, while the 4. _____ reflex involves a three-neuron reflex arc.

Color and label the components of the reflex arcs diagrammed below making any sensory components blue, integrative components green, and motor components red. If you need to refresh your memory, refer to Figure 7-14 in your textbook.

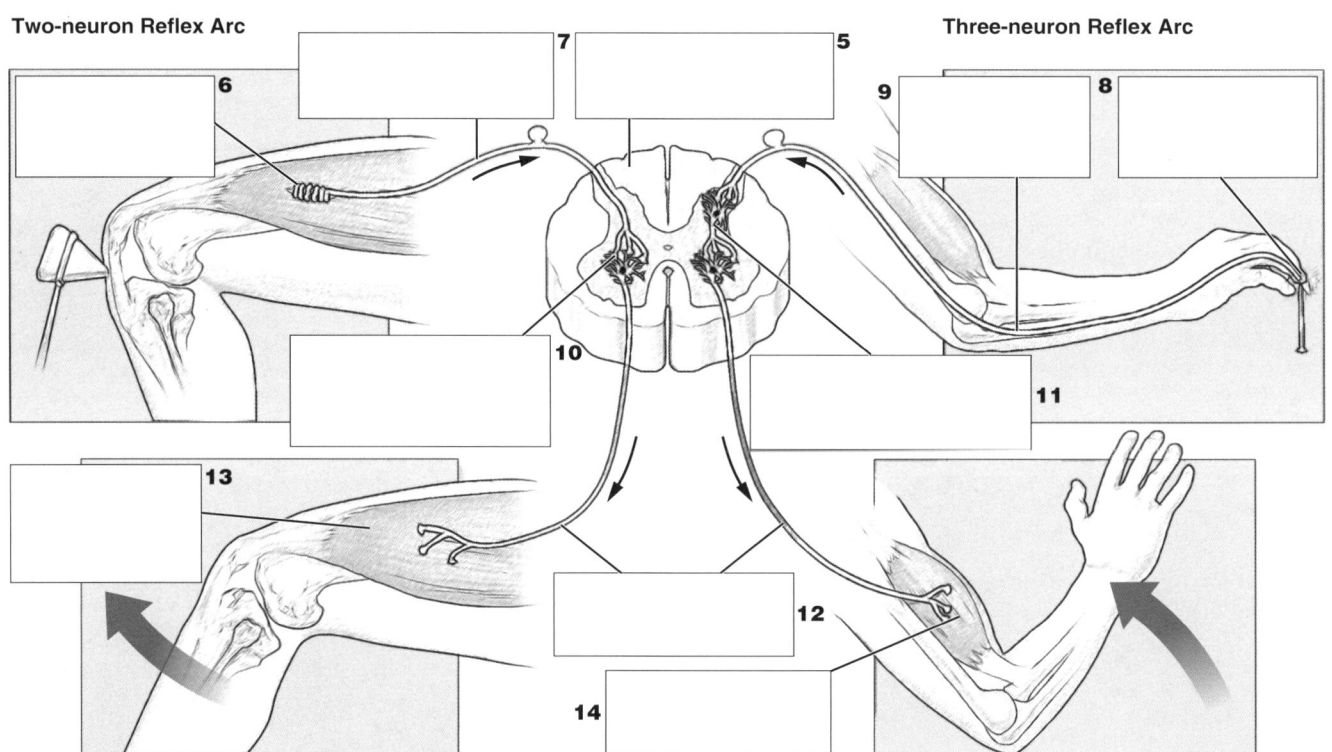

EXERCISE 8 • Sensory Receptors Table

Fill in the blanks to complete this table describing the different categories of sensory receptors, the stimulus each is sensitive to, and example(s) of the location for each category.

Receptor Category	Stimulus	Example Location
1.	Light	2.
Nociceptors	3.	4.
5.	6.	Joints and skeletal muscles
Mechanoreceptors	7.	8.
9.	Changes in chemical concentrations	10.
Thermoreceptors	11.	12.

EXERCISE 9 • Meninges Diagram

Color and label the diagram of the meninges covering the brain. If you need to refresh your memory, refer to Figure 7-20 in your textbook.

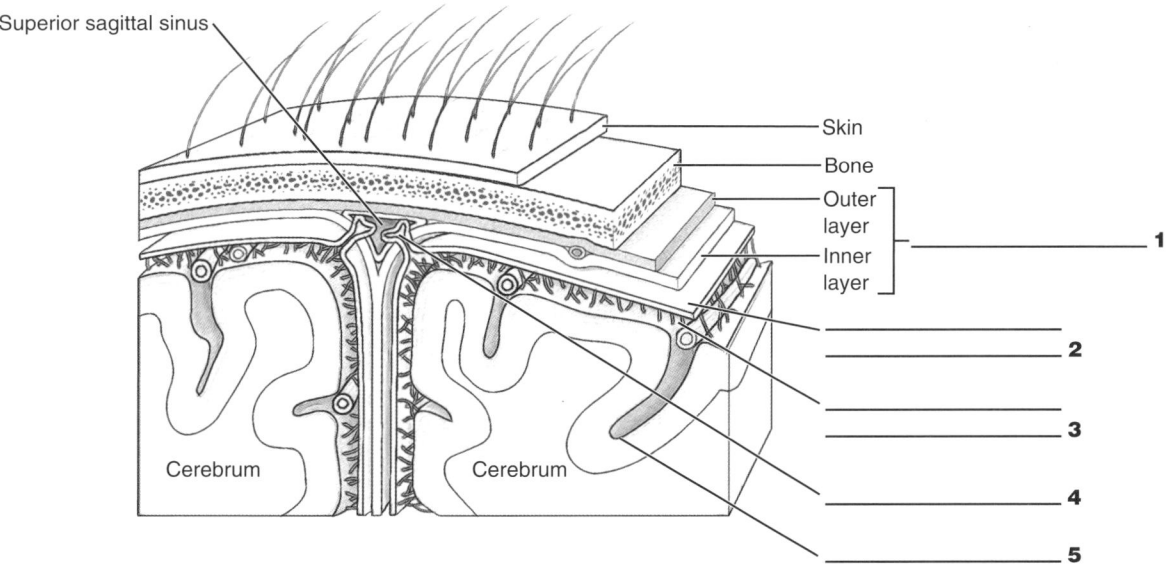

EXERCISE 10 • Nervous Terminology: Reviewing Synonyms

In the nervous system, structures are referred to by a variety of synonymous terms. For example, sensory neurons can also be referred to as **1.** _____ neurons because they transmit impulses toward the CNS, while **2.** _____ neurons are often called efferent neurons because they transmit impulses away from the CNS. Other structures that have several synonymous names include the spinal cord tracts and the nerve roots that split apart from the spinal nerves to attach to the cord. Use the diagram below to name the tracts and nerve roots and identify their synonyms.

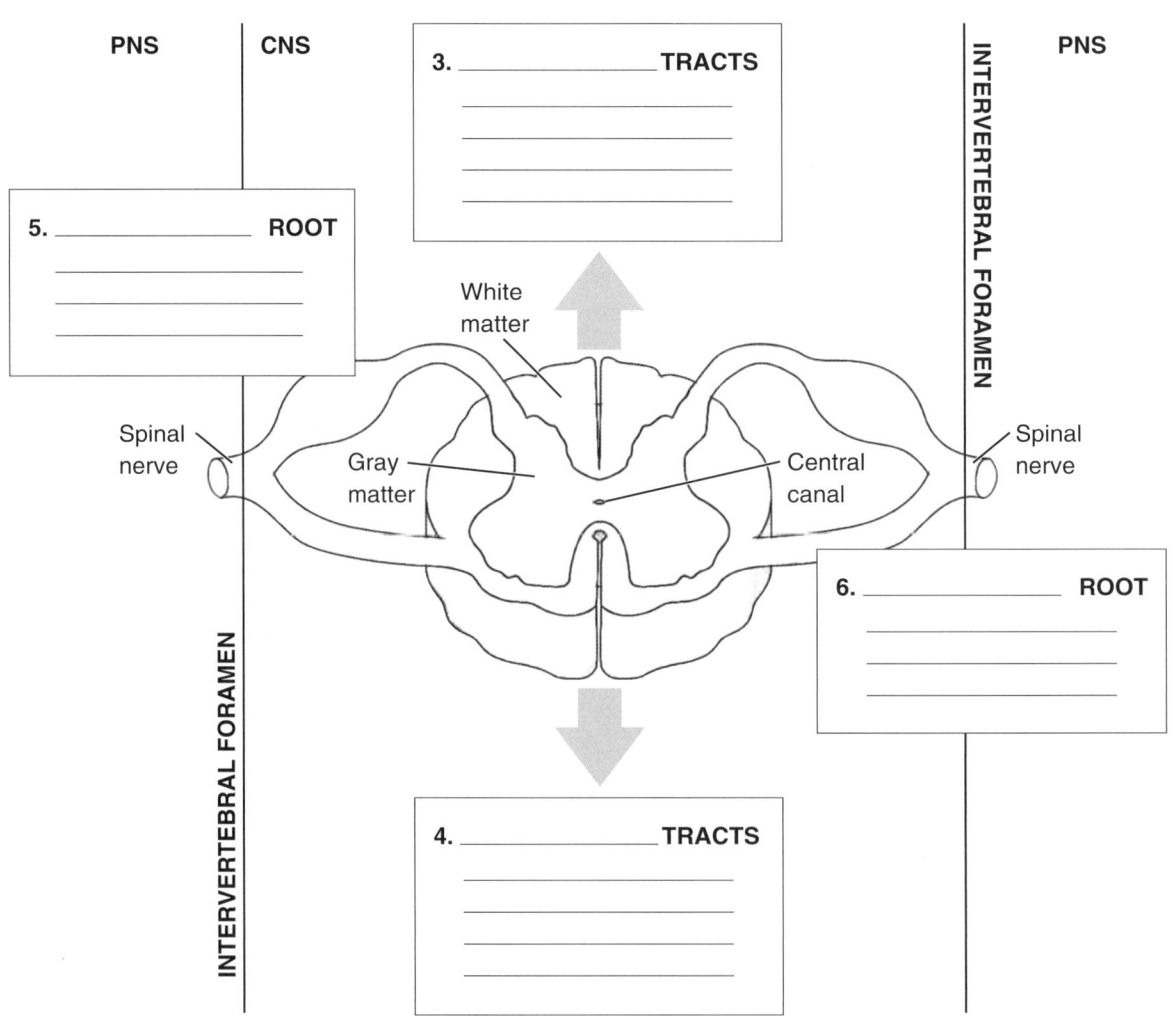

Chapter 7 The Nervous System 105

EXERCISE 11 • Spinal Cord Gray Matter Organization

The gray matter of the spinal cord is divided into three major regions or horns. Label these horns on the left side of the diagram below. The **1.** _____ horn receives sensory information, while the **2.** _____ and **3.** _____ horns contain the cell bodies and dendrites of motor neurons.

Color and label the four regions designated on the right side of the diagram to identify what information is received or sent from each region. If you need to refresh your memory, refer to Figure 7-22 in your textbook.

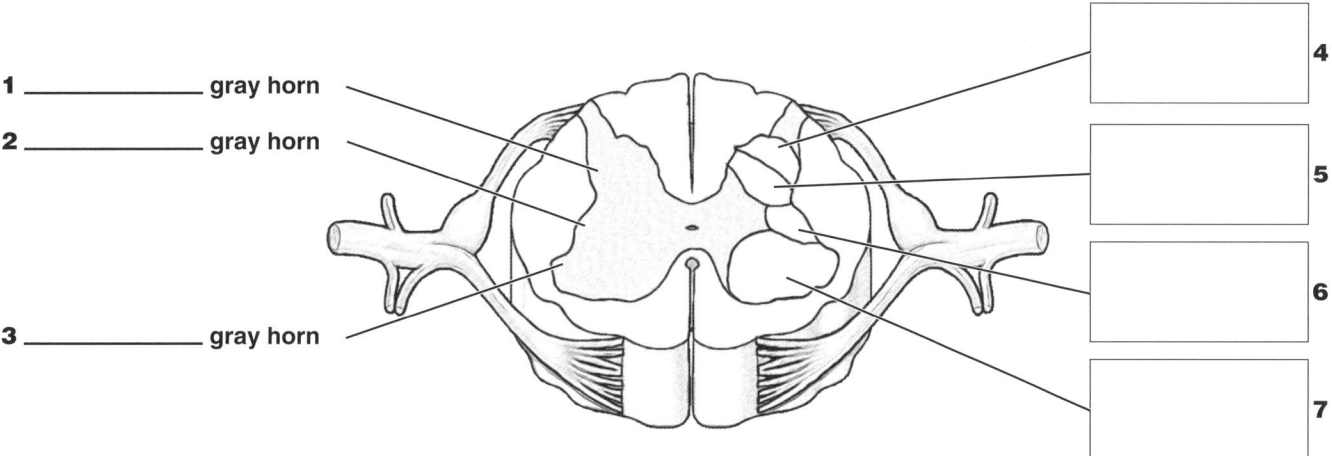

1 _____ gray horn
2 _____ gray horn
3 _____ gray horn

4
5
6
7

EXERCISE 12 • Matching Brain Parts and Their Functions

Color and label the parts of the brain identified on the diagram. Then, using the list provided, place the letter that best describes the function of each region next to its name. If you need to refresh your memory, refer to Figure 7-24 and the sections about the various brain regions in your textbook.

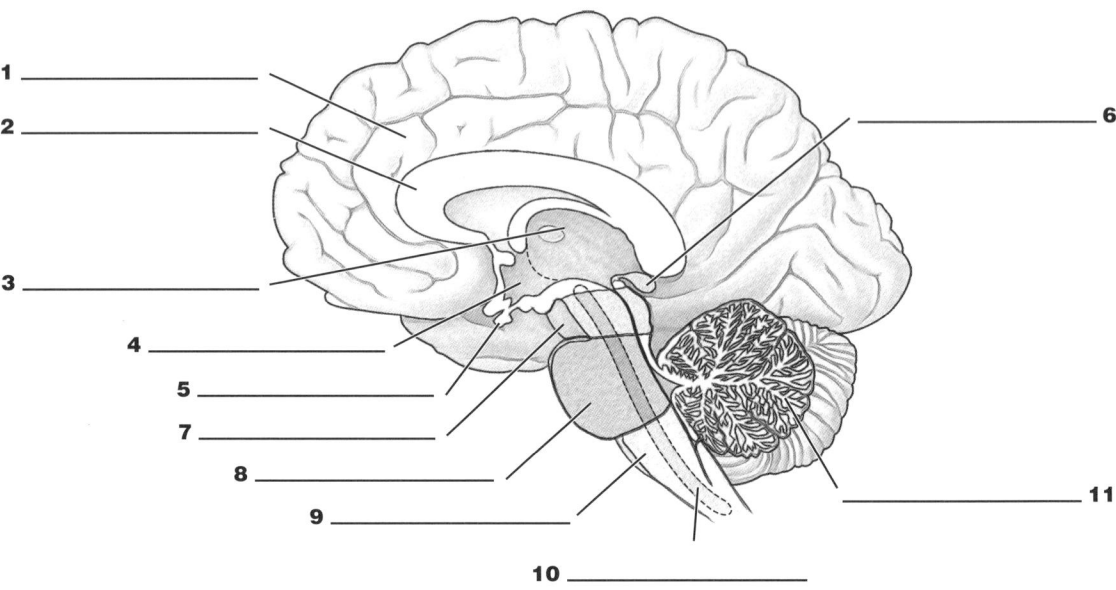

1. _____
2. _____
3. _____
4. _____
5. _____
6. _____
7. _____
8. _____
9. _____
10. _____
11. _____

1. Serves as a sensory clearing house
2. Controls reflexes including coughing, sneezing, and swallowing and contains the respiratory rhythmicity and cardiovascular centers
3. A white matter bridge that allows information to be shared between the cerebral hemispheres
4. Releases hormones that control other endocrine glands
5. Controls and coordinates muscle contractions for body movement, posture, and balance
6. Controls the ANS and links the nervous and endocrine systems
7. Manages conscious thought, creative thinking, and other complex processes
8. Forms important connections between the spinal cord, cerebellum, and cerebrum
9. Helps to coordinate muscle contractions and controls movements of the eyes, head, and neck in response to visual stimuli
10. Manages state of alertness and helps regulate resting muscle tone, digestion, urination, and sexual arousal
11. Secretes melatonin

EXERCISE 13 • Cerebral Structures

The cerebral cortex that covers the white matter of the cerebrum is characterized by its many folds or **1.** _____. Deep **2.** _____ divide the cerebrum into two **3.** _____. Shallow grooves called **4.** _____ divide each half into four **5.** _____.

Color and label the diagram below to identify the location of these structures. If you need to refresh your memory, refer to Figure 7-25 in your textbook.

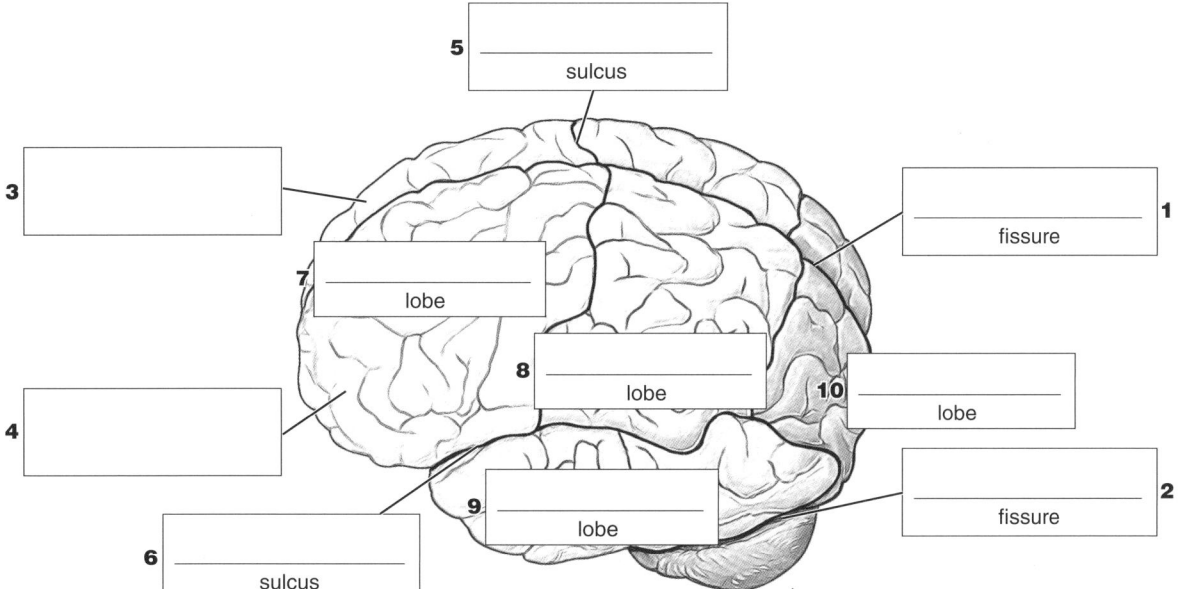

EXERCISE 14 • Pathways of the Nervous System

The CNS interprets and processes sensory information from the PNS and coordinates and controls motor commands to effectors. Neurons carrying sensory information form afferent pathways, while neurons transmitting motor information form efferent pathways. Place the number or letter from the diagram that matches each of the structures in the list below. Then, color the afferent pathways on the diagram blue and the efferent pathways red. If you choose, color the structures of the CNS and/or add more colors to distinguish the different types of PNS motor neurons on the diagram.

Sensory neurons _____
Somatic motor neurons _____
Sympathetic motor neurons _____
Parasympathetic motor neurons _____
Spinal cord _____
Cauda equina _____

Ascending tracts _____
Descending tracts _____
Cerebrum _____
Diencephalon _____
Brain stem _____
Cerebellum _____

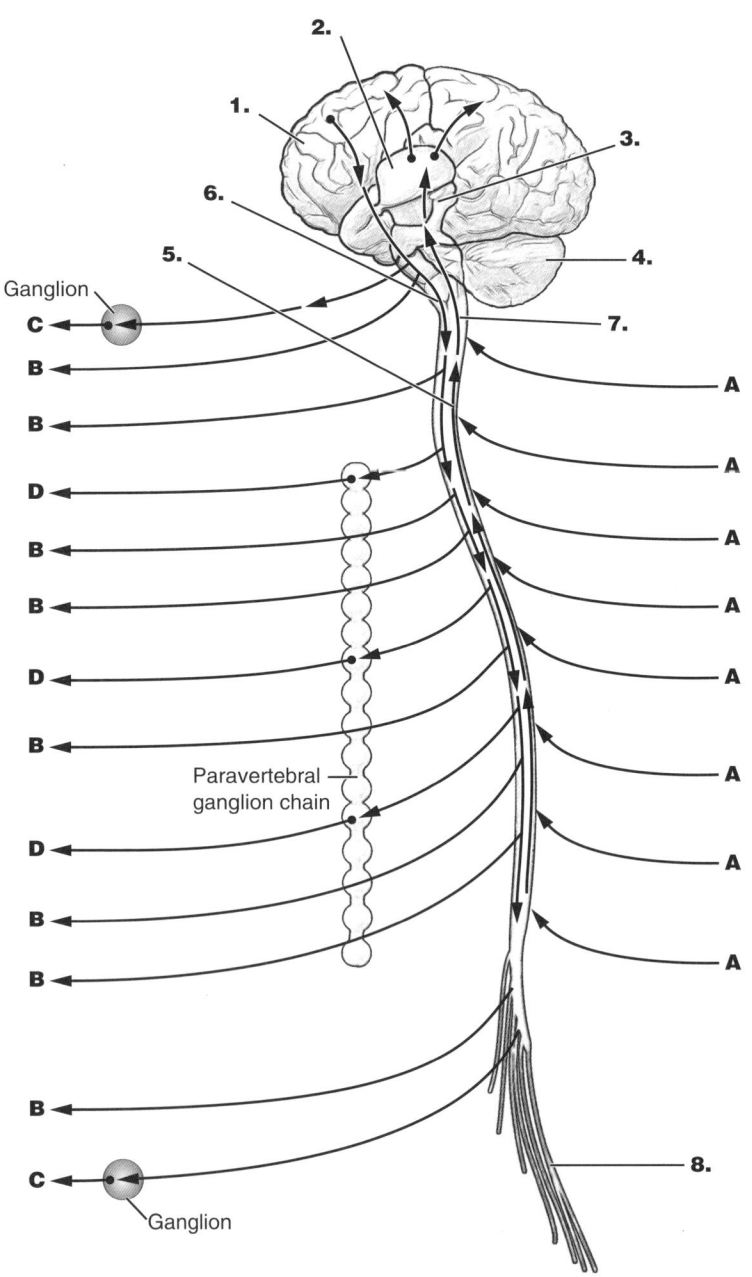

EXERCISE 15 • Comparing Somatic and Autonomic Motor Pathways

Use the Venn diagram below to compare and contrast the structural and functional characteristics of somatic and autonomic pathways. An example of one shared characteristic, that is, comprised of both sensory and motor pathways, has been placed in the area of overlap to get you started. Other characteristics to consider might include number of motor neurons in the divisions' pathways, types of effectors, neurotransmitters used by motor neurons, or nerves carrying the motor pathways (specific cranial or spinal nerves). If you need to review how to use a Venn diagram, refer to Chapter 6, Exercise 3.

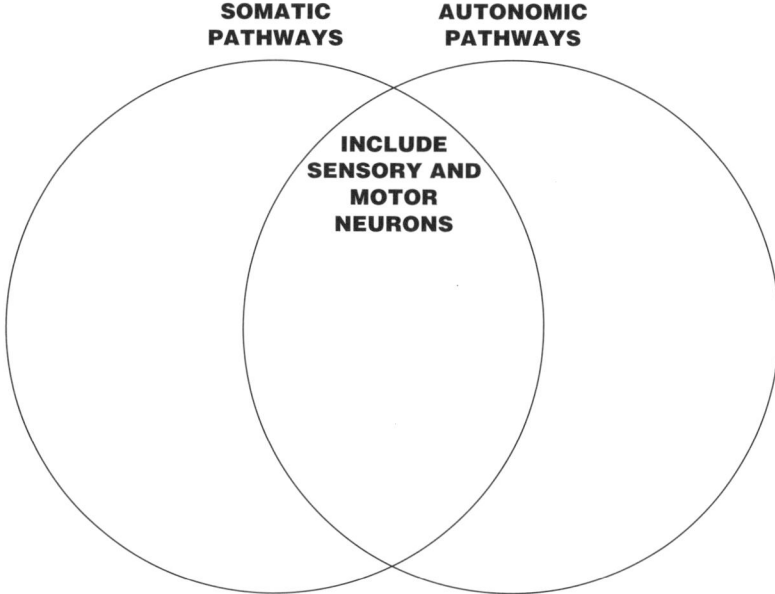

EXERCISE 16 • Structural Features of the ANS

Complete the following table that compares and contrasts the features and functions of the two branches of the ANS.

Characteristic	Sympathetic	Parasympathetic
Nickname for division based on general function or effect	1.	2.
Name of division based on nerves that carry the ANS motor pathways	3.	4.
Number of motor neurons in each ANS pathway	5.	6.
Location of ganglia	7.	8.
Widespread or targeted stimulation of effectors	9.	10.
Neurotransmitter released by the postganglionic neurons	11	12.

GROUP ACTIVITY 1 • Building a Model of the Spinal Cord

To better understand the structure of the spinal cord, you can build a simple 3D model using materials easily obtained from any craft store. While you can do this activity alone, it is often more helpful to do it with a group of people. Each person in your group will build a single cord segment. Then you can stack these segments together to form a portion of the spinal cord. For each segment, you will need:

- One 3" to 4" round disk of styrofoam, white clay, or white cardboard that is approximately 1" thick
- Gray-colored felt or paper
- Six blue pipe cleaners
- Six red pipe cleaners
- Glue
- Clear plastic wrap or tape

Follow these steps to create your model. You may find it helpful to refer to Figure 7-22A in your textbook.

1. Draw and cut a butterfly shape out of the gray-colored felt or paper to represent the gray matter of the spinal cord (don't forget the central canal). Glue it to the top of your disk to create a spinal cord segment. Once the gray matter is in place, be sure everyone in your group is clear where the anterior and posterior regions of their segment are located.
2. Using the blue pipe cleaners to represent sensory neurons, insert three sensory neurons on each side of the segment adjacent to the proper horn of gray matter. Twist a small loop in the pipe cleaners to represent the dorsal root ganglion.
3. Using the red pipe cleaners to represent motor neurons, insert three motor neurons on each side of the segment adjacent to the proper horn of gray matter.
4. Bring the three sensory neurons and three motor neurons on each side together to form a spinal nerve on either side of your spinal cord segment. Wrap your spinal nerve together with your plastic wrap or tape. Notice how the nerve divides close to the cord into dorsal and ventral roots.
5. Finally, stack your segments together to create a portion of the spinal cord. Be sure all your sensory neurons (blues) are on the dorsal side and the motor neurons (reds) are on the ventral side.

GROUP ACTIVITY 2 • Quiz Show

LEVEL I

	Neurons or Neuroglia	In the Periphery	Impulse Conduction	Parts of the Brain	Cranial Nerves
100	Most sensory neurons are this shape	The anatomic term for a bundle of neurons and their blood supply outside the CNS	This amount of stimulus needed to initiate an impulse	The posterior and inferior region of the brain	The number of cranial nerve pairs in the system
200	The cell that produces myelin in the PNS	The number of spinal nerve pairs	The polarity of a resting membrane potential; a neuron at rest	The cerebral lobe that is considered to be the general sensory region	The name for cranial nerve X
300	This is the primary function of ependymal cells	The anatomic name for the sensory nerve root	Increased membrane permeability allows this to rush into the neuron	The thalamus and hypothalamus are in this region	The French term for the painful syndrome of cranial nerve V
400	The plasma membrane of a Schwann cell	The directional term for a motor pathway on spinal nerves	The one-way direction of impulses in all neurons	The name for the region of the cerebrum that connects right and left hemispheres	Bell palsy is a pathology associated with this cranial nerve
500	The majority of these neurons are found only in the CNS	These are the effectors for somatic motor pathways	The anatomic point where the impulse begins to travel down an axon	The vital function reflex center of the brain stem	These first two cranial nerves are examples of sensory-only nerves

LEVEL II

	The ANS	Nerves & Plexuses	More Brain	The Spinal Cord	Sensory Receptors
200	The number of motor neurons in an autonomic pathway	This plexus innervates the entire upper extremity	The cerebral lobe for visual perception	The term that describes the direction of sensory information in the spinal cord	Touch, temperature, pain, and pressure are this type of sensory receptor
400	This division of the ANS is nicknamed the "feed and breed" division	The name of the nerve that innervates the diaphragm; a primary branch off the cervical plexus	This region is known as the emotional brain	The side of the spinal cord that carries motor information	The three major categories of proprioceptors
600	The location of the sympathetic chain ganglia	Major nerves branch off this plexus include the obturator, ilioinguinal, and femoral nerves	This is the function of the thalamus	The name of the CSF-filled opening in the middle of the gray matter	The three major types of proprioceptors in the body
800	The gray matter region of the spinal cord that is the origin of all ANS motor pathways	These are the primary nerve branches off the brachial plexus	These are the primary functions of the cerebellum	The innermost layer of the meninges	This is the proprioceptor responsible for stimulating the stretch reflex
1000	These are the three visceral effectors that have only sympathetic innervation	The peripheral nerve that innervates the SCM and upper trapezius	The limbic system structure that registers fear	The functions of the spinal cord	These specialized mechanoreceptors act as pressure receptors for some hollow organs

8 Neuromuscular and Myofascial Connections

Use this table to identify the study guide exercises and group activities that will help you explore or review each learning objective for this chapter.

No.	Learning Objective	Exercise	Study Group Activity
1	Discuss the importance of understanding key neuromuscular and myofascial connections in the practice of manual therapy.	1, 2	See Chapter 1, Activity 1
2	Describe the two neuronal loops utilized by muscle spindles to moderate muscle tension.	3	
3	Explain how manual therapists can use their knowledge of RI, SR, and GG to reduce muscle tension.	2	1
4	Describe the different physiologic mechanisms involved in the development of TeP and TrP and the implications those have on manual therapy choices.	4	1
5	Explain the concept of tensegrity as it applies to the human body.	1, 5	
6	Explain the general location and function of the layers, bands, and planes of the fascial system.	6	
7	Explain the functional importance of myofascial chains and how knowledge of these chains might affect therapeutic choices.		2
8	Explain the key mechanical properties of fascia and how knowledge of these properties might affect therapeutic choices.	1, 7	
9	Name the four types of mechanoreceptors found in fascia.	1, 8	
10	Discuss how knowledge of the mechanoreceptors and smooth muscle cells in fascia might affect therapeutic choices.		See Chapter 1, Activity 1
11	Describe the neuromuscular and neurofascial mechanisms related to maintaining posture, coordinating movement, and regulating muscle and motor tone.	1	3
12	Explain the difference between motor unit and muscle recruitment and between myofascial and kinetic chains.	9	

EXERCISE 1 • Neuromuscular and Myofascial Terminology Crossword

Use this crossword to review and test your knowledge of the anatomy and physiology terms from Chapter 8.

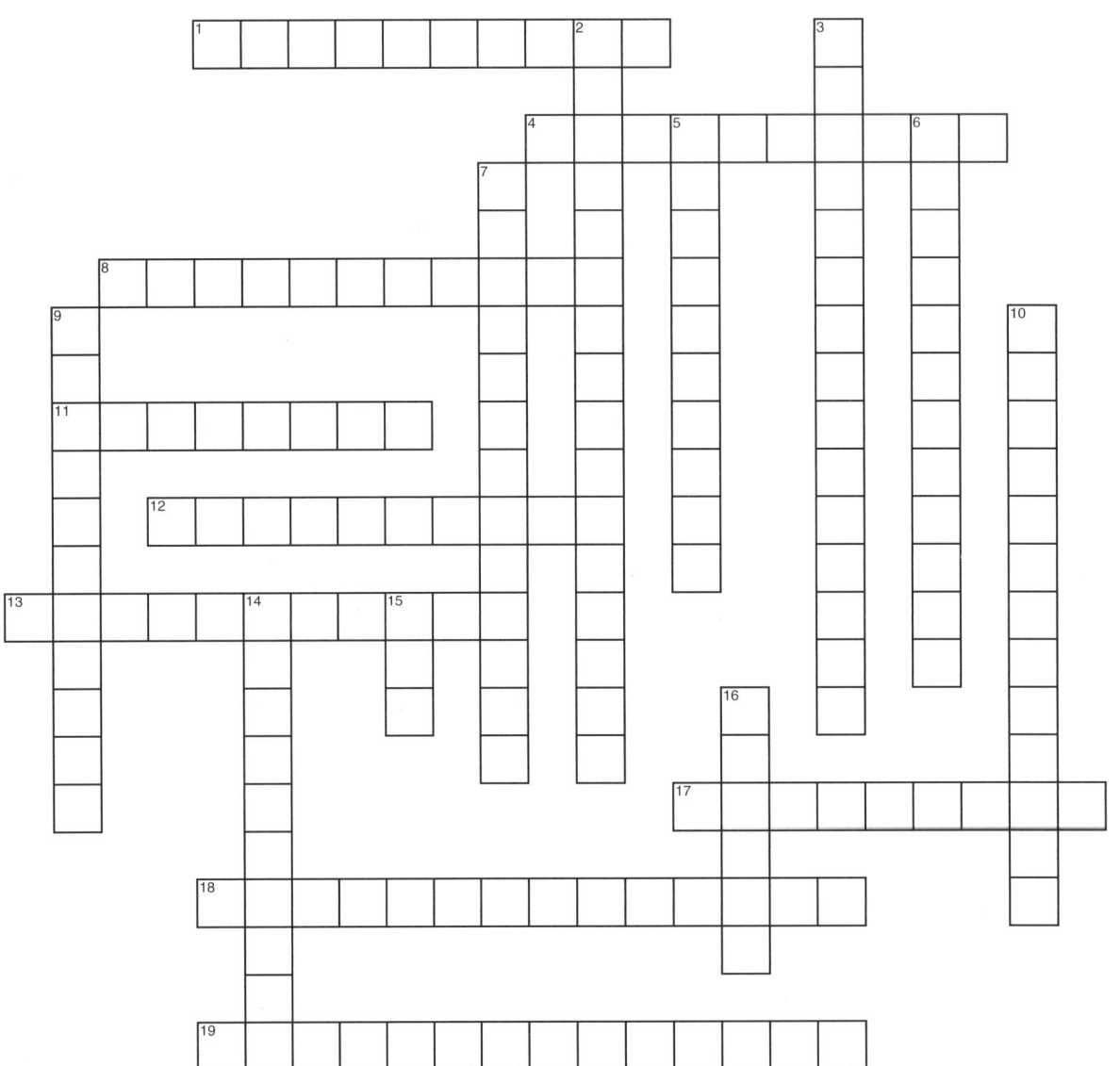

ACROSS

1. The ability of a substance to vacillate between gel and sol states.
4. Connective tissue layers that organize and surround individual muscles, bones, and organs.
8. Low grade tension created by smooth muscle cells within fascia that is regulated by the ANS.
11. Skeletal muscles that play an essential role in maintaining the body's upright position are called _____.
12. The superficial layer or tube of fascia.
13. The sense and awareness of movement.
17. Pre-tensioning of the muscle spindle that increases its sensitivity to rapid lengthening.
18. Sense and awareness of where body parts are positioned in space and in relationship to one another.
19. A very powerful GAG.

DOWN

2. Small electrical charge along a cell or tissue surface created by mechanical pressure.
3. The ability of tissues to extend and rebound rather than to stretch and recoil.
5. The ability of a substance to be molded or changed.
6. Most abundant myofascial sensory receptors.
7. Triple helix protein molecule found in collagen fibers.
9. Hypodermis is also _____ fascia.
10. Excessive muscle tension.
14. System in which tension between two opposing forces is balanced to create structural integrity.
15. A more liquid state.
16. Skeletal muscles whose primary role is to create movement are called _____.

EXERCISE 2 • Neuromuscular Reflexes Table

This table will help you organize the information about different neuromuscular reflexes and their implications for manual therapy. You may simply place the letter of the muscle reflex definitions and manual therapy applications into the proper row and column or rewrite the definitions or applications to fill in the table more completely. One manual therapy application has already been provided.

Definitions

A. The alpha neuronal pathway of muscle spindles is stimulated by lengthening or stretching of the extrafusal fibers and signals a reflexive contraction of the muscle.
B. The reflex mechanism that coordinates the effort between agonist and antagonist muscles. Reciprocal innervation (RI) between agonist and antagonist gives a simultaneous motor command for the agonist to contract and inhibition of contraction in the antagonist.
C. The gamma neuronal pathway of muscle spindles becomes hypersensitive to the rate of lengthening so that sudden lengthening of a muscle creates a "false stretch reflex" report that locks the muscle into a slightly shortened position. This response is especially pronounced if a muscle has been static or shortened for a period of time prior to rapid lengthening.
D. Golgi tendon organs that are sensitive to tension within skeletal muscle respond to the increased tension of an active muscle contraction by inhibiting its force.

Manual Therapy Application

E. Therapists employ a contract-relax method to a tight muscle that inhibits muscle tension to enhance stretch and gain improved range.
F. Therapists can reduce tension in tight muscles by engaging the antagonist of that muscle in an isometric contraction because it causes contraction of the tight muscle to be inhibited.
G. Static stretching (slow and gradual) is used to improve muscle length and ROM because it avoids stimulating a stretch reflex (SR) and possible tissue damage.

Type of Muscle Reflex	Definition	Manual Therapy Application
Stretch Reflex	1.	2.
Gamma Gain	3.	By shortening a muscle with TeP, and holding that position for ~ 90 s, therapists turn off the false SR report. Therapists must slowly and passively move the muscle back to normal resting length to avoid restimulation of the contraction.
Inverse Stretch Reflex	4.	5.
Reciprocal Innervation	6.	7.

EXERCISE 3 • Neuronal Loops

Complete the fill in the blank exercise and then color and label the diagram to identify the two types of muscle fibers and the neurons of the neuronal pathways associated with muscle spindles. Notice that the numbers in the diagram match the numbers in the fill in the blank exercise and colors for the different neurons are suggested. If you need to refresh your memory, refer to Figure 8-2 and the sections on neuromuscular reflexes in your textbook.

Muscle spindles are proprioceptors that sense 1. _____ of muscle fibers and signal a reflexive 2. _____ of the muscle called the 3. _____ _____. Muscle spindles have two distinct portions linked to different neuronal pathways that innervate different types of muscle fibers. The alpha loop is made up of the 4. _____ _____ neuron (blue) looped around the central region of the muscle spindle and the 5. _____ _____ neuron (red) that innervates 6. ____ fibers within the muscle. The alpha loop is the reflex arc for the 7. _____ _____. In addition, the alpha neurons are also part of the sensory and motor pathways used by the primary motor centers of the cerebrum and cerebellum to 8. _____.

The second reflex arc, called the 9. _____ _____, is comprised of a 10. _____ _____ neuron (purple) attached toward the ends of the spindle and the 11. _____ _____ neuron (orange) that innervates the 12. _____ fibers. This reflex arc regulates the 13. _____ of the muscle spindle by adjusting its 14. _____ and _____. In other words, when stimulated to contract via this neuronal loop, the 14. _____ within the muscle spindle increases, effectively increasing the proprioceptor's 15. _____ to any lengthening of the muscle. This phenomenon is called 16. _____ _____.

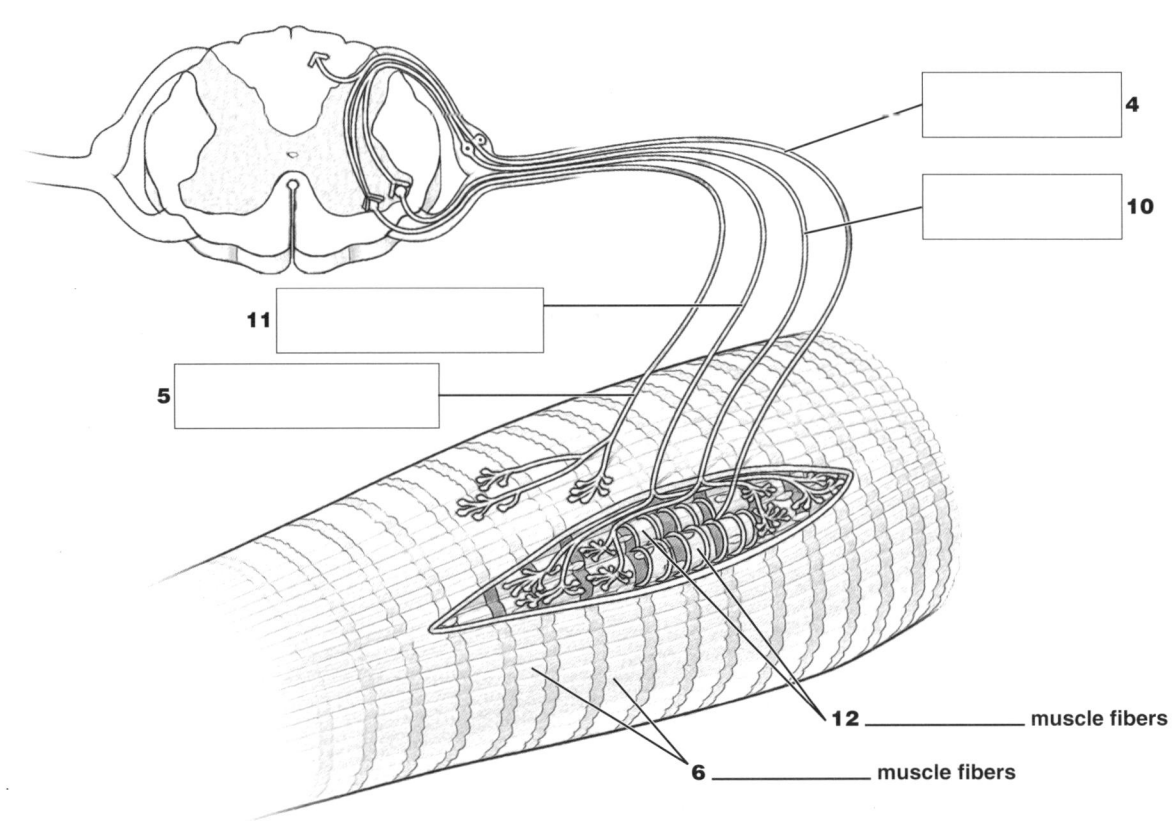

EXERCISE 4 • Trigger Versus Tender Points

Identify each statement below as characteristic of trigger points (TrP), tender points (TeP), or both (B).

_____ 1. Point may or may not be palpable
_____ 2. Point is hypersensitive to mechanical pressure
_____ 3. Caused by high gamma-gain in the muscle spindle
_____ 4. Has a palpable nodule in a taut band of muscle
_____ 5. Digital pressure reproduces pain complaint in a predictable pattern
_____ 6. Caused by chemical irritation of motor end plate
_____ 7. Causes muscle to be hypersensitive to stretch
_____ 8. Digital pressure creates no referred pattern of pain
_____ 9. Causes muscle to be resistant to stretch
_____ 10. "Calcium spill" into sarcomere leads to actin-myosin bonding
_____ 11. Often silent until compressed
_____ 12. Treatment requires repositioning of muscle

EXERCISE 5 • Tensegrity

The term tensegrity describes how the 1. _____ between two opposing forces can be balanced to create structural 2. _____. In the musculoskeletal system, gravity creates a 3. _____ force on the bones of the skeleton, while the muscles and fascia that connect and functionally integrate the skeleton exert 4. _____ on the bones and joints to maintain 5. _____.

The musculoskeletal system is not the only example of tensegrity in the human body. For example, the functional integrity of the nervous system relies on both convergent and divergent pathways. Convergent pathways allow for a single control decision to be made from multiple pieces of information, while divergent pathways allow many regions of the brain or effectors to respond to a singular piece of information. What other examples of tensegrity can you think of in the human body or in your life? Make this a group activity by sharing your responses with your classmates and teacher.

EXERCISE 6 • Fascial Layers, Bands, and Planes

Use the lists provided to label and identify the different layers, bands, and planes of fascia by color in each of the diagrams. If you need to refresh your memory, refer to Figures 8-7, 8-10, and 8-11 in your textbook.

Fascial Layers

Each layer of fascia creates a **1.** _____ or organizing **2.** _____ for its structures. All four sleeves merge together at the **3.** _____ _____.

- Axial fascia
- Meningeal fascia
- Pannicular fascia
- Visceral fascia

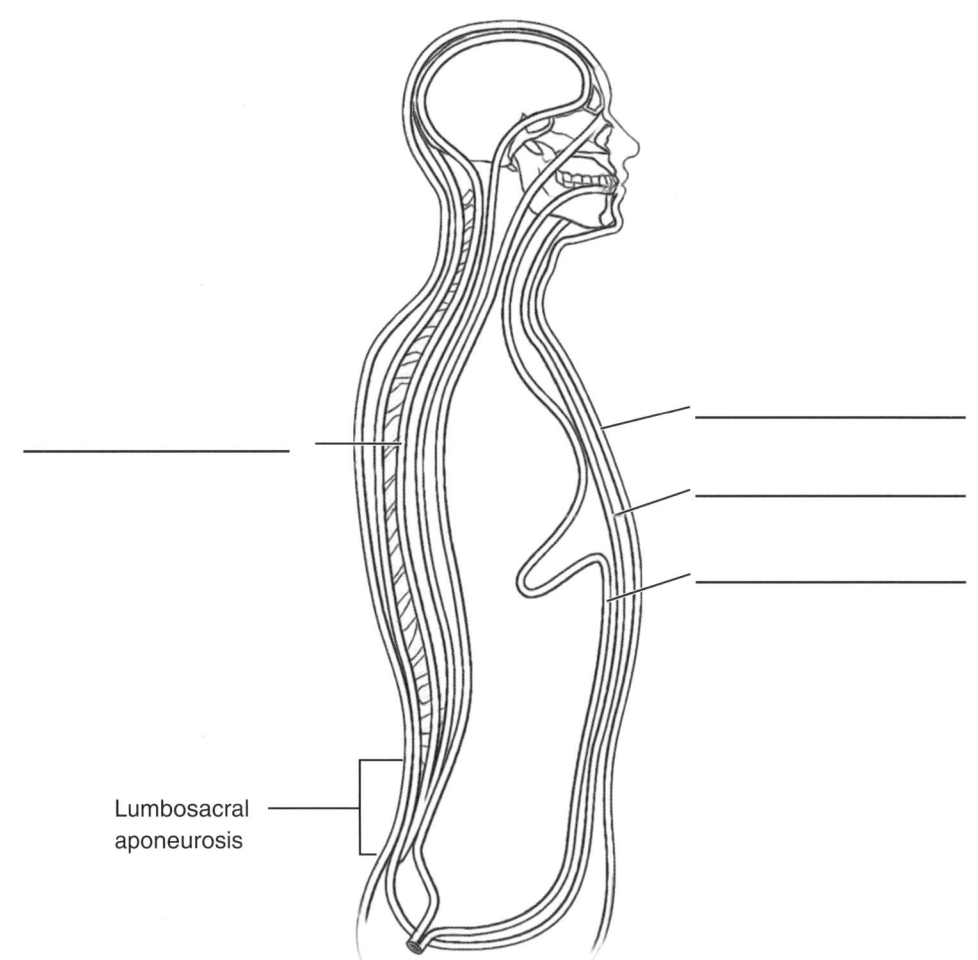

Lumbosacral aponeurosis

Fascial Bands

Fascial bands are **4.** _____ _____ _____ within the normal subcutaneous contours of the torso that firmly anchor the softer rounder anterior torso to the vertical, semirigid spine. Though their precise location varies from one individual to another, each band can be correlated to a specific **5.** _____ _____. They generally **6.** _____ slightly, following individual body contours instead of following a straight horizontal line.

- Chest
- Chin
- Collar
- Eye
- Groin
- Inguinal
- Umbilical

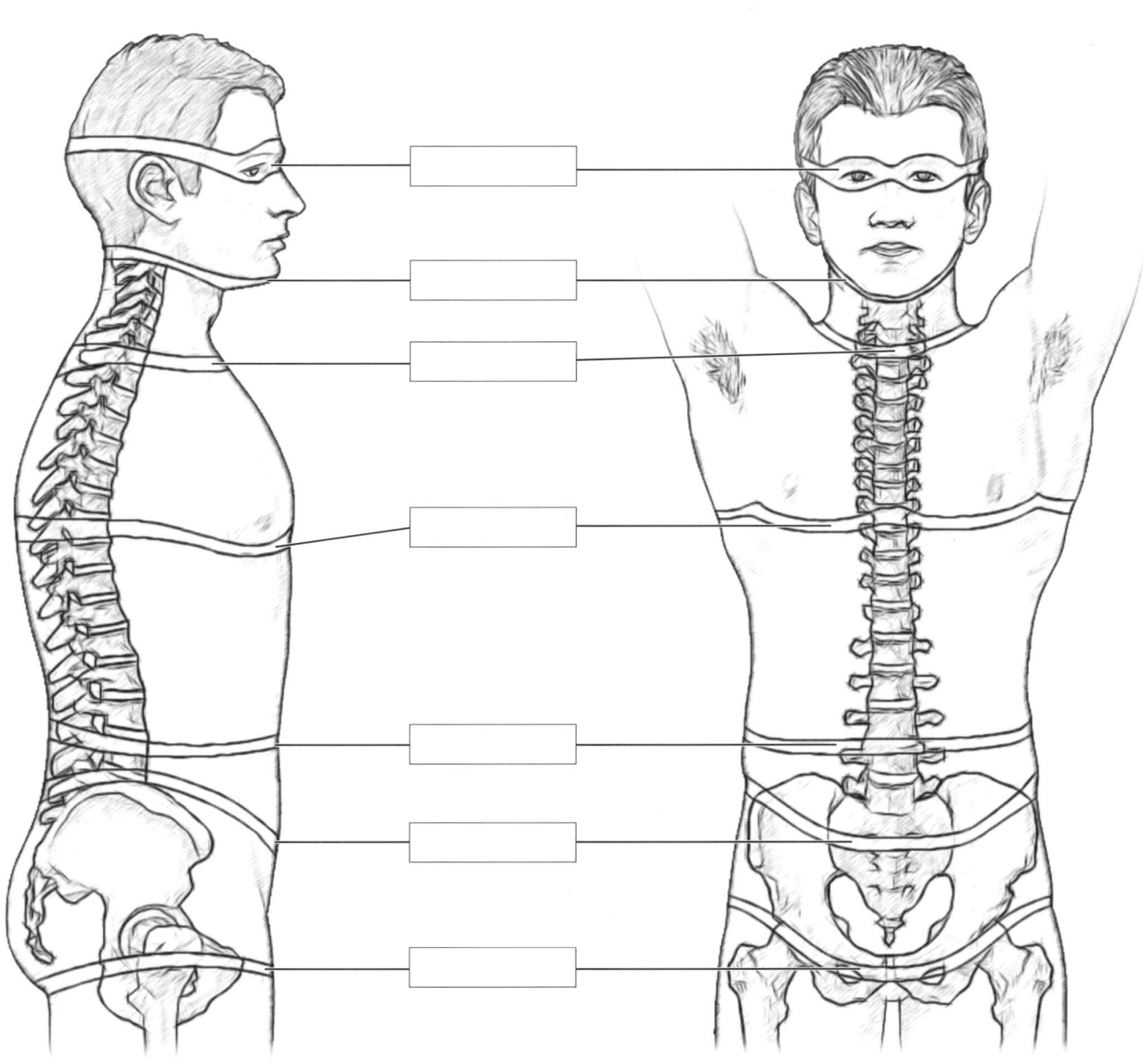

Fascial Planes

Fascial planes are horizontal structural components of the **7.** _____. These planes are thickened sheets of fascia inside **8.** _____ that provide structural **9.** _____ to the torso and support the major **10.** _____, _____, and _____.

- Cranial base
- Diaphragm
- Pelvic floor or diaphragm
- Thoracic inlet

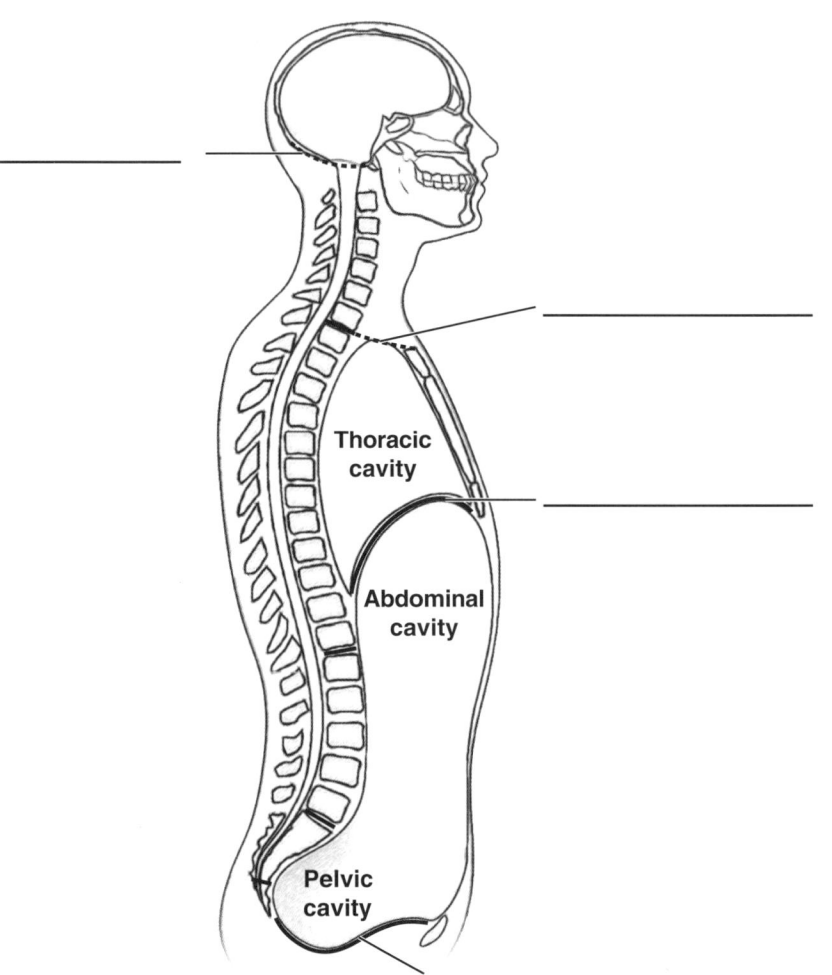

Chapter 8 Neuromuscular and Myofascial Connections

EXERCISE 7 • Mechanical Properties of Fascia

Each mechanical property of fascia has implications for the application of many manual therapy techniques. Complete the table below by defining each of the mechanical properties and describing the implications the physical property has on the pace, pressure, duration, and/or movement utilized in manual therapy.

Mechanical Property	Definition	Implication for Pace, Pressure, Duration, and/or Movement
Viscoelasticity	1.	Decrease pace to allow for unwinding of tropocollagen; increased duration to allow complete unwinding; movement and pressure specific to technique and tissue being addressed
Thixotropy	2.	4.
Piezoelectricity	3.	5.

EXERCISE 8 • Fascial Receptors

Identify each statement below as characteristic of one of the four fascial mechanoreceptors. Use the following abbreviation to indicate your choices: Golgi organs (GO), pacinian receptors (P), Ruffini receptors (R), and interstitial myofascial receptors (IMF). If you need to refresh your memory, refer to Table 8-2 in your textbook.

_____ 1. Located in spinal ligaments, as well as the epi-, peri-, and endomysium of muscle

_____ 2. Specifically responsive to lateral and tangential stretch

_____ 3. Stimulation causes decreased motor tone in related skeletal muscle

_____ 4. Stimulation causes increased vagal activity that results in global relaxation and less emotional arousal

_____ 5. Responsive to rapid pressure changes and vibrations

_____ 6. Responsive to rapid and sustained pressure changes

_____ 7. Only fascial mechanoreceptor found in the dura mater

_____ 8. Input from these sensory receptors is key proprioceptive feedback for kinesthesia

_____ 9. 50% of these mechanoreceptors are high threshold units and the other 50% are low threshold units

_____ 10. Receptors at musculotendinous junction sense tension due to muscle contraction, while others in this category are only sensitive to strong stretch

EXERCISE 9 • Concepts in Posture, Balance, and Coordinated Movement

Match each of these terms to their proper definition.

_____ 1. Muscle tone

_____ 2. Phasic muscle

_____ 3. Muscle recruitment

_____ 4. Motor tone

_____ 5. Neurofascial loops

_____ 6. Motor unit recruitment

_____ 7. Fascial tone

_____ 8. Postural muscle

A. Organizational pattern of stimulation and co-activation of muscle groups regulated by the cerebellum to produce complex coordinated movements

B. Skeletal muscle whose primary role is to create movement

C. Skeletal muscle that plays an essential role in maintaining the body's upright position

D. Low-grade tension created by smooth muscle cells within the fascia that is independent of motor tone in surrounding skeletal muscles; regulated by the ANS

E. Increasing the number of motor units stimulated to increase the force of a muscle; also known as graded response

F. A consistent state of low-grade tension generated through tonic contractions; palpated as firmness in the muscle

G. Natural firmness of a muscle created by its fluid and connective tissue elements

H. Reflexive neuronal pathways connecting the ANS to smooth muscle cells in the fascia

GROUP ACTIVITY 1 • Making Manual Therapy Choices

Manual therapists often use physiologic rationale to make appropriate therapeutic choices for treatment of specific client complaints. This exercise will help you develop your critical thinking skills as you identify techniques and physiologic principles at play in specific client scenarios. Begin this exercise by completing the table provided. First, select the technique(s) you would use to address the situation described in the scenario. Next, identify which neuromuscular principle your chosen technique is based on, and name the muscle or muscle group that you would target. You may do this portion of the exercise individually, in teams, or as one group. Once the table is complete, discuss your choices with one another. Finally, take turns demonstrating how you would apply each of the technique(s) you chose. Depending how far you are along in your manual therapy training, your group can have a lively discussion on how each of you might integrate these techniques into a full-hour session. To help you, abbreviations for the techniques and neuromuscular principles are provided below.

Techniques

Reciprocal Inhibition
Contract-Relax/Facilitated Stretch
Static stretch
Positional Release/Tender Point Deactivation

Neuromuscular Principles

Stretch Reflex
Inverse Stretch Reflex
Gamma Gain
Reciprocal Innervation

Scenario	Technique	NM Principle	Muscle/Muscle Group
A client gets a hamstring cramp while lying supine on the massage table.	1.	2.	3.
The client's complaint is chronic tension and aching in his or her posterior neck. The assessment shows a forward head, a few TeP in the suboccipital and pectoral muscles, and general tension in the interscapular muscles.	4.	5.	6.
Your very active client suffered an Achilles tendon strain last week and has come to you complaining that his or her entire posterior leg feels tight and stiff. This is causing some general back pain and he or she is not sleeping well.	7.	8.	9.

GROUP ACTIVITY 2 • Applying Knowledge of Myofascial Chains and Bands

For each of the scenarios, discuss which myofascial chains, fascial bands, and muscle groups you would prioritize for the client in your manual therapy session. To extend the learning from this exercise, explain your choices and sketch out a time line for a full treatment session of 1 to 1½ hours.

Scenario 1:
The client has come to you for relief of pain in his or her right foot from a diagnosed case of plantar fasciitis. Your review of the medical history reveals he or she has also had a moderate hamstring strain and an inguinal hernia repair on that same side.

Scenario 2:
This female client's primary complaint is chronic tension and ache in her mid-back. Medical history shows she had a C-section childbirth 8 years ago and a hysterectomy 2 years ago. In addition to the surgical scars, you also notice two taut bands of tissue running horizontally around the torso during your assessment. One starts at the level of the xyphoid and the other is around the umbilical.

GROUP ACTIVITY 3 • Discussing Concepts of Posture, Balance, and Coordinated Movement

Look back at the neuromuscular and myofascial concepts described in Exercise 9. Mind map a discussion on how these neuromuscular and neurofascial mechanisms are related to maintaining posture, coordinating movement, and regulating muscle tension. If you need to refresh your memory on how to mind map a discussion, refer to Group Activity 1 in Chapter 1 of this study and review guide.

9 The Endocrine System

Use this table to identify the study guide exercises and group activities that will help you explore or review each learning objective for this chapter.

No.	Learning Objective	Exercise	Study Group Activity
1	List the functions of the endocrine system and discuss their importance in relation to the practice of manual therapy.	3	See Chapter 1, Activity 1
2	Name and locate the major endocrine glands.	1, 2	1, 2
3	Compare and contrast the communication and control functions of the nervous and endocrine systems.	3	2
4	Explain the mechanisms of action for both water- and lipid-soluble hormones and identify which process is the second-messenger mechanism.	1, 4	1, 2
5	Explain negative feedback and the primary methods of stimulating hormone release.	1, 5	2
6	Name the hormones secreted by each of the endocrine glands, and describe the primary action of each.	1, 6, 7	1, 2
7	Explain the physiologic processes involved in the body's stress response.	1, 8	2
8	Discuss the changes that occur in endocrine function as the body ages.		See Chapter 1, Activity 1

EXERCISE 1 • Endocrine System Crossword

Use this crossword to review and test your knowledge of the anatomy and physiology terms from Chapter 9.

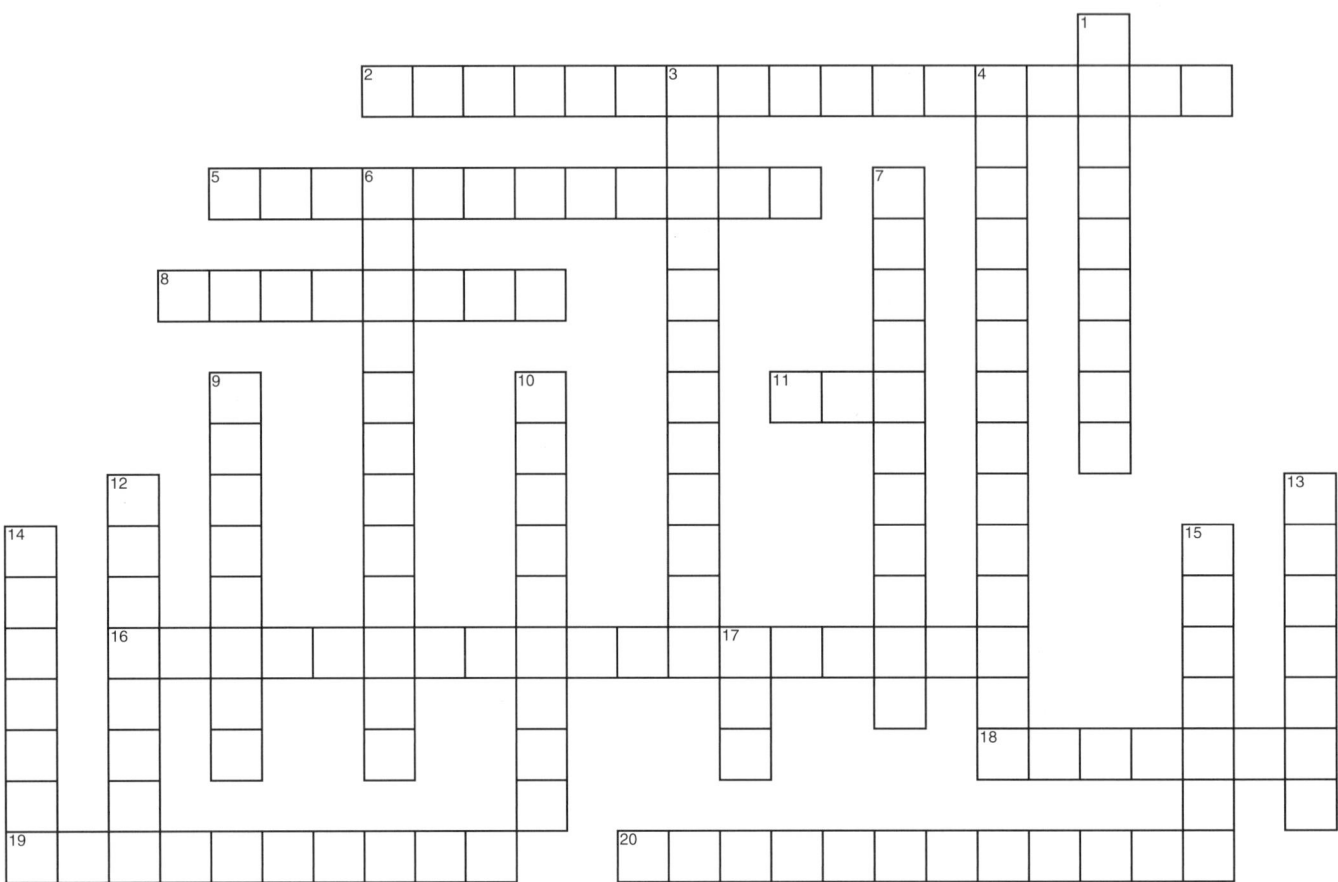

ACROSS

2. Aldosterone is an example of one of these hormones released from the outer layer of the adrenal cortex.
5. Another name for growth hormone.
8. Most hormone levels are regulated via this kind of feedback mechanism.
11. Rate of oxygen consumption of the body at rest.
16. Stimulates endocrine activity when stress stimulus is sustained beyond the ability of the alarm response to manage.
18. Lipid-soluble hormone made from cholesterol.
19. The pancreatic islets are also called the islets of _____.
20. These hormones require a second messenger to affect their target.

DOWN

1. Master gland attached to the hypothalamus.
3. These hormones do not require a second messenger to affect their target; includes steroid hormones.
4. Group of hormones that include adrenaline and noradrenaline.
6. Effect created by two hormones that work against one another.
7. Effect created when two hormones work together to enhance or intensify a target's response.
9. Most important glucocorticoid.
10. Any hormone secreted by the adrenal cortex.
12. Steroid that acts as a male sex hormone.
13. A compound comprised of a chain of 3–49 amino acids.
14. Synonym for suprarenal.
15. Specialized chemical messenger released by endocrine glands into the blood.
17. Also known as vasopressin.

Chapter 9 The Endocrine System 127

EXERCISE 2 • Locating Endocrine Glands

Color and identify each of the endocrine glands in the diagram below.

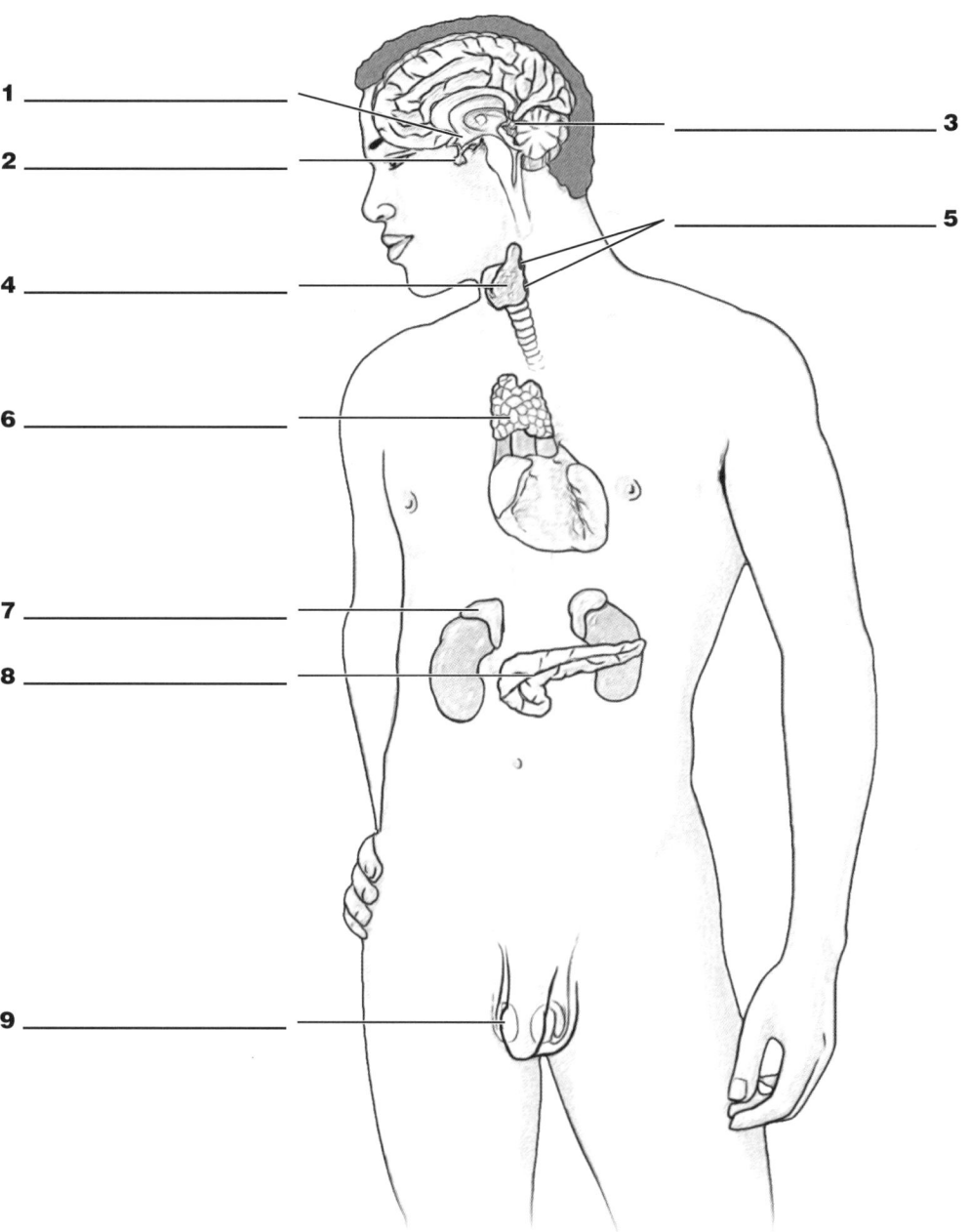

1. _____
2. _____
3. _____
4. _____
5. _____
6. _____
7. _____
8. _____
9. _____

EXERCISE 3 • Comparing the Communication Systems

Complete the table to compare and contrast important features and functions of the endocrine and nervous systems.

Characteristic/Function	Endocrine System	Nervous System
Primary organs of system connected and exclusive to the system. (yes or no)	1.	2.
Speed of communication	3.	4.
Rate and type of physiologic changes controlled by the system	5.	6.
Anatomic connections between the systems	7.	8.
Method of signaling effector change	9.	10.

EXERCISE 4 • Mechanisms of Hormone Action

Completing the blanks, as well as coloring and labeling the diagrams in this exercise will help you walk step-by-step through the two mechanisms of hormone action. You may want to do the fill-in exercise first and then color the diagrams or vice versa. Since the answers for the fill-in exercise and the labels for the diagrams match, you may also choose to move back and forth between the two portions of the exercise. No matter how you choose to work, if you need to refresh your memory refer to Figures 9-4 and 9-5, and the section on mechanisms of hormone action in your textbook.

There are two broad categories of hormones: 1. _____ _____ and 2. _____ _____ hormones. 3. _____ _____ hormones are recognized by receptors on the 4. _____, which bond with the hormone. This connection between hormone and receptor activates a 5. _____ _____ _____ which initiates the conversion of ATP in the cytoplasm into 6. _____. The presence of this substance activates proteins within the cell that produce a designated 7. _____ _____. This sequence of events is called the 8. _____ _____ _____. In contrast, 9. _____ _____ hormones are more direct because they are able to pass through the 10. _____ _____ to bond with receptors in the 11. _____. This forms a hormone-receptor complex that passes through the 12. _____ _____ and activates a process in which specific genes (segments of 13. _____) are copied onto an 14. _____ molecule that then directs the production of a new 15. _____ by the ribosomes. This substance alters the metabolic activity of the cell.

This is a diagram of the **8** _____ - _____ _____.

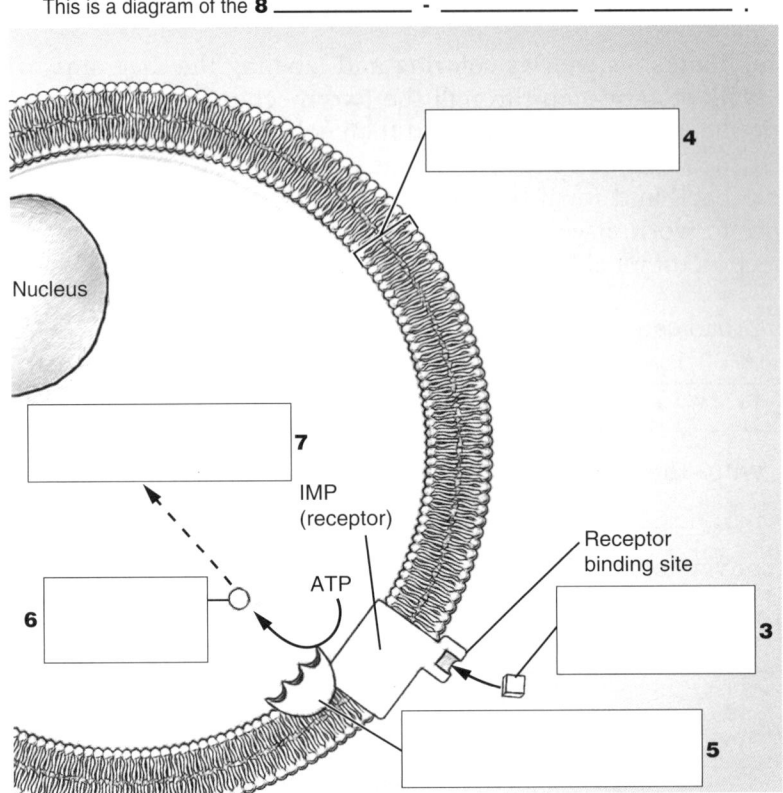

This is a diagram of direct mechanism used by **9.** _____ - _____ hormones.

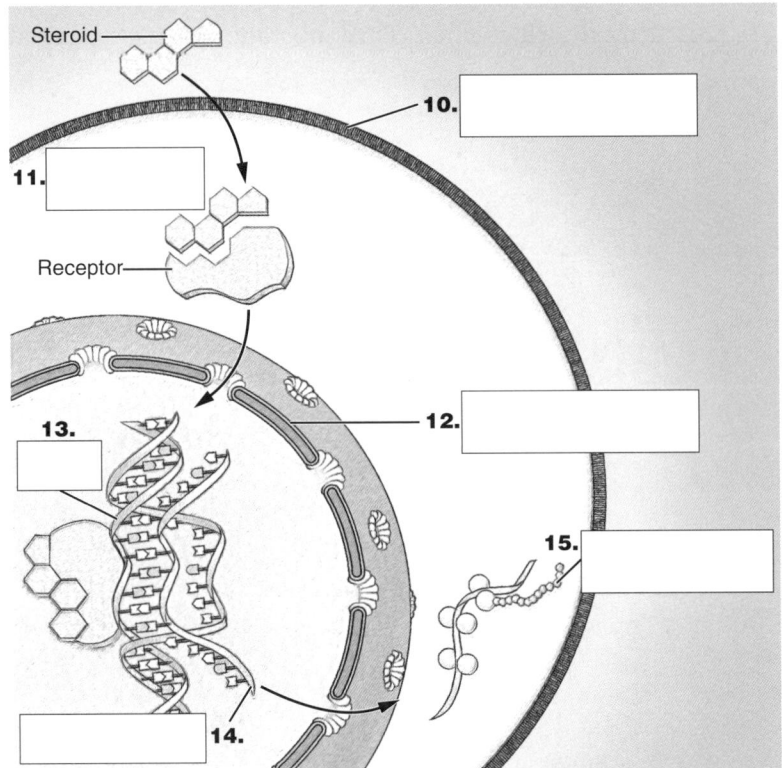

EXERCISE 5 • Stimulating and Regulating Hormone Activity

Most hormone levels and activity are regulated through negative feedback mechanisms. Color and label the diagram below to identify the components of the feedback loop. If you need to refresh your memory, refer to Figure 9-6 in your textbook.

- endocrine gland
- physiologic response
- stimulus
- negative feedback
- hormone
- target cells or organ

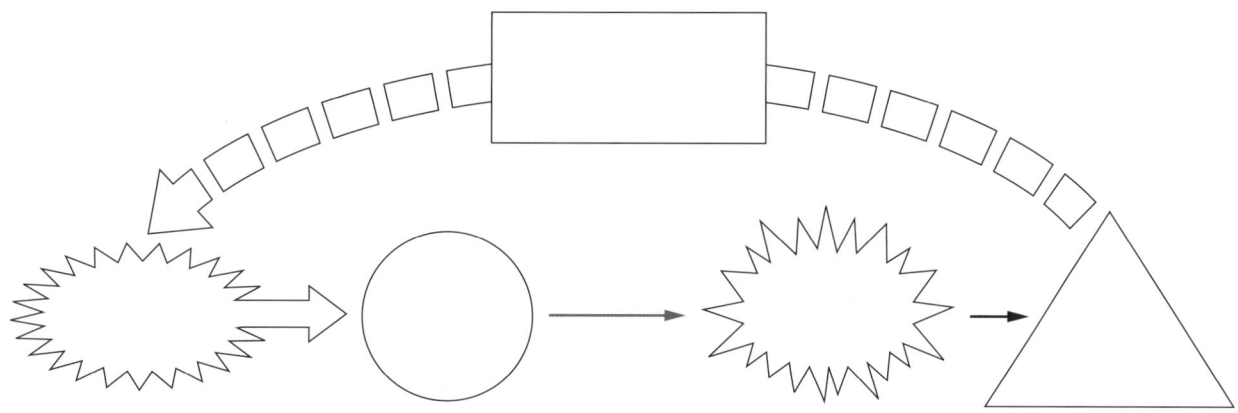

List three types of stimuli that activate endocrine glands and provide at least one example of each.

1. _____ EX. _____ _____

2. _____ EX. _____ _____

3. _____ EX. _____ _____

EXERCISE 6 • Glands and their Hormones

List the hormones secreted for each endocrine gland identified in the diagram. The parenthetical numbers let you know how many hormones you should be able to list.

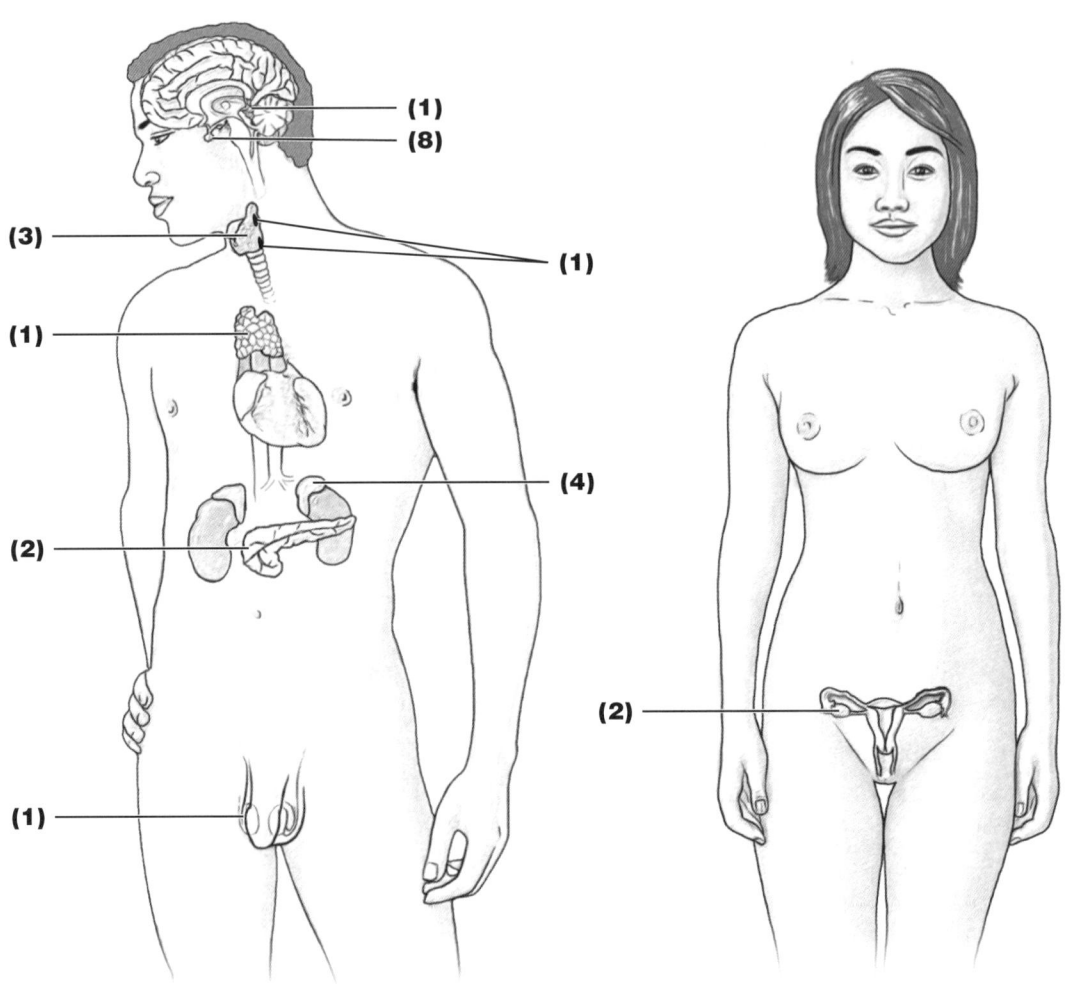

Pineal:

Pituitary (anterior):

Pituitary (posterior):

Thyroid:

Parathyroids:

Thymus:

Adrenal (cortex):

Adrenal (medulla):

Ovaries:

Testes:

EXERCISE 7 • Matching Hormones and Physiologic Responses

Match each of these hormones with its physiologic effect.

_____ 1. ACTH
_____ 2. Glucagon
_____ 3. PTH
_____ 4. Testosterone
_____ 5. Thymosin
_____ 6. LH
_____ 7. Cortisol
_____ 8. GH
_____ 9. Prolactin
_____ 10. Adrenaline
_____ 11. Oxytocin
_____ 12. Estrogen
_____ 13. Calcitonin
_____ 14. Progesterone
_____ 15. Thyroxine(T_4)
_____ 16. Insulin
_____ 17. Aldosterone
_____ 18. Melatonin

A. Increases Na$^+$ retention and thus water to increase blood pressure; decreases K$^+$ in blood
B. Increase blood glucose and anti-inflammatory process, especially during stress response
C. Increase blood glucose; increase metabolism; prolong body changes initiated by alarm response during stress
D. Maturation of ova; development and maintenance of secondary sex characteristics; prepares uterus for implantation
E. Development and maintenance of secondary sex characteristics; sperm production
F. Promotes growth of uterine lining and decreases uterine contractions to support pregnancy
G. Accelerates conversion of glycogen and other nutrients to glucose to increase glucose level in blood
H. Accelerates transport of glucose into cells to decrease glucose level in blood
I. Promotes maturation of T-cells
J. Stimulates bone resorption to increase calcium level in blood, and production of calcitriol to increase Ca^{2+} absorption in digestive tract
K. Inhibits bone resorption and accelerates calcium uptake to decrease calcium level in blood
L. Increases metabolism
M. Triggers sleep
N. Stimulates uterine contraction and release of milk
O. Stimulates growth and increases metabolism
P. Stimulates milk production
Q. Increased secretion of hormones from testes and ovaries
R. Increased secretion of glucocorticoids from the adrenals

EXERCISE 8 • Diagramming Stress

Color and complete the flow chart below to outline the three stages of stress and the physiologic responses associated with each. If you need to refresh your memory, refer to Figure 9-17 in your textbook.

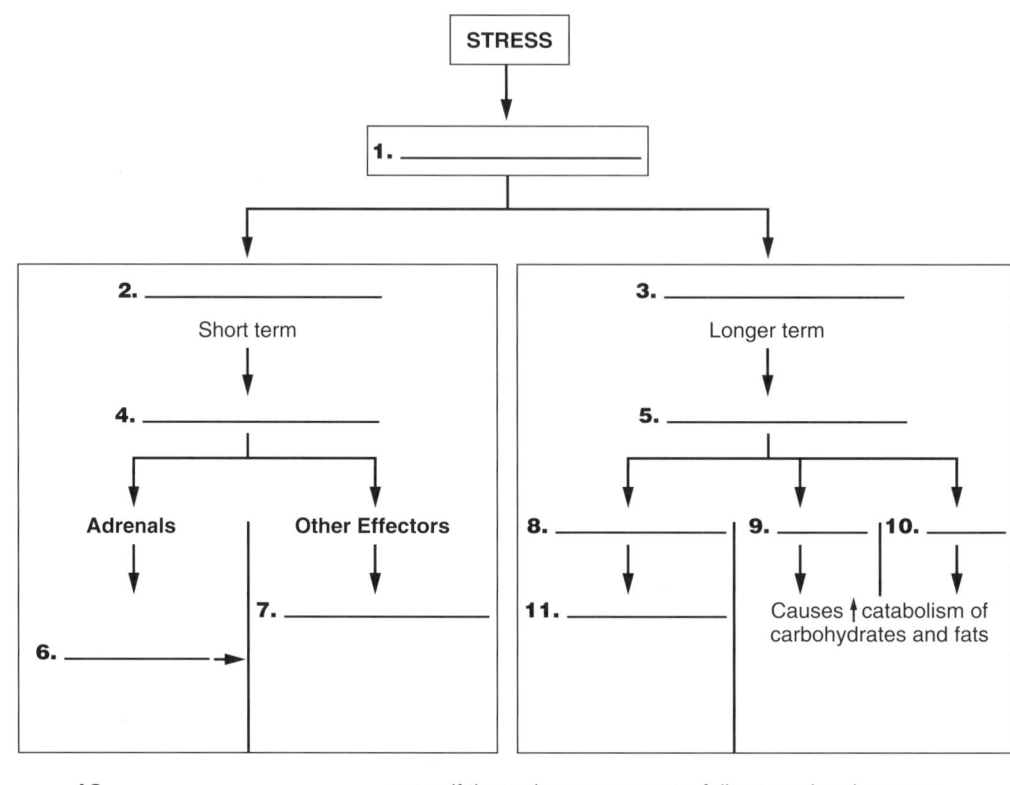

12. _____ – occurs if the resistance response fails to combat the stress.

GROUP ACTIVITY 1 • Endocrine Concept Map

You may recall that a concept map is an organizing tool that goes further than a mind map by asking you to show relationships between linked items. Concept maps can help you show and explain a hierarchy or web of information. Look back at the example provided in Chapter 3, Exercise 7. Notice how it shows a flow of information from big ideas to smaller details. Each connecting line or stem is accompanied by a descriptive phrase or linking words that describe the connection represented by the stem. As a group activity, concept maps provide lots of opportunities for discussion and clarification. They allow members of a group to show connections between independent pieces of information in a fun and graphic way. You can develop maps together or work individually and share your maps to see where your thinking differs.

For the endocrine system, use all the glands, hormones, and physiologic responses to create your concept map(s). For specific directions, refer back to Chapter 3.

GROUP ACTIVITY 2 • The Pyramid Game

This group activity was introduced back in Chapter 1. If you need to refresh your memory on how to develop and play this game refer back to Group Activity 3 in that chapter. Some suggested topics for your Endocrine System Pyramid Game could include:

- The tropic hormones
- The adrenal hormones
- The gonadotropins
- Hormones that affect blood glucose
- Posterior pituitary hormones
- Methods of hormone action
- Types of hypothalamus links to the pituitary
- Hormones that increase metabolism and growth
- Hormones that increase blood pressure
- Types of stimuli that activate the endocrine glands

Have fun brainstorming your own categories!

PRACTICE EXAM UNIT 4 • Chapters 7–9

1. The positive feedback mechanism is used to regulate levels for which of these hormones?

   A. Calcitonin
   B. TSH
   C. Adrenaline
   D. Oxytocin

2. The target-specific method by which most hormones alter the metabolic activities of their target cells is called what?

   A. First messenger
   B. Second messenger
   C. Direct intervention
   D. Indirect intervention

3. The mineralocorticoid hormones are secreted by the

   A. adrenal cortex.
   B. posterior pituitary.
   C. adrenal medulla.
   D. adrenal hypophysis.

4. What region of the brain contains the thalamus and hypothalamus?

   A. Cerebral cortex
   B. Medulla oblongata
   C. Midbrain of the brainstem
   D. Diencephalon

5. Glands, abdominal organs, and smooth muscle tissue are all examples of

   A. somatic effectors.
   B. visceral receptors.
   C. autonomic effectors.
   D. endocrine organs.

6. What other terms are synonymous with sensory pathway?

   A. Efferent and ventral tract
   B. Efferent and descending tract
   C. Afferent and posterior tract
   D. Descending tract and unipolar pathway

7. The neuromuscular reflex that inhibits the antagonist of a contracting muscle is called

   A. all-or-none.
   B. reciprocal inhibition.
   C. reciprocal relaxation.
   D. contract–relax mechanism.

8. What hormone stimulates reabsorption of Na⁺ from urine and secretion of K⁺ from the blood into the urine?

    A. Aldosterone
    B. Glucocorticoids
    C. ADH
    D. Cortisol

9. Which component of connective tissue gives them their thixotropic nature?

    A. Mast cells
    B. Ground substance
    C. Elastin fibers
    D. Collagen fibers

10. What are the functions of the cerebellum of the brain?

    A. It maintains muscle tone, posture, and balance and coordinates voluntary muscle activity.
    B. It carries out all cognitive processes, maintains consciousness, and coordinates movement.
    C. It senses and corrects postural imbalances, maintains muscle tone, and coordinates muscle recruitment.
    D. It is the body's primary motor center and integration center for general sensory input.

11. Tension of the intrafusal fibers in a muscle spindle is regulated by which reflex loop?

    A. Alpha
    B. Beta
    C. Gamma
    D. Delta

12. The tropic hormones are secreted by which endocrine gland?

    A. Adrenal cortex
    B. Posterior pituitary
    C. Hypothalamus
    D. Anterior pituitary

13. Which hormone is released by the pancreas when blood sugar levels are high?

    A. Glucagon
    B. Insulin
    C. Glycogen
    D. Glucosamine

14. The majority of hormones are classified as being

    A. steroidal.
    B. fat soluble.
    C. water soluble.
    D. prostaglandins.

15. The epimysium, perimysium, and endomysium of skeletal muscle collectively form which of the four fascial tubes in the body?

    A. Pannicular
    B. Axial
    C. Menigeal
    D. Visceral

16. What is the first step in neuronal impulse conduction, once threshold stimulus has been applied to the neuron?

    A. Polarization
    B. Depolarization
    C. Repolarization
    D. Neurotransmitter release

17. Which nerve is often compressed and irritated in association with the frequent tension headaches?

    A. Accessory
    B. Trigeminal
    C. C-7
    D. Cranial VII

18. A group of nerve roots that innervate the head and neck is the definition for what?

    A. Cranial nerves
    B. Cervical nerves
    C. Cervical nerve plexus
    D. Brachial nerve plexus

19. The four largest horizontal planes of fascia in the body are the thoracic inlet, pubic floor, and

    A. meninges and thoracic outlet.
    B. cranial base and diaphragm.
    C. diaphragm and dura mater.
    D. cranial sutures and transverse abdominus.

20. What cellular component is considered the "second messenger" that stimulates the target cell response to a hormone?

    A. ADP
    B. IMPs
    C. RNA
    D. cAMP

21. What term is used to describe the action of one hormone increasing the sensitivity of the target organ to another hormone?

    A. Permissive effect
    B. Synergistic effect
    C. Antagonistic effect
    D. Hypersensitizing

22. The three types of stimuli that activate the endocrine glands include neurologic stimulus, hormonal stimulus, and

    A. emotional stimulus.
    B. psychogenic stimulus.
    C. changes in blood concentrations.
    D. changes in respiratory rate.

23. What is the effect of the primary hormone released by the pineal gland?

    A. Regulation of appetite
    B. Regulation of our circadian rhythm
    C. Stimulation of metabolism
    D. Shifting water and sodium reabsorption

24. What type of neurons is found only in the CNS?

    A. Multipolar
    B. Sensory
    C. Motor
    D. Integrative neurons

25. What part of a neuron contains the vesicles that store and release the neurotransmitters?

    A. Synaptic bulbs
    B. Nodes of Ranvier
    C. Axon
    D. Cell body

26. What is the function of the ependymal cells in the nervous system?

    A. Produce myelin in PNS
    B. Transmit impulses between sensory and motor neurons
    C. Carry out phagocytosis in the brain
    D. Produce cerebrospinal fluid

27. What adjustment is made in the fascial tissue when it is subjected to sustained and repeated tension?

    A. It becomes less extensible to withstand the repeated stress.
    B. The collagen fibers become more elastic.
    C. More chains of tropocollagen are added to the collagen fibrils.
    D. There is a thixotropic shift to a more "gel" state.

28. What are the three mechanical properties of fascia?

    A. Viscoelasticity, recoil, and compression
    B. Viscoelasticity, thixotropic, piezoelectricity
    C. Piezoelectricity, autoregulatory, rhythmicity
    D. Thixotropic, autonomic, self-propagating

29. What is meant by the term fascial plasticity?

    A. It refers to the stiff plastic feeling of fascial planes when in their sol state.
    B. It denotes the changeable, responsive, and adaptive nature of fascia.
    C. It refers to the rich network of nerves that create piezoelectricity in fascia.
    D. It means that all fasciae have a limited capacity to stretch and rebound.

30. Which of the following is a key characteristic of a tender point?

    A. The localized spasm is due to a neurologic signal.
    B. It is always found in a taut band of tissue.
    C. Moderate pressure over the point causes a predictable pattern of pain around it.
    D. It is palpable as a ropy or gritty knot in the muscle.

31. What characteristic do all 31 pair of spinal nerves share?

    A. All use the same neurotransmitter, acetycholine.
    B. Each is a two-neuron pathway.
    C. They are all mixed nerves.
    D. The motor neurons on each spinal nerve pass through the paravertebral ganglia.

32. Which of the mechanoreceptors found in fascia is the most abundant of all the fascial sensory receptors?

    A. Pacinian corpuscles
    B. Golgi receptors
    C. Interstitial myofascial receptors
    D. Ruffini organs

33. Muscle spindles and Golgi tendon organs are examples of specialized mechanoreceptors called

    A. interstitial myofascial receptors.
    B. proprioceptors.
    C. nociceptors.
    D. kinesthetic receptors.

34. What is the function of cerebrospinal fluid?

    A. Shock absorption, nutrition, physical barrier between pathogens in blood and the CNS organs
    B. Chemical defense between the brain and blood, insulates the organs of CNS, excretes waste to the outside of the meninges
    C. Shock absorption, primary neurotransmitter of the CNS, medium for nutrient waste exchange in the meninges
    D. Forms the blood–brain barrier, serves as the plasma for all the blood vessels in the meninges, insulates the brain and spinal cord

35. Which autonomic effects have only sympathetic innervation?

    A. Heart, lungs, and stomach
    B. Blood vessels, intestines, and pancreas
    C. All smooth muscle, fascia, and adrenals
    D. Adrenals, smooth muscle in blood vessels, and sweat glands

10 The Cardiovascular System

Use this table to identify the study guide exercises and group activities that will help you explore or review each learning objective for this chapter.

No.	Learning Objective	Exercise	Study Group Activity
1	List the functions of the cardiovascular system and discuss their importance as they relate to the practice of manual therapy		See Chapter 1, Activity 1
2	Identify the key components of plasma and explain the functional purpose of each	1, 2	1
3	Name the three types of blood cells and explain the function of each	1, 2	1
4	Name the types of blood vessels and describe the distinguishing characteristics of each	1, 3, 4	1
5	Identify and locate the primary arteries and veins and name those that might be affected by manual therapy	5, 6	1
6	Describe the tissues and functional contribution of each layer of the heart	1, 7	1
7	Identify the chambers, valves, and great vessels of the heart in the order that blood moves through them	1, 8	1
8	Explain the conduction system of the heart, how it creates the cardiac cycle, and mechanisms that regulate heart rate	1, 9, 10	1
9	Name the two divisions of cardiovascular circulation and describe blood flow through each	1, 11	1
10	Explain the primary influences on arterial, capillary, and venous blood flow and how they differ	12	1
11	Define blood pressure and explain how it is regulated and influenced and how the body responds to blood pressure fluctuations	1, 13	1
12	List and describe the Starling forces that create fluid exchange in the capillary beds	1, 14	1
13	List the three stages of tissue healing and describe the key physiologic events of each	1, 15	1
14	Describe changes that occur in the cardiovascular system as the body ages		See Chapter 1, Activity 1

EXERCISE 1 • Cardiovascular Crossword

Use this crossword to review and test your knowledge of the general anatomy and physiology terms from Chapter 10.

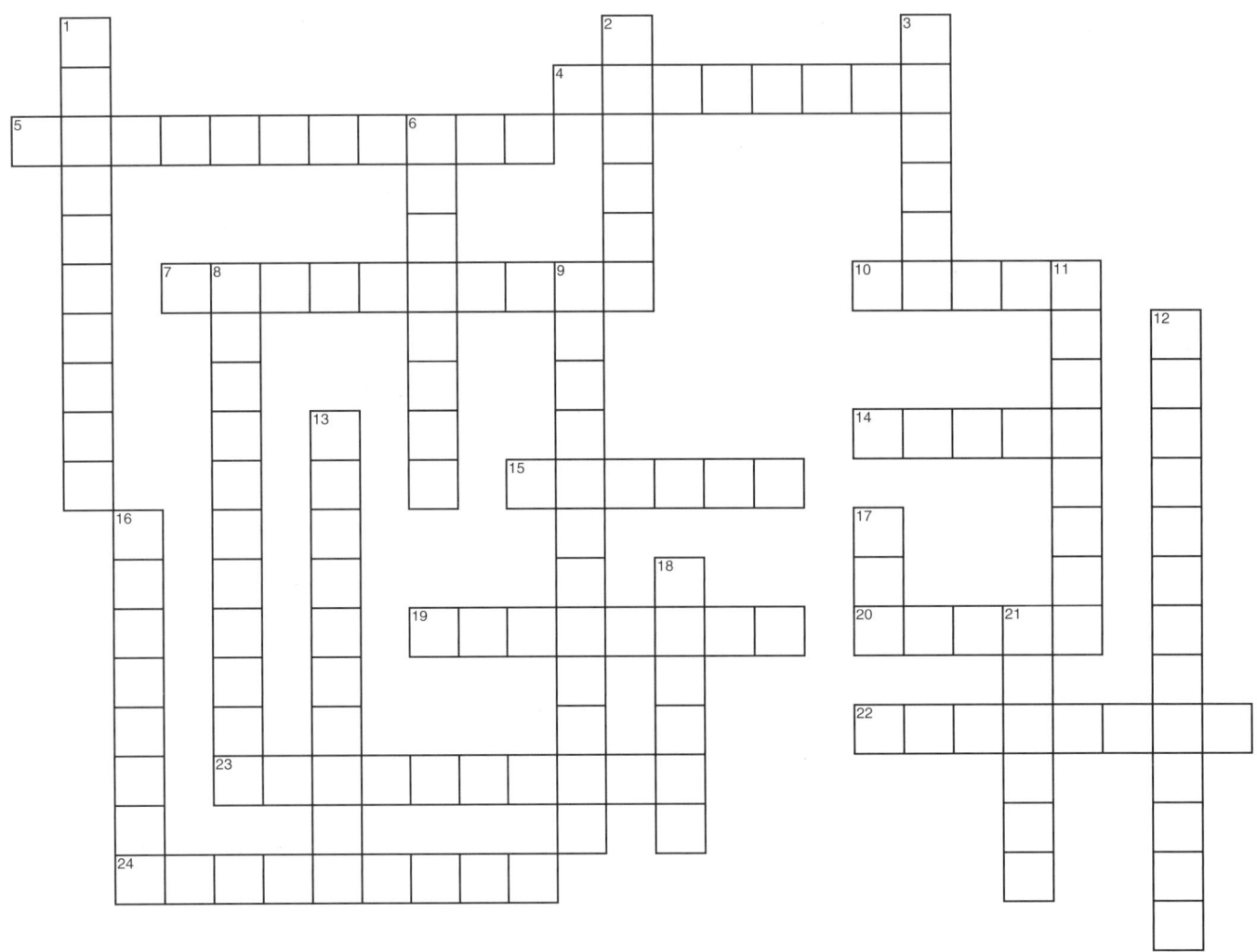

ACROSS

4. Relaxation state in which the chambers of the heart dilate as they fill with blood.
5. Process of blood clotting.
7. The elasticity of blood vessels, the size of lumens, and blood viscosity all contribute to _____ resistance within the cardiovascular network.
10. In the pulmonary circuit, these vessels carry oxygen-rich blood.
14. Excess collection of fluid in the interstitium.
15. Blood vessel that carries blood away from the heart.
19. Thrombocyte.
20. The rhythmic expansion of an artery in response to ventricular contraction.
22. Bluish appearance of the skin due to tissues not receiving enough oxygen.
23. Also known as the visceral pericardium.
24. Reflexive contraction of muscles surrounding an injured area to help keep the area still and protected.

DOWN

1. The thick muscular layer of the heart.
2. Valve located between the left atrium and ventricle.
3. Small vein.
6. Local decrease in blood volume or flow.
8. RBC.
9. An organized network of _____ cardiac muscle cells create the conduction system of the heart.
11. Also known as the proliferative stage of healing.
12. Blood cell production in the red bone marrow.
13. The Starling forces at the arteriole end of the capillary bed produce net _____.
16. Blood clot.
17. Force created by blood pressing out against the wall of the capillary.
18. Fluid component of blood.
21. The heart's pacemaker.

EXERCISE 2 • Matching Blood Components

Match the plasma components and formed elements below with the descriptions and characteristics offered.

_C_ 1. Water
_I_ 2. Hemoglobin
_E_ 3. Erythrocytes
_H_ 4. Thrombocytes
_B_ 5. Globulins
_F_ 6. Leukocytes
_A_ 7. Albumins
_J_ 8. Neutrophils
_D_ 9. Fibrinogen
_G_ 10. Lymphocytes

A. The most abundant type of protein found in plasma
B. Plasma proteins such as antibodies and complements
C. 90% of plasma is made up of this key component
D. Plasma protein that forms thin initial threads of a blood clot
E. Formed element present in the highest numbers in blood
F. Round cells with a prominent nucleus
G. Specialized agranular leukocytes
H. Formed elements essential for blood clotting
I. RBC protein that binds and carries O_2 and CO_2
J. Along with other granular leukocytes this formed element plays a role in inflammation and tissue healing

EXERCISE 3 • Blood Vessel Structure

Place the name of the blood vessels shown within the numbered boxes of the diagram provided. Then, color and label the lettered items in the diagram to identify the layers of the vascular walls and other distinctive structural features of the blood vessels. If you need to refresh your memory, refer to Figure 10-3 in your textbook.

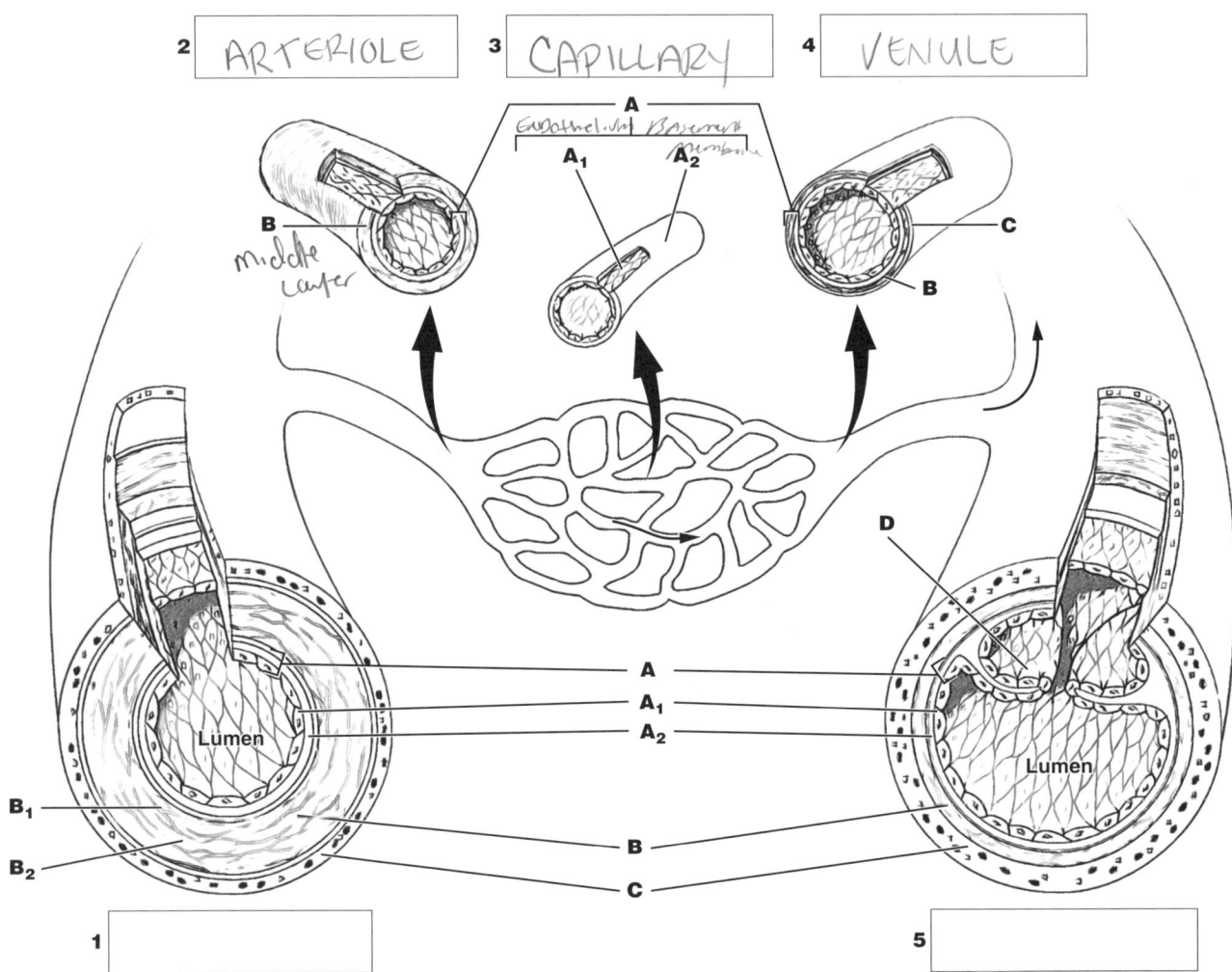

2. ARTERIOLE
3. CAPILLARY
4. VENULE

EXERCISE 4 • Comparing and Contrasting Blood Vessels

Use the Venn diagram below to identify similarities and differences between arteries, capillaries, and veins. If you need to refresh your memory about structural characteristics and specific functions of the blood vessels, refer to Table 10-2 and the sections describing blood vessels in your textbook. To review instructions on how to use a Venn diagram, look at Chapter 6, Exercise 3 in this study and review guide. Notice, a characteristic common to all three types of vessels has been provided to help get you started.

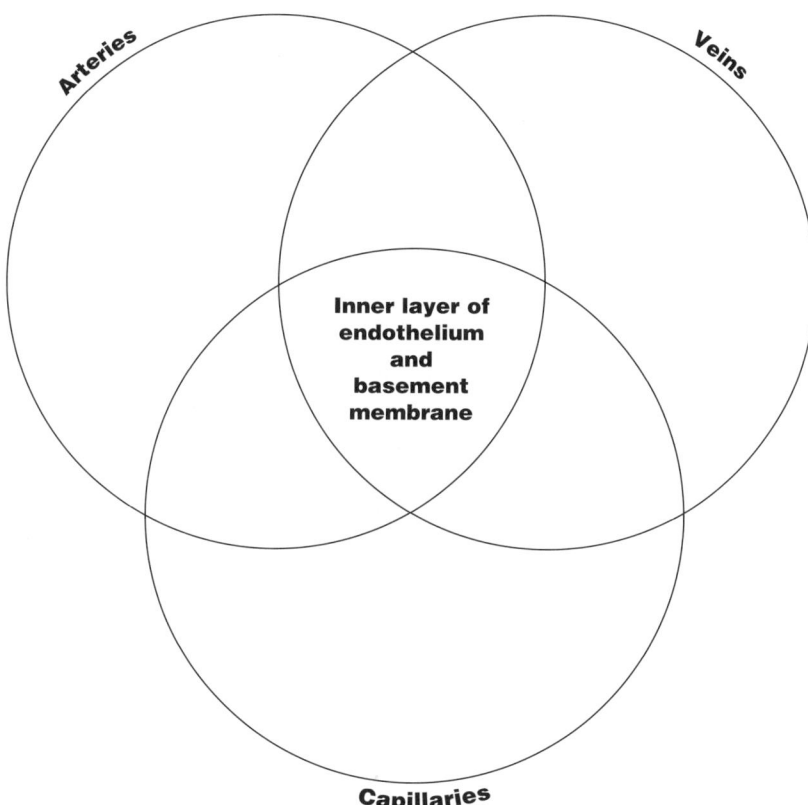

EXERCISE 5 • Primary Arteries of the Body

Match the artery with the letter identifying it on the diagram. Identify the common pulse points with a circle both on the diagram and list. Refer to Figure 10-4 in your textbook if you need to refresh your memory.

_____1. Temporal
_____2. Brachial
_____3. Dorsal pedis
_____4. Common iliac
_____5. Radial
_____6. Femoral
_____7. Renal
_____8. Facial
_____9. Subclavian
_____10. Ulnar
_____11. Descending aorta
_____12. External carotid
_____13. Popliteal
_____14. Brachiocephalic trunk
_____15. Abdominal aorta
_____16. Common carotid
_____17. Axillary
_____18. Posterior tibial

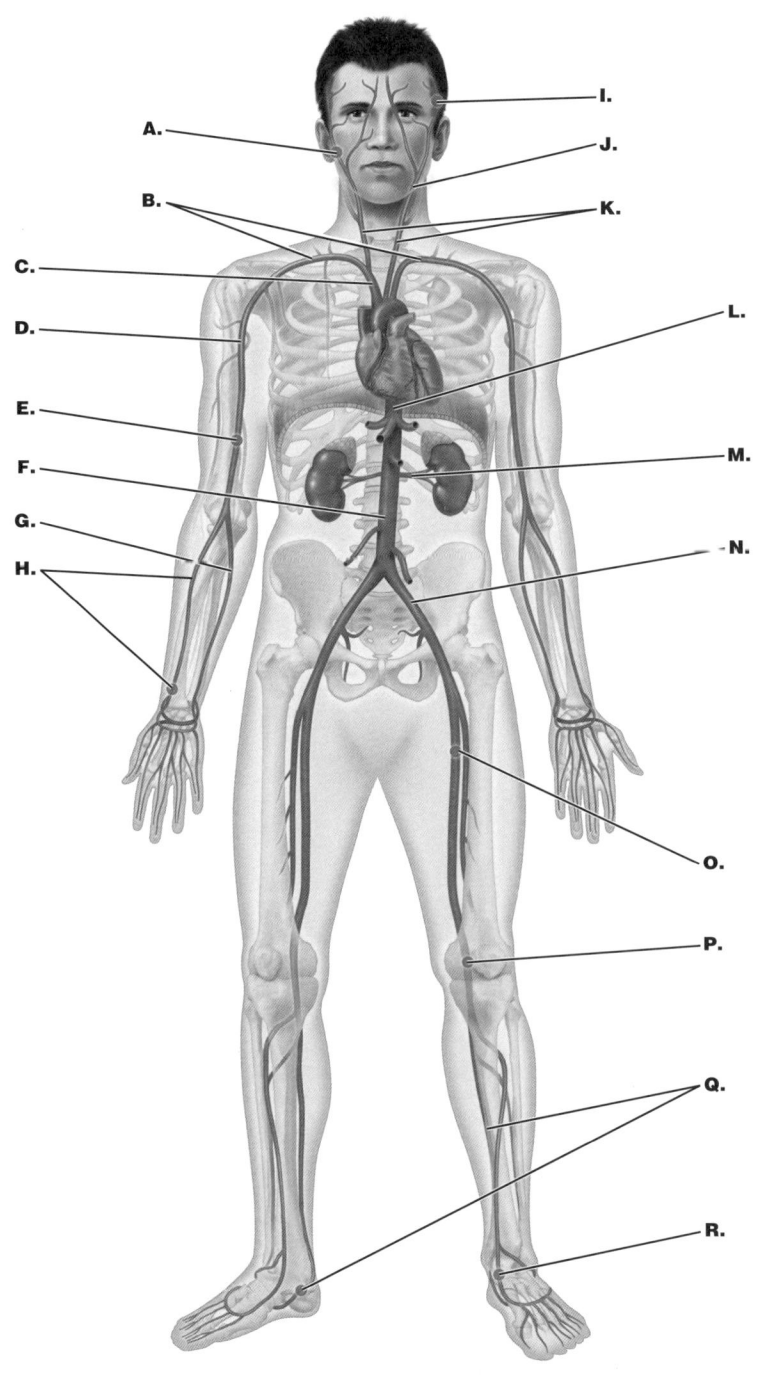

Chapter 10 The Cardiovascular System

EXERCISE 6 • Primary Veins of the Body

Match the vein with the letter identifying it on the diagram.

_____ 1. Popliteal
_____ 2. Brachiocephalic
_____ 3. Superior vena cava
_____ 4. Inferior vena cava
_____ 5. Radial
_____ 6. Ulnar
_____ 7. Femoral
_____ 8. Internal iliac
_____ 9. Subclavian
_____ 10. Cephalic
_____ 11. Palmar arches
_____ 12. Digital
_____ 13. Brachial
_____ 14. Internal jugular
_____ 15. External jugular
_____ 16. Axillary
_____ 17. Median cubital
_____ 18. Basilic
_____ 19. Saphenous
_____ 20. Dorsal venous arch

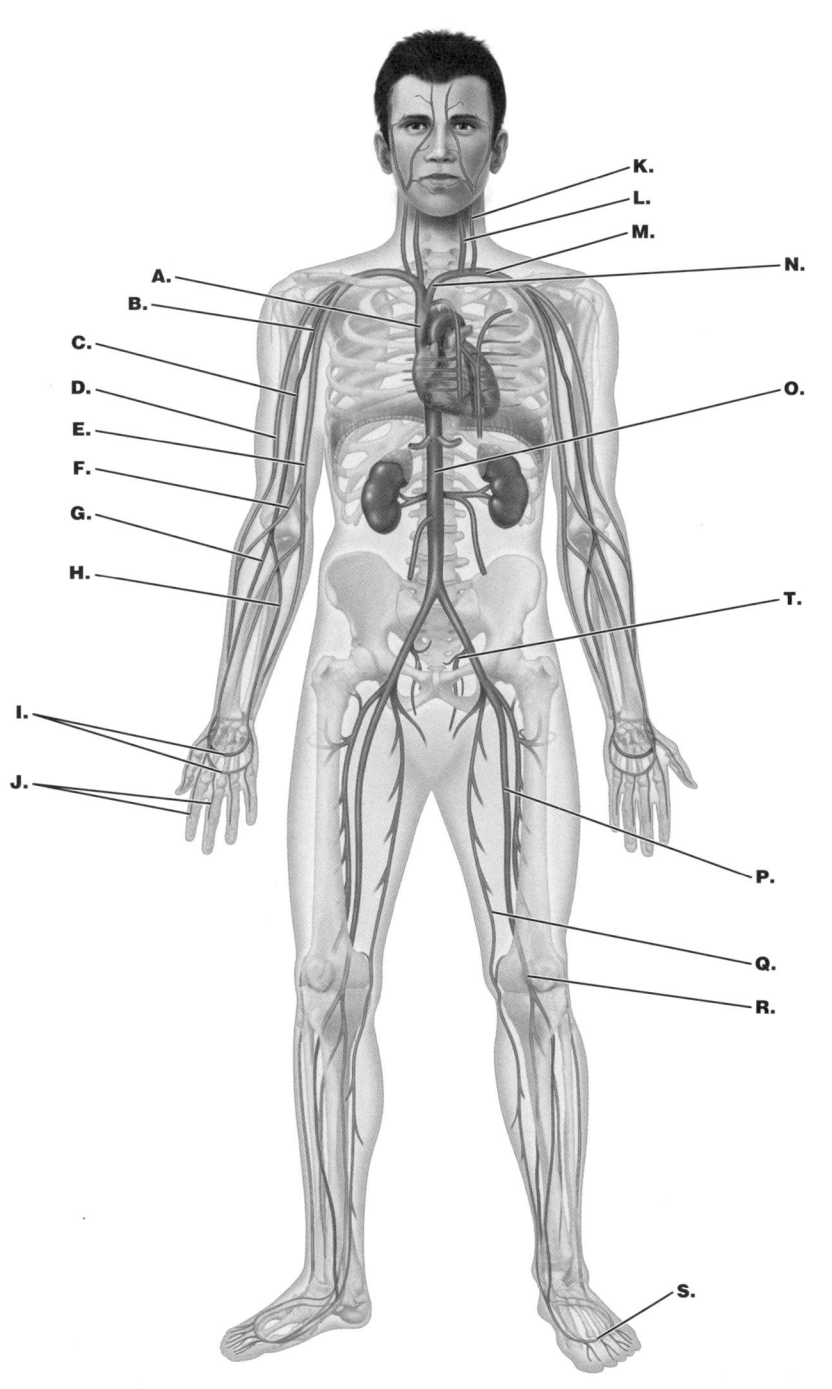

EXERCISE 7 • The Layers of the Heart

Using the diagram provided, color and label the layers of the heart wall and the sack surrounding the heart. Bracket the layers that actually form the heart wall. If you need to refresh your memory, refer to Figure 10-7 in your textbook.

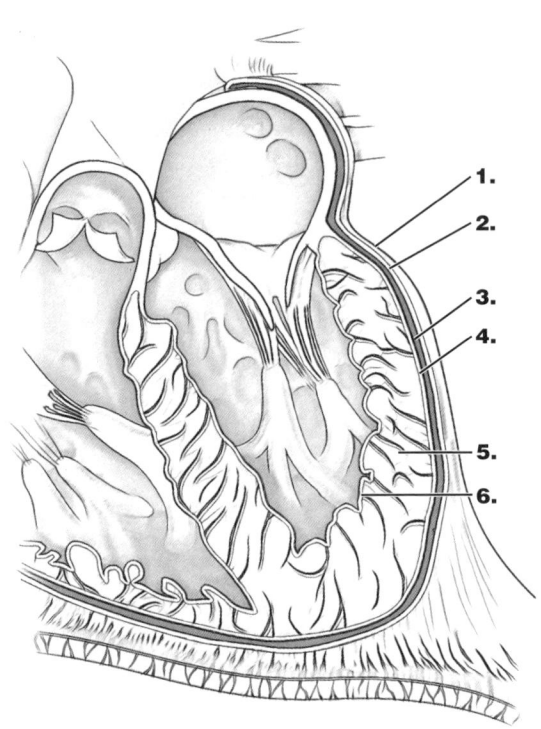

1.
2.
3.
4.
5.
6.

EXERCISE 8 • Blood Flow through the Heart

Color and label the great vessels and structures of the heart identified in the diagram below. If you need to refresh your memory, refer to Figure 10-8 in your textbook.

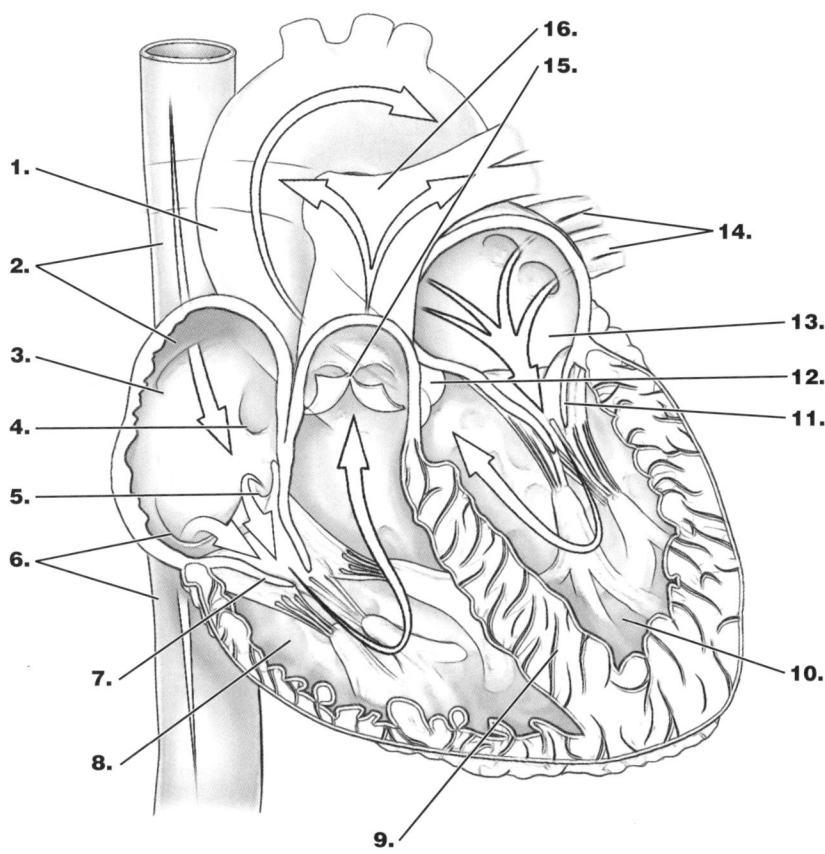

Beginning with the right atrium (#1), number the following list to designate the order a blood cell would circulate through each structure.

___1___ Right atrium
_____ Left atrium
_____ Right ventricle
_____ Left ventricle
_____ Bicuspid valve
_____ Tricuspid valve
_____ Aortic valve
_____ Pulmonary valve
_____ Aorta
_____ Vena cavae
_____ Pulmonary veins
_____ Pulmonary arteries
_____ Systemic capillaries
_____ Lung capillaries

EXERCISE 9 • The Conduction System of the Heart

Complete the matching exercise to identify the components of the heart's conduction system.

_____ 1. Atrioventricular node   A. Pacemaker; initiates signal
_____ 2. Purkinje fibers   B. Carries signal to the intraventricular septum
_____ 3. AV bundle   C. Convey signal to apex of the heart
_____ 4. Bundle branches   D. Delays signal to allow contraction of atria
_____ 5. Sinoatrial node   E. Carry signal up through the ventricles

Now, color and complete the diagram to outline the path a signal passes across the heart to coordinate contraction. If you need to refresh your memory, refer to Figure 10-10B in your textbook.

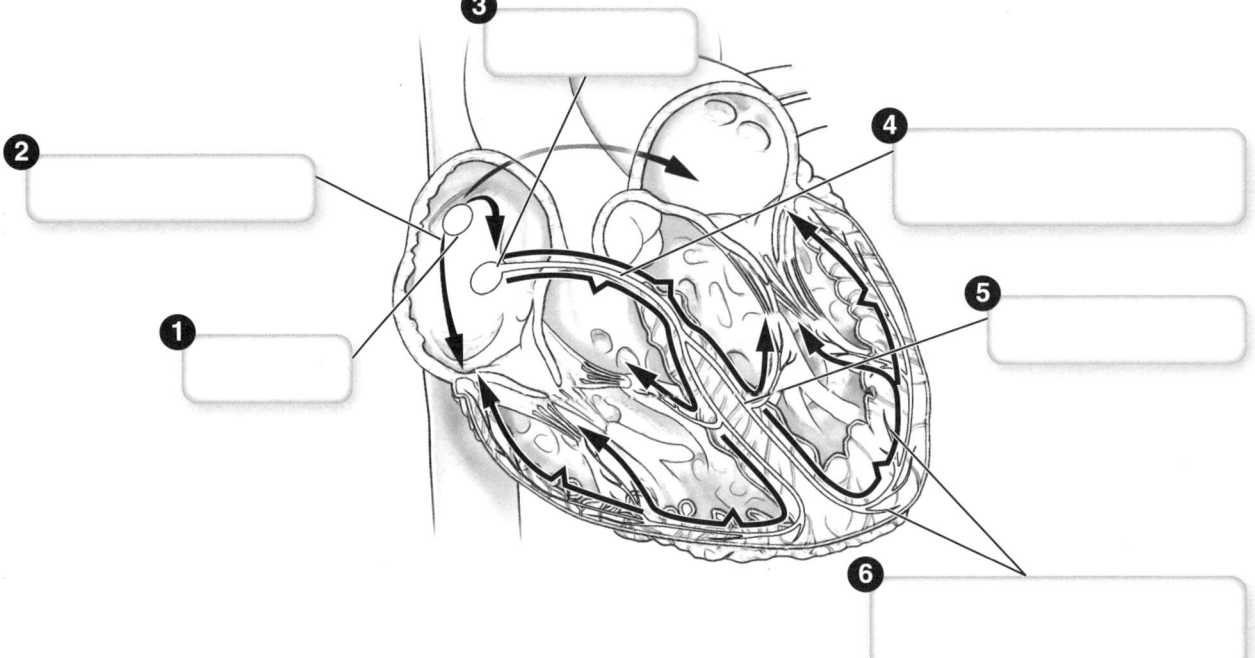

EXERCISE 10 • The Cardiac Cycle

Complete the description of each stage of the cardiac cycle by circling the contraction state of the atria and ventricles, the position of the valves, and describing the flow of blood.

Relaxation Phase

    Atria are relaxed/contracted
    Ventricles are relaxed/contracted
    Semilunar valves are open/closed
    AV valves are open/closed
    Blood flows from _____ to _____

Atrial Systole

    Atria are relaxed/contracted
    Ventricles are relaxed/contracted
    Semilunar valves are open/closed
    AV valves are open/closed
    Blood flows from _____ to _____

Ventricular Systole

    Atria are relaxed/contracted
    Ventricles are relaxed/contracted
    Semilunar valves are open/closed
    AV valves are open/closed
    Blood flows from _____ to _____

EXERCISE 11 • Cardiovascular Circulation

Color and label the schematic representation of cardiovascular circulation. Use the list of terms provided for your labels. Notice that the right and left sides of the heart are already designated. Color blood vessels that carry oxygenated blood red while making vessels that carry deoxygenated blood blue. Color sites of gas exchange half and half. If you need to refresh your memory, refer to Figures 10-8B and 10-12 in your textbook.

Pulmonary circuit
Systemic circuit
Aorta
Pulmonary arteries
Pulmonary arterioles
Pulmonary capillaries
Pulmonary veins
Pulmonary venules
Superior and inferior vena cavae
Systemic arterioles
Systemic capillaries
Systemic venules

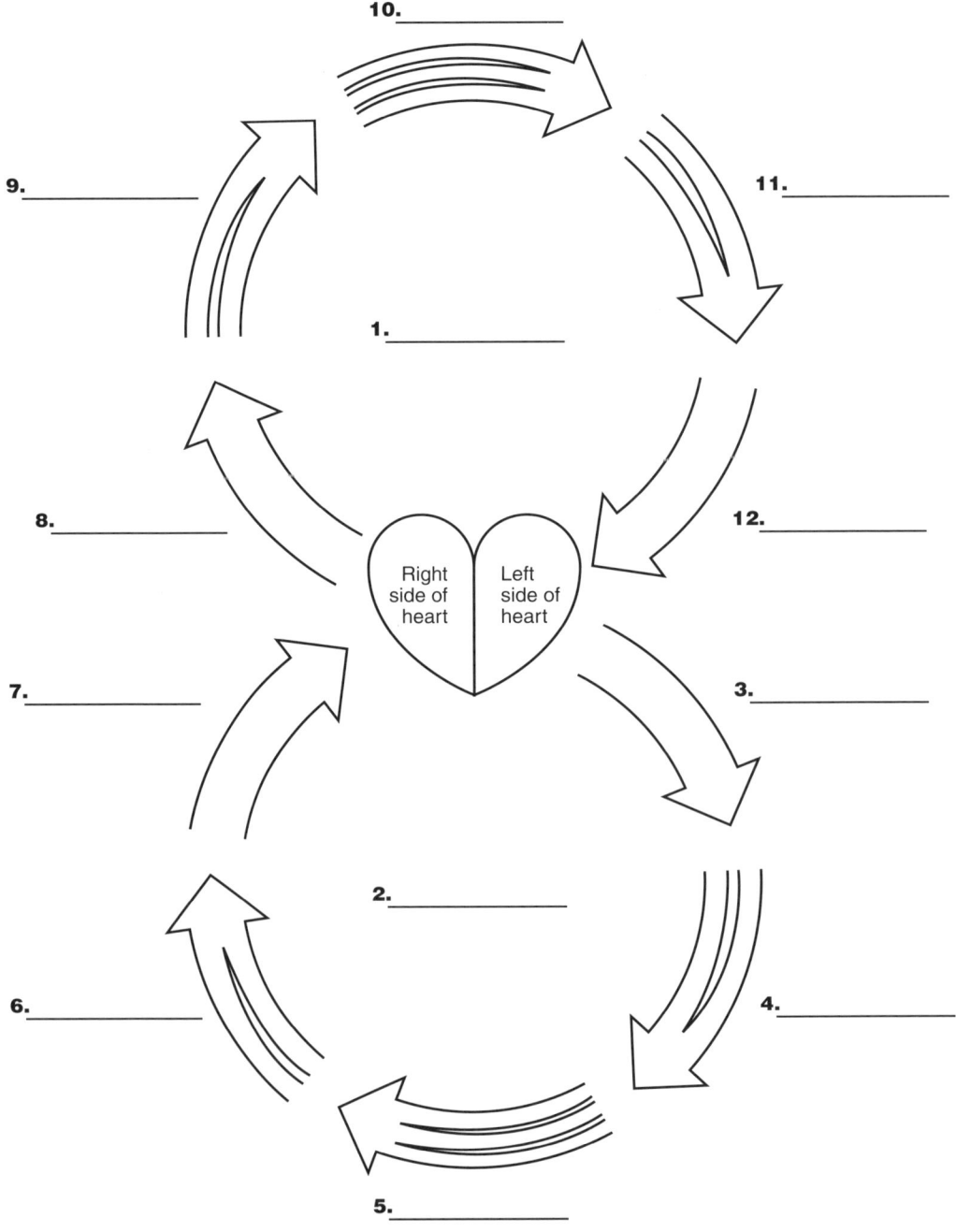

EXERCISE 12 • Blood Flow

Blood moves through the different vessels of the cardiovascular network through a variety of forces.

- Arterial blood flow is driven by the combined forces of 1. _____ _____ and 2. _____ _____.

- Blood flow into the capillaries is controlled by the 3. _____ _____ that constrict and dilate to control both the 4. _____ and the 5. _____ of blood flow into the capillaries.

- Venous flow is driven by 6. _____ _____ _____ that apply external compression to the veins. 7. _____ _____ _____ assist venous flow by creating shorter segments for blood to travel. In the ventral cavities the driving force for venous flow is the 8. _____ _____.

EXERCISE 13 • Blood Pressure Regulation

Blood pressure is a measurement of the 1. _____ _____. This measurement consists of two numbers, stated in terms of millimeters of mercury (mm Hg). The higher number is the 2. _____ pressure, which represents the pressure generated during 3. _____ _____. The 4. _____ pressure is a lower number that represents the pressure in the arteries when the 5. _____ _____. Blood pressure changes occur throughout the day to meet circulatory demands. Mark each example listed below with either a ≠ to indicate a factor that would increase blood pressure or a ▯ to indicate a factor that would decrease blood pressure.

_____ 6. Increased viscosity of the blood

_____ 7. Hardening of the arteries

_____ 8. Relaxation

_____ 9. Physical exertion

_____ 10. Use of medications to thin the blood

_____ 11. Aldosterone release from the adrenals

_____ 12. Increased elasticity of the vascular wall

EXERCISE 14 • Capillary Flow

Capillary exchange between blood and the interstitium involves the movement of particles or solutes, as well as fluids. Solutes move through the wall of the capillary via 1. _____ and include substances such as 2. _____, _____, and _____. Fluid is exchanged through a combination of two hydrostatic and two osmotic pressures collectively referred to as 3. _____ _____. The two 4. _____ pressures are:

- 5. _____ _____ pressure or 6. _____ created by blood inside the capillary pushing outward against its wall.

- 7. _____ _____ pressure or IFP created by 8. _____ _____ pressing inward against the capillary wall.

The two 9. _____ pressures are:

- 10. _____ _____ pressure or 11. _____, the osmotic pressure created by the 12. _____ content of the blood inside the capillary.

- 13. _____ _____ pressure or IOP, an osmotic pressure created by the 14. _____ _____ content of interstitial fluid.

The movement of plasma and its dissolved solutes out of the blood and into the interstitium is called 15. _____, while 16. _____ refers to the movement of fluid and substances back into the capillary bed. Both 17. _____ and _____ create filtration, whereas 18. _____ and _____ are the forces involved in reabsorption. In healthy tissue, the dominant Starling force at the arteriole end of the capillary bed is CFP causing 19. _____ to occur at the arteriole side of the capillary bed. When fluid filters out of the capillary it increases the concentration of plasma proteins within the blood. This elevates the POP at the venule end of the capillary bed and causes 20. _____ to occur at the venule side of the capillary. If filtration greatly exceeds reabsorption 21. _____ results.

EXERCISE 15 • Stages of Tissue Healing

Complete the table by filling in the key physiologic events that occur during each stage of the tissue healing process.

Stage of Healing	Key Physiological Events
Acute	Hemorrhage & 1. _____
	2. _____ & muscle spasm
	3. _____ _____ _____
	4. _____ _____
Subacute	Increased numbers of 5. _____
	Decreased numbers of 6. _____
	7. _____ begins with the lay down of
	8. _____ tissue
Maturation	9. _____ remodeling based on demonstrated lines of
	10. _____

GROUP ACTIVITY 1 • Quiz Show

Here are sample quiz show boards for the cardiovascular system. If you need to review the rules of this game, refer to Group Activity 1 in Chapter 5.

LEVEL I

	Formed Elements	The Vascular Network	Oh My Heart	Cardiac Conduction	Pressure and Flow
100	This is the anatomic name for red blood cells	The name for blood vessels that carry blood <u>away</u> from the heart	This the fibrous sac that surrounds the heart	The general route of conduction is from this chamber to that chamber	"Normal" blood pressure for an average sized male
200	Blood contains the highest number of this formed element	These vessels serve as the site for nutrition & waste exchange	This valve separates the right atrium from left ventricle	The anatomic name for the "pacemaker"	The major influence on venous flow
300	This formed element has several varieties of granular and agranular cells	The name of the smaller vessels that carry blood <u>out</u> of the capillary beds	This is the common term for both valves between ventricles & arteries	This is the name of the fibrils that stimulate contraction of the ventricular walls	Besides blood pressure, the major influence on blood flow in arteries
400	This special molecule on RBC's is how they carry oxygen	The anatomic name for the opening in the middle of a blood vessel	This heart chamber pumps blood into the aortic artery	This is the anatomic name for the bundle is His that also describes it's general location	The term for the blood pressure reading during ventricular relaxation
500	The anatomic name for platelets	These are the 2 structural features that distinguish veins from arteries	This chamber receives blood returning to the heart from systemic circulation	This term describes cardiac muscle by it's ability to pass action potentials from one fiber to another	The term for the blood pressure reading during ventricular contraction

Chapter 10 The Cardiovascular System

LEVEL II

	Arteries	Veins	Capillary Exchange	Tissue Healing	Potpourri
200	The name of the first major artery branch off the aortic arch	The large veins that return blood to the heart	The name of the physician who ID'd the forces that create and regulate capillary exchange	This is the second stage of blood clotting	The proper physiologic term for the process of blood clotting
400	These arteries deliver blood to the upper extremities	The large vein on medial lower extremity & is most prone to the pathology of varicose vein	These circular muscle control the volume of blood entering the capillaries	The term for the fluid that continues to pool in the injured tissue even after clotting	The physio-logic term for blood cell production
600	This is the location where pulse in the abdominal aorta can be palpated	This vein starts in lateral cubital & travels full lateral brachium before joining subclavian	The region of the capillary bed where filtration occurs	The stage of healing in which tissue repair actually begins	This category of plasma proteins includes antibodies and complements
800	The short artery that connects the femoral to the anterior & posterior tibialis arteries	Unlike most veins, these carry oxygen rich blood	The dominant force that drives capillary filtration	This fragile repair tissue is laid down in the subacute stage of healing	In addition to hormones & ion levels, this is the 3rd mechanism that monitors & regulates heart rate
1,000	The artery that delivers blood to the intestines	This vein carries blood into the liver for cleansing	The dominant force that drive reabsorption	The key physiologic process throughout the maturation stage of healing	In addition to nervous system and hormones, it is the 3rd method of regulating peripheral circulation

11 The Lymphatic System

Use this table to identify the study guide exercises and group activities that will help you explore or review each learning objective for this chapter.

No.	Learning Objective	Exercise	Study Group Activity
1	Discuss the importance of understanding the separate roles of the lymphatic system, fluid return and immune response, as they relate to manual therapy practices		See Chapter 1, Activity 1
2	Name the primary components of lymph	1	
3	Identify the five types of lymph vessels and describe the key structural features of each	1, 2, 4	
4	Explain the general structure and functions of a lymph node	1, 3	
5	Explain the process of interstitial fluid uptake and distinguish this process from lymph flow	1, 5	1
6	Describe the key internal and external mechanisms that create and influence lymph flow	1, 5, 6	1
7	Name and locate the primary lymphatic catchments and watersheds of the body	1, 4, 7	
8	Explain the different routes for lymph flow back into cardiovascular circulation for the torso, upper and lower extremities	1, 8	
9	Compare and contrast the three major categories of edema	1, 9	

EXERCISE 1 • Lymphatic System Crossword

Use this crossword to review and test your knowledge of the general anatomy and physiology terms from Chapter 11.

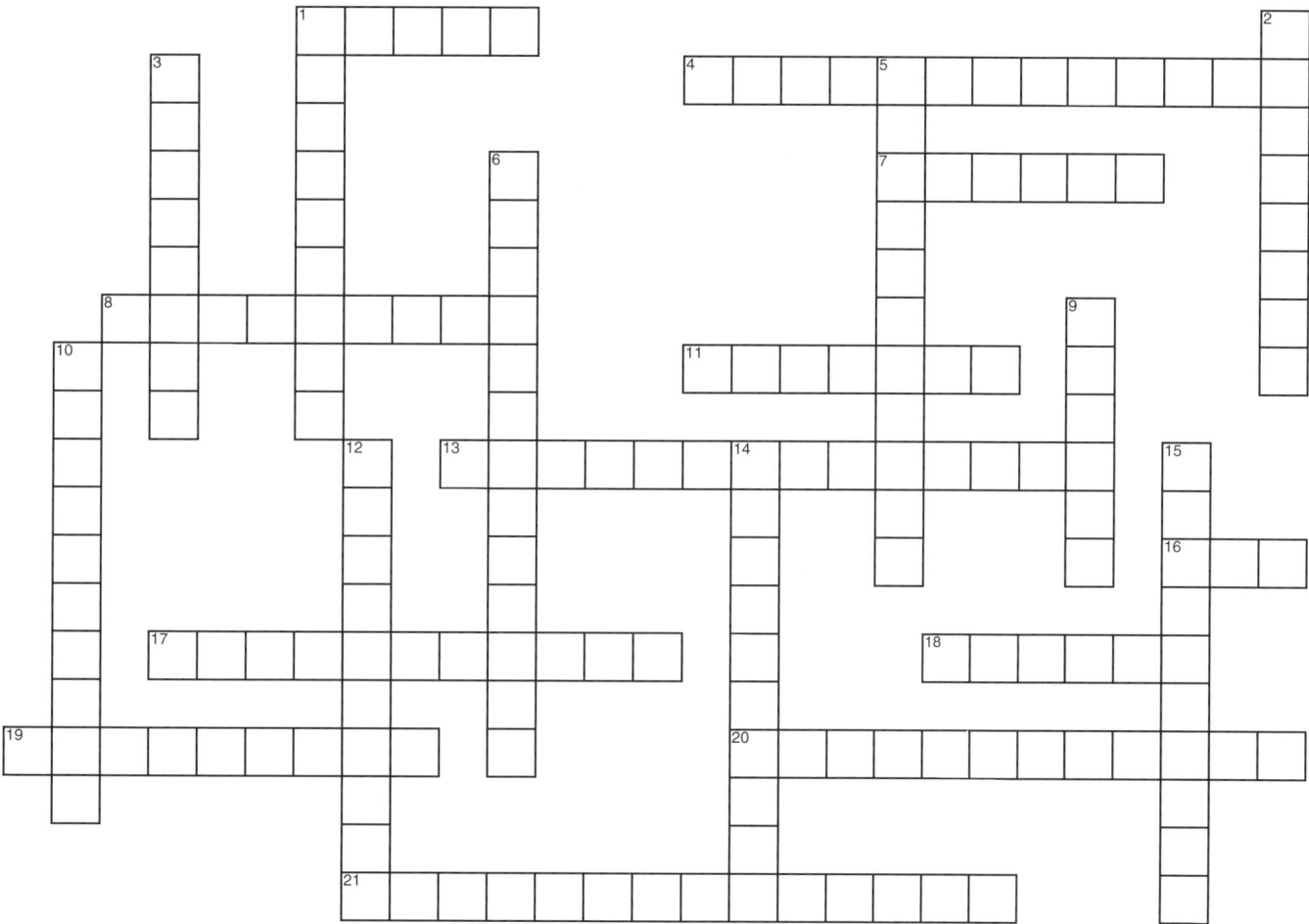

ACROSS

1. Lymph is mostly this substance with dissolved electrolytes.
4. Fluid outside the cells is called _____ fluid.
7. Segment of the primary lymphatic vessel.
8. Lymph node bed.
11. This type of edema is related to cardiovascular dysfunctions.
13. The first capillaries in the lymphatic network.
16. Rhythmic contractions of the angions are regulated by the _____.
17. Specialized WBCs found in high concentrations in lymph.
18. Movement of excess interstitial fluid into lymphatic capillaries is called edema _____.
19. An important external influence on lymph flow is deep _____.
20. Collects lymph from the left upper and both lower quadrants of the body.
21. This junction is also called the lymphatic terminus.

DOWN

1. Zone between two lymphotomes.
2. These large molecules are too large to be reabsorbed into the blood and are returned to circulation via lymph.
3. Specialized lymph capillaries in the the intestines for lipid absorption.
5. An end-to-end arrangement of lymph vessels.
6. Enlarged sac at the base of the thoracic duct that serves as a collecting well.
9. This transportation system is a _____ system.
10. The 10% of capillary filtrate returned to circulation via the lymphatic system is this type of load.
12. Primary lymphatic vessels.
14. Specific lymphatic drainage region.
15. These projections divide the interior of a lymph node into sinuses.

EXERCISE 2 • The Lymphatic Vessels

Complete the table, filling in key structural and functional information about the vessels of the lymphatic network. Notice the table is organized from the smallest to the largest vessels.

Lymphatic Vessel	Location & Structure	Function
1.	Located in 2. _____ 3. _____ or snub-nosed 4. _____ attached to a basement membrane 5. _____ attached to cells to hold vessel in place and pull cells outward for fluid uptake	Entry point for fluid uptake into vascular network
Collecting capillaries	Located in superficial 6. _____ Wall is several layers of epithelial cells 7. _____ at junctions with initial vessels	Collect lymph from several 8. _____
9. _____	Superficial vessels located in the dermis; deeper vessels are subdermal or in deep fascia Divided into 10. _____ by one-way intralymphatic valves Spiraled 11. _____ layer	Collect lymph from several 12. _____ Pump lymph through lymph nodes and towards larger trunks
Lymphatic or 13. _____ trunks	Located deep and alongside 14. _____ Intralymphatic valves spaced at wider intervals than in lymphangia	Collect lymph from specific 15. _____ or _____
Deep ducts	Located deep within the tissue or ventral cavities 16. _____ is an enlarged collecting well at the base of 17. _____	18. _____ collects all lymph from right upper quadrant and returns it to the right 19. _____ Thoracic duct collects all lymph from 20. _____ _____ and returns it to the left subclavian vein

EXERCISE 3 • Structure and Function of a Lymph Node

Lymph nodes are small specialized **1.** _____ _____ interspersed along the length of the **2.** _____. They are scattered both along the lymphatic pathway and also found in clusters called **3.** _____ _____ _____ or **4.** _____. Lymph nodes function as **5.** _____, removing particulate matter such as **6.** _____, along with **7.** _____ from lymph as it passes through. Additionally, lymph nodes contain numerous **8.** _____ _____ _____ called **9.** _____ making them important sites for the specific immune responses.

Color and label the diagram to review the structure of a lymph node. If you need to refresh your memory, refer to Figure 11-13 in your textbook.

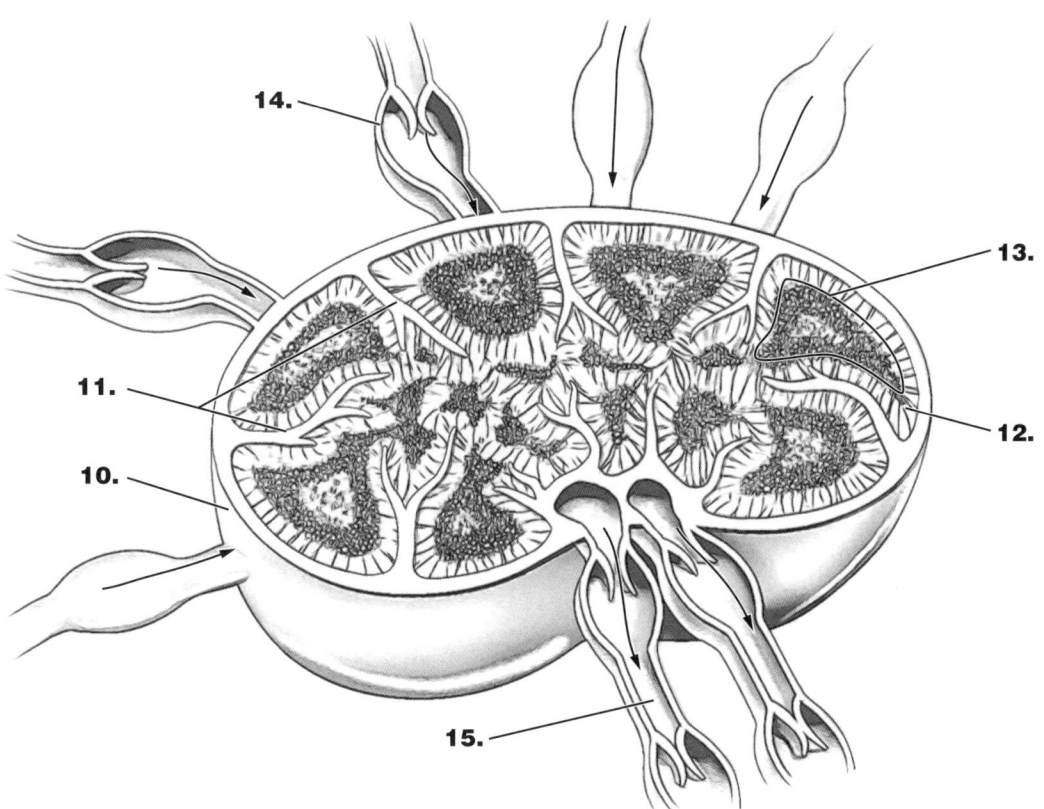

EXERCISE 4 • The Lymphatic Network

Color and label the diagrams of the lymphatic network provided. Be sure to use different colors to differentiate the lymphatic from the venous structures. If you need to refresh your memory, refer to Figure 11-3 in the textbook.

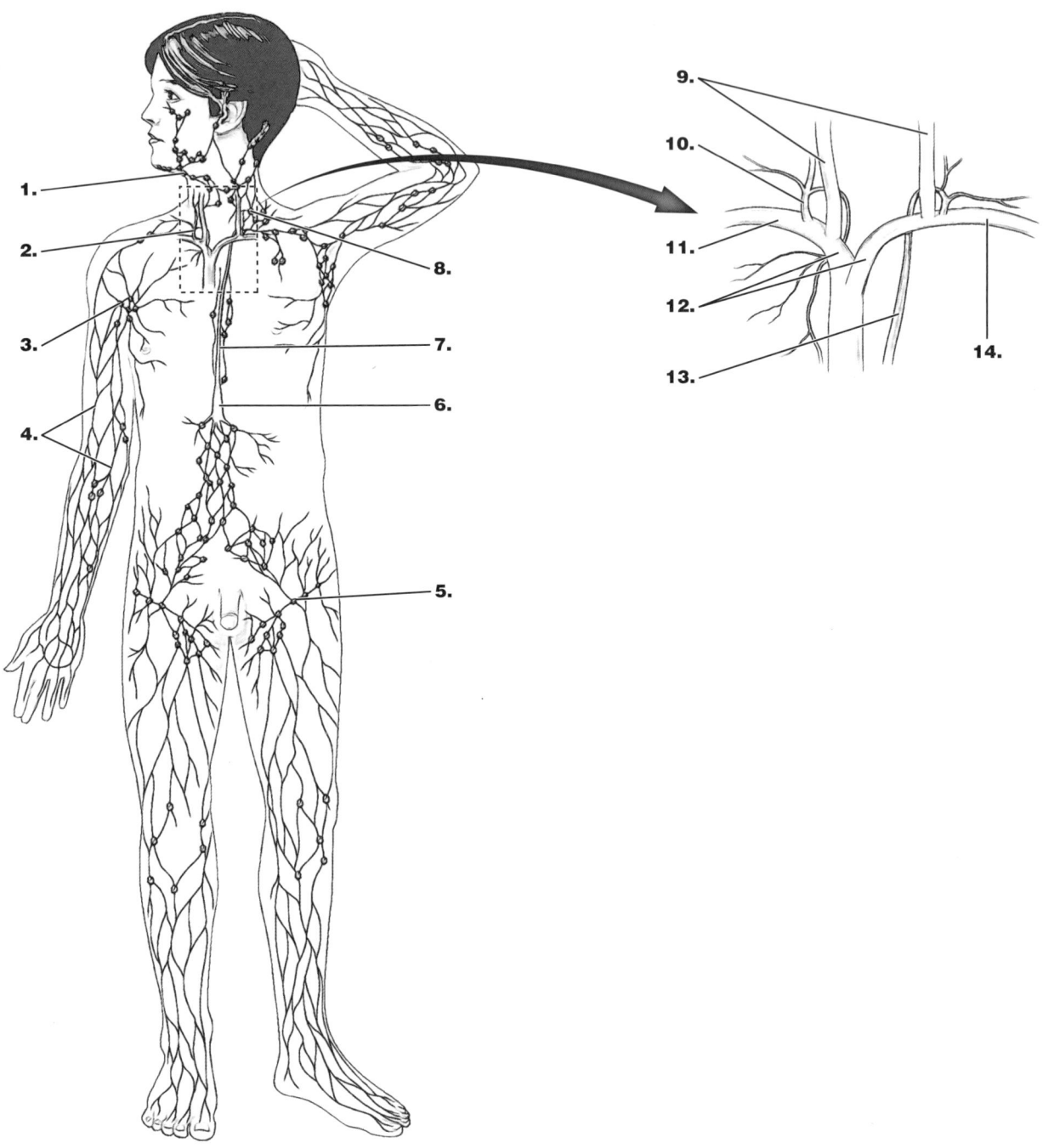

EXERCISE 5 • Edema Uptake vs. Lymphatic Flow

While interdependent, the processes of edema uptake and lymphatic flow are two different processes each facilitated by different structural characteristics and physiologic mechanisms. Mark each of these physiologic processes or structural features as either EU to indicate it is a primary influence on edema uptake, or LF if more related to lymph flow.

_____ 1. The 10% of capillary filtrate that must be returned to circulation via the lymphatic system.

_____ 2. Autonomic nervous system stimulation of smooth muscle contraction within the lymphangia.

_____ 3. External manipulation of tissue to move superficial fluid across a watershed.

_____ 4. External manipulation of tissue that applies a light stretch and release of the epidermis.

_____ 5. When interstitial fluid volumes increase, anchor filaments pull epithelial flaps of initial vessels open.

_____ 6. Anastomoses.

_____ 7. Negative pressure inside the lymphatic system.

_____ 8. No valves in initial vessels.

_____ 9. One-way valves inside the lymphangia.

_____ 10. Edema creates increased hydrostatic pressure in the interstitium.

EXERCISE 6 • Mechanisms of Lymph Flow

Complete the concept map to identify the physiologic mechanisms that create and support lymph flow.

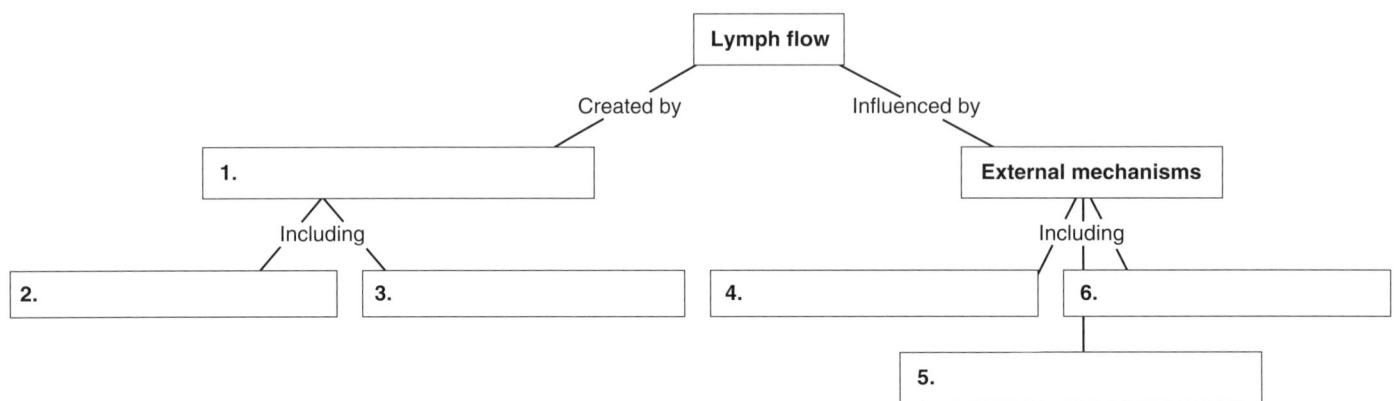

Chapter 11 The Lymphatic System

EXERCISE 7 • Catchments and Watersheds

Color and label the diagrams to identify the major catchments and watershed lines of the body. To refresh your memory or check your work, refer to Figures 11-14 and 11-16 in the textbook.

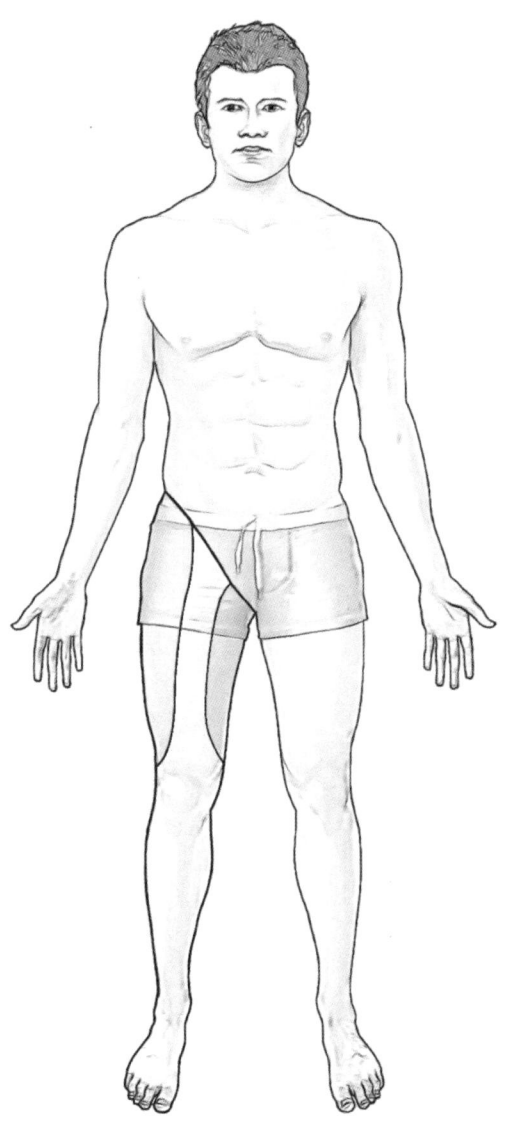
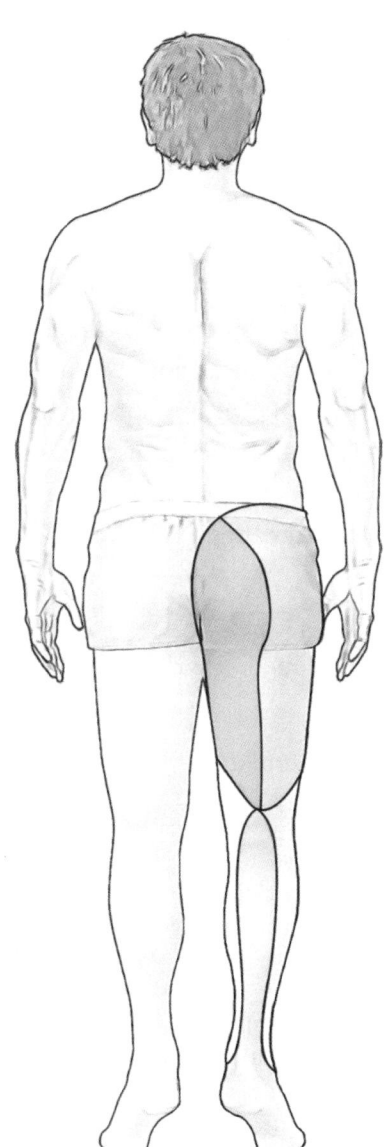

EXERCISE 8 • Routes of Lymph Flow

Use the list of lymphatic structures to outline routes of lymphatic flow. Beginning with edema uptake in the specific regions identified, place the letter of the structures into their proper sequence. Note that some structures may be a part of multiple routes.

A. Thoracic duct
B. Right lymphatic duct
C. Terminus
D. Axillary catchment
E. Inguinal catchment
F. Cisterna chyli
G. Popliteal catchment
H. Anterior thigh lymphotomes
I. Anterior leg lymphotomes
J. Posterior leg lymphotomes
K. Medial arm lymphotomes
L. Lateral arm lymphotomes

Edema uptake
@ anterior thigh   → 1. ___ → 2. ___ → 3. ___ → 4. ___ → 5. ___

Edema uptake
@ right medial wrist → 1. ___ → 2. ___ → 3. ___ → 4. ___

Edema uptake
@ calf   → 1. ___ → 2. ___ → 3. ___ → 4. ___ → 5. ___ → 6. ___

Edema uptake
@ right ribcage   → 1. ___ → 2. ___ → 3. ___

Edema uptake
@ left lateral elbow → 1. ___ → 2. ___ → 3. ___ → 4. ___

Edema uptake
@ anterior ankle   → 1. ___ → 2. ___ → 3. ___ → 4. ___ → 5. ___ → 6. ___

EXERCISE 9 • Types of Edema

Complete the table that compares and contrasts the different types of edema.

Type of Edema	Definition	Examples/Etiology
Primary Lymphedema	1.	2.
3.	Edema due to damage to lymphatic system	• Surgery 4. 5.
6.	7.	• Hypertension • Obesity or Pregnancy 8.
Traumatic Edema	9.	10.

GROUP ACTIVITY 1 • Manual Therapy and Lymph Flow Discussion

Use the concept map from Exercise 6 to support a discussion about lymph flow. Spend time explaining how each mechanism physiologically creates or influences lymph flow. Then describe how manual therapy could be used to support each mechanism of lymph flow.

12 Immunity and Healing

Use this table to identify the study guide exercises and group activities that will help you explore or review each learning objective for this chapter.

No.	Learning Objective	Exercise	Study Group Activity
1	Explain the function of the immune system and discuss its relationship and importance to manual therapy practices.		See Chapter 1, Activity 1
2	Explain the difference between primary and secondary lymphoid tissues.	1, 2	
3	Name, locate, and describe the general function of the primary and secondary lymphoid tissues.	1, 2	
4	Explain the difference between nonspecific defenses and specific immune responses.	1	
5	List the nonspecific immune defenses of the body and explain how each mechanism works.	1, 3, 5	
6	Name and describe the roles of the primary lymphocytes involved in antibody-mediated and cell-mediated immune responses.	1, 4, 5	
7	Discuss the difference between naturally and artificially acquired immunity and give examples of active and passive forms of each.	1, 6	
8	Discuss the immune system changes that commonly occur with aging.		See Chapter 1, Activity 1
9	Define the field of study known as psychoneuroimmunology and explain what implications this discipline may bring to the practice of manual therapy.	1	1

EXERCISE 1 • Immunity Crossword

Use this crossword to review and test your knowledge of the anatomy and physiology terms from Chapter 12.

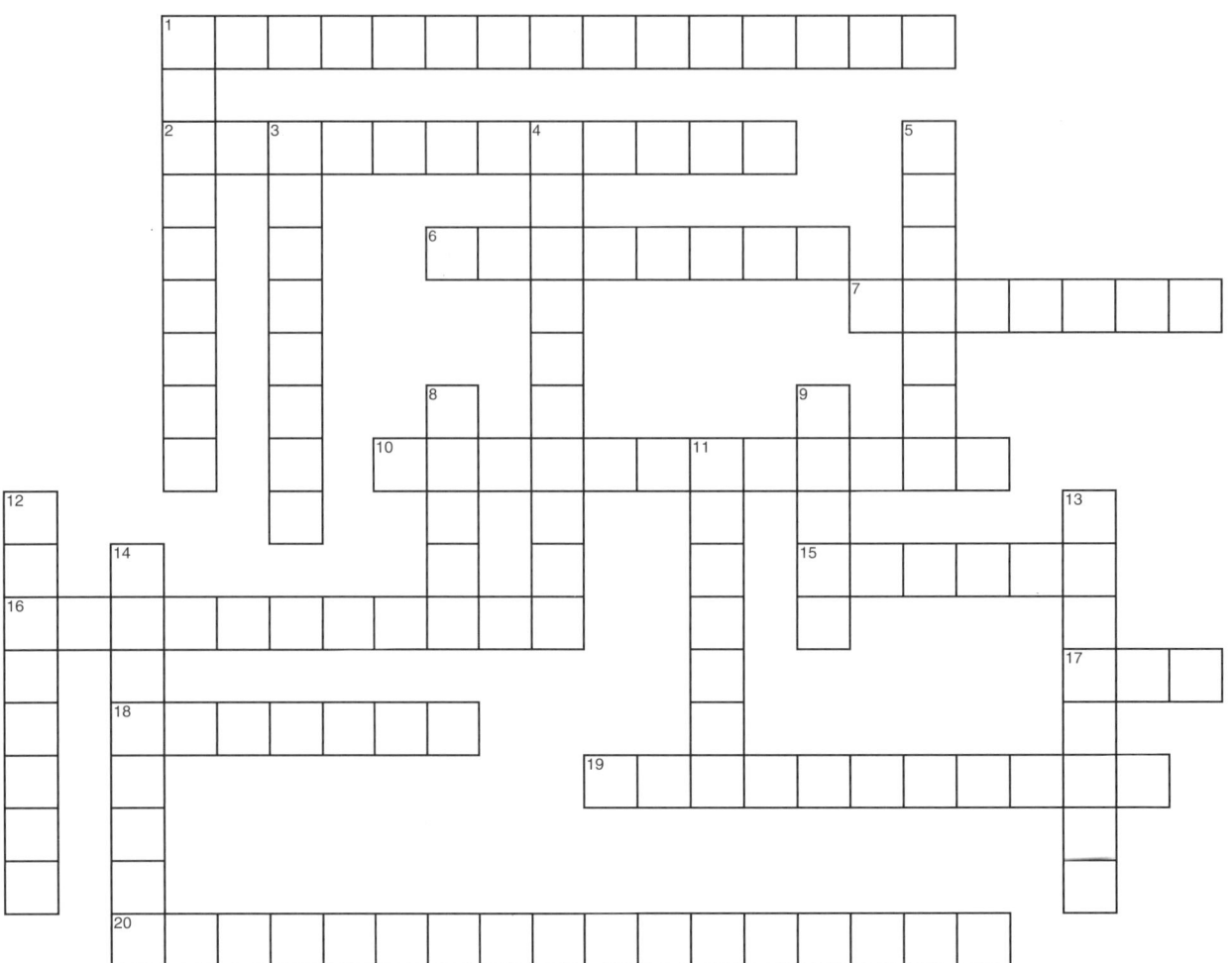

ACROSS

1. Specialized lymphocyte that inhibits or shuts down the body's specific immune response when it is no longer needed.
2. Disease resistance produced through the activation of T cells is _____ immunity.
6. Cell-signaling molecule.
7. Lymphoid tissues where lymphocytes are produced.
10. Small masses of lymphoid tissue located within the mucous membrane of the lower portion of the small intestine.
15. A peptide molecule that binds to receptor proteins in the plasma membrane of target cells to stimulate cellular activity.
16. A plasma protein that binds iron when activated by a pathogen to make it unavailable to bacteria.
17. The study of the communication links between the nervous, endocrine, immune, and digestive systems.
18. Antibody-mediated immunity is also known as _____ immunity.
19. A group of general body defenses that are not directed at any particular pathogen; innate immune defense.
20. Disease resistance obtained without medical intervention.

DOWN

1. The lymph nodes, spleen and MALTs are considered this type of lymphoid tissue.
3. Tissues that contain mature lymphocytes.
4. Cytokine that inhibits the spread of viral infection from infected to uninfected body cells.
5. A minute organism, including many types of pathogens such as bacteria and viruses.
8. Elevated core body temperature.
9. Specialized lymphocyte involved in antibody-mediated immunity.
11. Any substance that elicits a specific immune response.
12. A plasma protein released by plasma B cells that can bind with an antigen to neutralize or kill it; immunoglobulin.
13. Synonym for specific immune response.
14. Disease-causing agent such as bacteria, virus, allergen, or microbe.

EXERCISE 2 • Lymphoid Tissues

Label the following as either primary (P) or secondary (S) lymphoid tissues. Then match each with its description.

_____ 1. Red bone marrow

_____ 2. Lymph node

_____ 3. Spleen

_____ 4. Thymus

_____ 5. Tonsils

_____ 6. Peyer patches

_____ 7. Appendix

_____ 8. Adenoids

A. MALTs located in the mouth and throat

B. Filters blood, stores and releases lymphocytes

C. Filters lymph, stores and releases lymphocytes

D. Site of T lymphocyte maturation

E. MALTs in lower small intestine

F. Also known as the pharyngeal tonsils

G. Site of lymphocyte formation

H. Small twisted tube attached to the cecum

EXERCISE 3 • Nonspecific Immune Defenses

The nonspecific or **1.** _____ immune defenses of the body are a group of **2.** _____ responses, that are neither stimulated by, nor directed toward, **3.** _____ of pathogen or foreign invader. For each nonspecific defense listed, provide a general description and specific examples where appropriate. The first bullet has been completed to get you started. If you need to refresh your memory, refer to Table 12-1 in your textbook.

- Physical barriers—Mechanical barriers such as the skin and mucous membranes that physically block microbes from entering the body.
- Chemical barriers—_____
  _____
  _____

- Internal antimicrobial proteins—_____
  _____
  _____

- Phagocytes—_____
  _____
  _____

- Natural killer cells—_____
  _____
  _____

- Inflammation—_____
  _____
  _____

- Fever—_____
  _____
  _____

EXERCISE 4 • Specific Immune Responses

Specific or 1. _____ immune responses are acquired over time through 2. _____ to specific pathogens. These immune defenses involve 3. _____ and _____ lymphocyte responses to 4. _____ pathogenic agents each with a recognizable chemical marker or 5. _____ that identifies it as a 6. _____ _____ and stimulates an 7. _____ _____. For each unique 8. _____, there is a lymphocyte with a corresponding 9. _____ _____ on its plasma membrane. The response initiated by 10. _____ cells is an 11. _____ _____ or humoral response, while that initiated by 12. _____ cells is a 13. _____ _____ response. In most cases, both specific immune responses are stimulated by any particular pathogen.

Color and label the diagram to illustrate the specific immune responses. Color the cells activated and produced through the two different specific immune responses different colors. If you need to refresh your memory, refer to Figures 12-5 through 12-7 in the textbook.

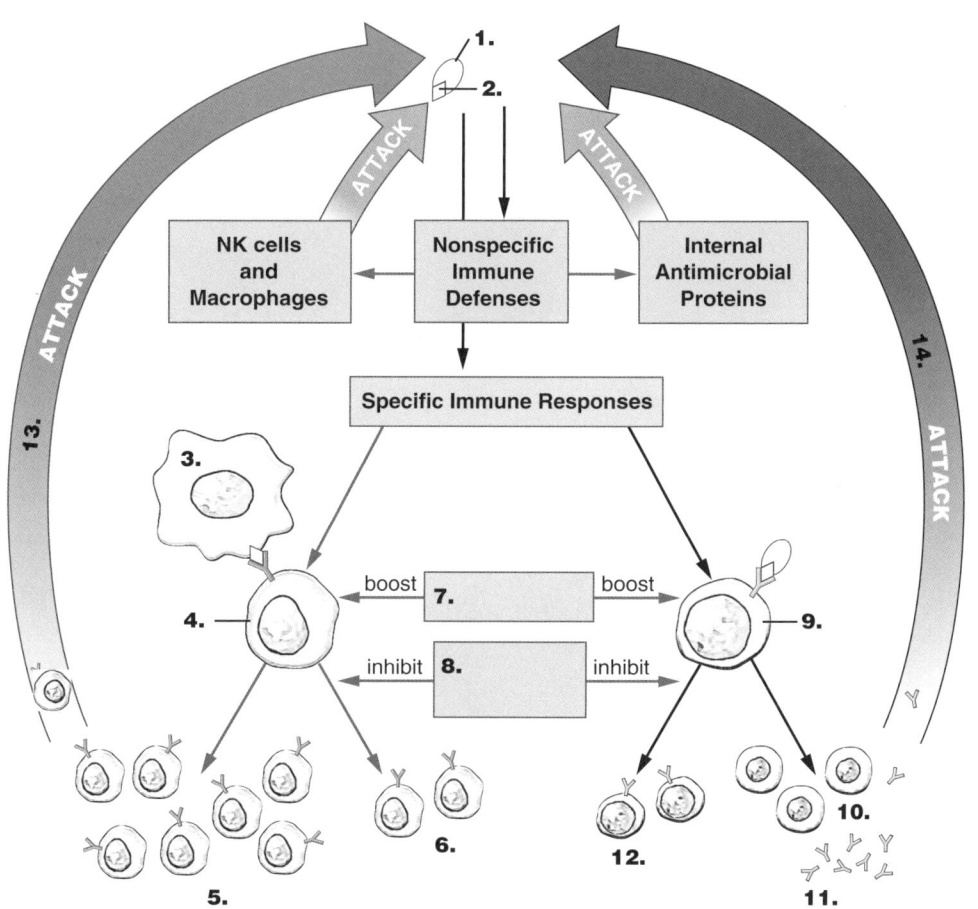

EXERCISE 5 • A Story of Immunity

Taking the steps of a physiologic process and turning them into a story can help with understanding and recall. In addition, writing the story can be a creative way to review and organize information either individually or together as a group. The following provides one example of how a story about the body's immune response might begin. Have fun completing this story, or if you are not inspired by this beginning, write a different story altogether.

Once upon a time, there was a small and prosperous village called Wellsville. This village was often visited by artisans, peddlers, and tradesmen of nearby towns with whom they exchanged goods and services. One foggy day, a stranger wearing a cloak and carrying a staff with strange markings upon it arrived at the walls of Wellsville seeking entrance into the town...

EXERCISE 6 • Gaining Immunity

Mark the following statements about naturally and artificially acquired immunity as T for true and F for false.

_____ 1. Being immune to chicken pox after having it as a child is an example of naturally acquired immunity.

_____ 2. Immunizations are examples of artificially acquired immunity.

_____ 3. Immunity gained through actually having a disease like mumps is considered passively acquired natural immunity.

_____ 4. A mother passing immunity to her infant through nursing is considered an active form of naturally acquired immunity.

_____ 5. Getting a tetanus shot is an example of artificially acquired passive immunity.

_____ 6. Getting an annual flu shot is an example of naturally acquired passive immunity.

_____ 7. After a child has measles, he or she has a lifelong immunity to the disease through naturally acquired active immunity.

_____ 8. A polio vaccination is an example of artificially acquired active immunity.

GROUP ACTIVITY 1 • PNI Discussion

Have a group discussion on psychoneuroimmunology and mind map that discussion as you have other group discussions in previous chapters. Here are some ideas to spur your discussion:

- Have each member of the group give an example from their own life in which "gut instincts" played a significant role, or they just "knew it" in their gut. Try and be as descriptive as possible about the thoughts, emotions, past experiences, and beliefs that went along with that. Then describe how that "gut instinct" affected their health or way they felt.

- Have each person offer their thoughts on this statement: "Regardless of how a peptide molecule is categorized (neurotransmitter, hormone, cytokine, etc.) and which system, organ, or tissue releases it, the ligand is capable of stimulating any cell that possesses a receptor for it." Does this support or help you explain your thoughts or experiences with the healing power of manual therapy?

- Have each group member talk about their belief, skepticism, questions, and experiences with what they understand with the body-mind-spirit connections.

PRACTICE EXAM UNIT 5 • Chapters 10–12

1. Which formed element in blood plays a key role in blood clotting?

    A. Erythrocytes
    B. Thrombocytes
    C. Leukocytes
    D. Fibrocytes

2. What is the name of the vein that carries blood from the intestines to the liver for cleansing?

    A. Hepatic
    B. Mesenteric
    C. Portal
    D. Splenic

3. What structure serves as the major site for immune functions and filtration of lymph?

    A. Spleen
    B. Lymph nodes
    C. Thymus
    D. Cisterna chyli

4. What is the fastest route for removing edema from the ankle?

    A. Direct it into the popliteal catchment
    B. Move it up the anterior leg
    C. Direct it into the patellar catchment
    D. Move it across the peroneal watershed

5. Where is the lymphatic terminus located?

    A. Lateral to the clavicular head of sternocleidomastoid muscle
    B. At the distal end of the thoracic duct
    C. Just medial to the sternal head of the sternocleidomastoid muscle
    D. Lateral to the subclavius muscle insertion

6. Which heart chamber receives blood from the pulmonary veins?

    A. Left atrium
    B. Left ventricle
    C. Right ventricle
    D. Right atrium

7. Systemic circulation begins when blood leaves the _____ _____ of the heart and enters the _____ artery.

    A. right ventricle; pulmonary
    B. right atrium; systemic
    C. left ventricle; aorta
    D. left atrium; subclavian

8. Nonspecific or general immune defenses include the actions of which of these immune cells?

   A. Helper T cells
   B. B cells
   C. NK cells
   D. Phagocytes

9. Transmission of antibodies from the mother to the child is an example of what type of immunity?

   A. Artificially acquired active
   B. Naturally acquired passive
   C. Artificially acquired passive
   D. Naturally acquired active

10. What type of lymphocytes are the ones primarily responsible for the cell-mediated immune response?

    A. All B cells
    B. All T cells
    C. Suppressor B cells
    D. Phagocytes

11. The three regulatory mechanisms for heart rate include ANS control from the cardiovascular centers in the brainstem; changes in blood levels of sodium, calcium, and potassium; and

    A. hormone secretions that increase general metabolic rate.
    B. cardiac control centers in the parasympathetic ganglia.
    C. limbic system regulation of basal metabolism.
    D. chemoreceptor monitoring and regulation of blood pH.

12. What is the term for the capillary exchange process where nutrients and fluid flow out of blood and into the interstitium?

    A. Nutrient diffusion
    B. Osmosis
    C. Capillary absorption
    D. Filtration

13. Study of the links between the nervous, endocrine, digestive, and immune systems is called what?

    A. Neuroendocrinology
    B. Psychoneuroimmunology
    C. Gastroneuroimmunology
    D. Psychosomatic endocrinology

14. What type of T lymphocyte directly destroys the antigen?

    A. NK cells
    B. Suppressor T cells
    C. Cytotoxic T cells
    D. Helper T cells

15. What is the function of primary lymphoid tissues?

    A. Site of B-lymphocyte maturation
    B. Production of the lymphocytes
    C. Primary site of immune responses
    D. Production of antibodies

16. What term correctly identifies edema caused by obesity, hypertension, venous insufficiency, and pregnancy?

    A. Primary lymphedema
    B. Traumatic edema
    C. Secondary lymphedema
    D. Dynamic edema

17. Which of these changes would cause blood pressure to increase?

    A. Vasoconstriction
    B. Vasodilation
    C. Hemorrhage
    D. Use of a diuretic medication

18. The lymphatic system's function of fluid return is reliant on what physiologic mechanism for movement?

    A. Diffusion
    B. Osmosis
    C. Siphon principle
    D. Filtration pressure

19. Examples of secondary lymphoid tissues and organs include lymph nodes, thymus,

    A. tonsils, and red bone marrow.
    B. bone marrow, and cisterna chyli.
    C. cisterna chyli, and spleen.
    D. Peyer patches, and tonsils.

20. In healthy individuals, which Starling force is the driving factor for capillary reabsorption?

    A. Capillary fluid pressure
    B. Interstitial fluid pressure
    C. Interstitial oncotic pressure
    D. Plasma oncotic pressure

21. What are the three defining characteristics of the specific immune responses?

    A. Specificity, system wide, reproducible
    B. Specificity, lymphocyte responses, creates memory
    C. Inflammation, phagocytosis, creates memory
    D. Fever, antibody production, all leukocytes engaged

22. What stage of tissue healing is marked by an increase in the number of fibrocytes and decrease in the number of leukocytes?

    A. Acute
    B. Subacute
    C. Maturation
    D. Secondary edema formation

23. What local tissue changes occur when histamine is released by mast cells, basophils, and platelets in the area of tissue trauma?

    A. Vasodilation and increased capillary permeability
    B. Vasoconstriction and decreased capillary permeability
    C. Proliferation of phagocytes and capillary reabsorption
    D. Capillary spasm and formation of platelet plug

24. Edema uptake, or the formation of lymph, occurs when the initial vessels are opened, and the interstitial fluid pressure is _____ intralymphatic pressure.

    A. lower than
    B. the same as
    C. higher than
    D. maintained by

25. What is the other anatomic name for the mitral valve?

    A. Tricuspid
    B. Bicuspid
    C. Pulmonary
    D. Semilunar

13 The Respiratory System

Use this table to identify the study guide exercises and group activities that will help you explore or review each learning objective for this chapter.

No.	Learning Objective	Exercise	Study Group Activity
1	List the functions of the respiratory system and discuss their importance as they relate to the practice of manual therapy.		See Chapter 1, Activity 1
2	Name the major organs of the system and describe the functions of each.	1–3	
3	List the organs that make up the upper and lower respiratory tracts and describe the structure of each.	1, 2, 4	
4	Explain the respiratory processes of ventilation and respiration.	1, 6	2
5	Name and locate the skeletal muscles involved in ventilation and describe how each contributes to this action.	1, 5	2
6	Explain the key physiologic processes involved in internal and external respiration.	1, 6	
7	Explain how oxygen and carbon dioxide are transported in blood.	1, 6	
8	Describe the physiologic processes involved in respiratory control and regulation.		1

EXERCISE 1 • Respiratory System Crossword

Use this crossword to review and test your knowledge of the general anatomy and physiology terms from Chapter 13.

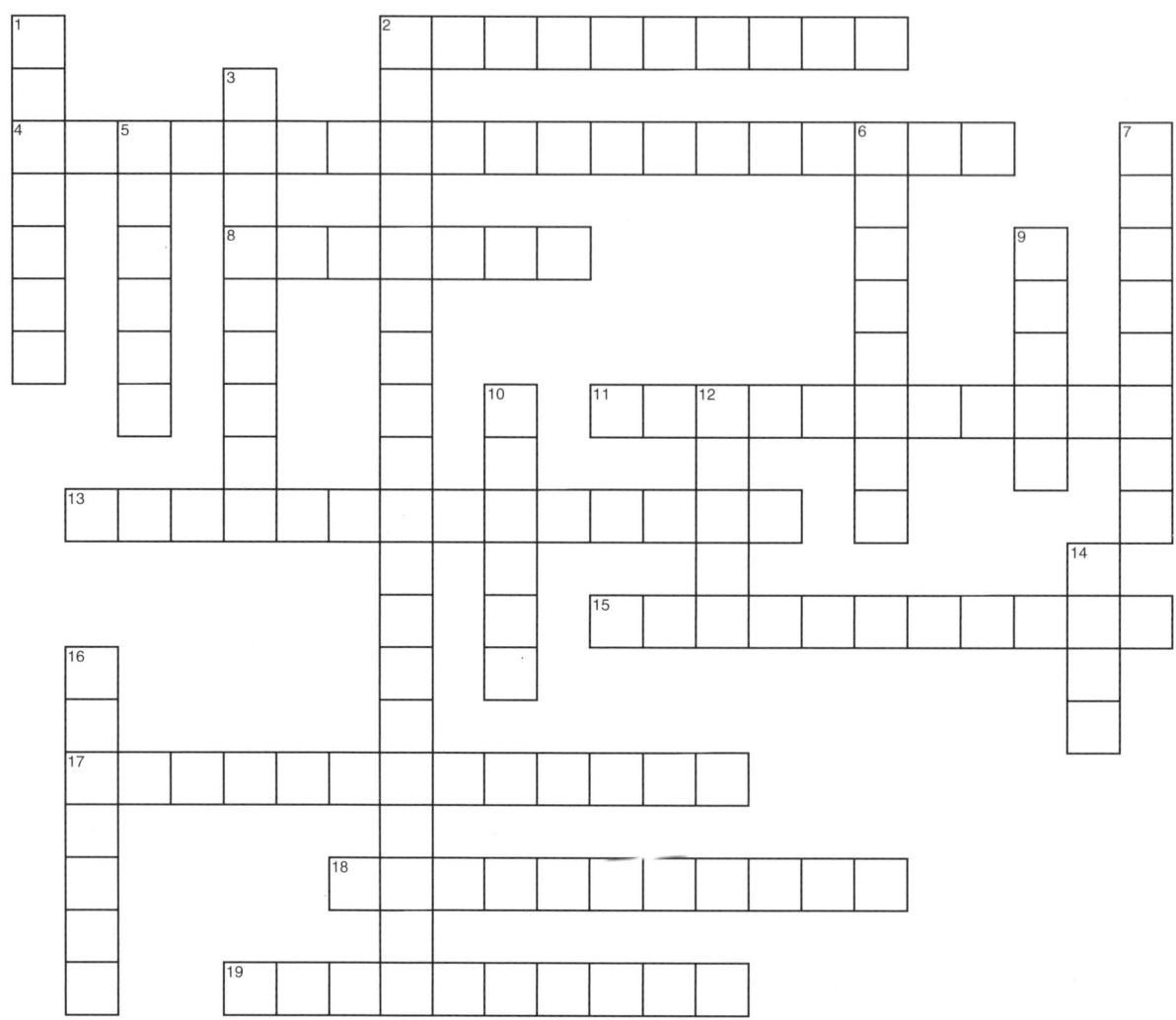

ACROSS

2 Expelling air from the lungs; expiration.
4 Formed by the alveolar and capillary walls.
8 Passageway for air and food between the nose and larynx.
11 Movement of air into and out of the lungs.
13 Type of receptors that sense changes in oxygen and carbon dioxide blood levels.
15 Exchange of oxygen and carbon dioxide across the respiratory or cell membrane.
17 Primary method of transporting oxygen in the blood.
18 Most CO_2 is converted into _____ ions for transport back to the lungs.
19 Smallest air passageway of the bronchial tree.

DOWN

1 Nerve that innervates the diaphragm.
2 Gas exchange between the air in the alveoli of the lungs and the bloodstream.
3 Primary muscle of respiration.
5 Cartilage and bony divider that separates the nasal cavity.
6 Air sac in the lungs at the end of the bronchial tree.
7 Muscles of respiration that insert on the 1st and 2nd ribs.
9 Beat and help remove particulate matter from air passages.
10 A serous membrane that lines the thoracic cavity and surrounds the lungs.
12 Nostrils.
14 Respiratory regions are found in the medulla oblongata and _____.
16 Space between the vocal cords of the larynx.

Chapter 13 The Respiratory System

EXERCISE 2 • Respiratory Structures

Color the diagram of the respiratory system and label each of the specific structures. If you need to refresh your memory, refer to Figure 13-1 in the textbook.

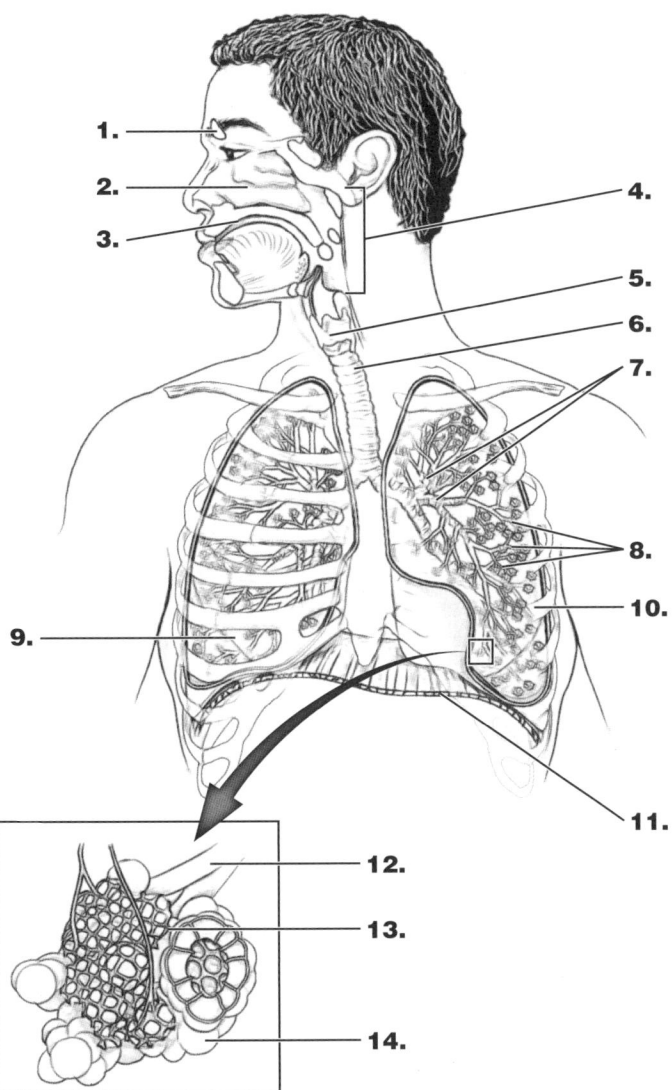

EXERCISE 3 • Matching Respiratory Organs

Match each the respiratory structures with their proper location or function.

_____ 1. Pharynx

_____ 2. Nasal conchae

_____ 3. Sinuses

_____ 4. Trachea

_____ 5. Lungs

_____ 6. Alveoli

_____ 7. Bronchioles

_____ 8. Primary bronchi

_____ 9. Pleura

_____ 10. Larynx

_____ 11. Respiratory membrane

_____ 12. Respiratory cilia

A. Windpipe; passageway for air from pharynx to the bronchial tree

B. Hair-like projections in the respiratory mucosa that help trap small inhaled particles

C. Voice box; situated between the pharynx and trachea

D. Throat or posterior region of the mouth; serves as a common passageway for food and air

E. Scroll-shaped bony shelves in the nasal cavity that "ruffle" air to enhance olfaction and help humidify it

F. The first branches of the trachea that carry air into the lungs

G. Serous membrane that produces a lubricating fluid to decrease resistance for lung expansion

H. Mucous membrane–lined cavities in the frontal, maxillary, and ethmoid bones that humidify and warm air

I. Smallest branches of the bronchial tree

J. A thin membrane formed by the alveolar and capillary walls; produces surfactant to keep alveoli open

K. The largest organs of the respiratory system that fill the thoracic cavity on either side of the heart

L. Tiny air sacs; where respiration occurs

EXERCISE 4 • Upper or Lower Respiratory Tract

Identify the following structures with a U if they are a part of the upper respiratory tract, or an L if part of the lower respiratory tract.

_____ 1. Alveolar duct

_____ 2. Respiratory membrane

_____ 3. Lungs

_____ 4. Trachea

_____ 5. Larynx

_____ 6. Primary bronchi

_____ 7. Pharynx

_____ 8. Epiglottis

_____ 9. Sinuses

_____ 10. Nasal conchae

EXERCISE 5 • Muscles of Ventilation

Place each of the muscles listed below on the table provided according to their location and/or action on the ribcage. Also, identify each as either a muscle of inhalation or exhalation by placing it in the correct column. Note that this will leave eight cells blank on the table. If you need to review the information about muscles of ventilation, check Figure 13-10 in the textbook.

Diaphragm

External intercostals

Internal intercostals

Pectoralis minor

Rectus abdominus

Scalenes

Serratus anterior

Sternocleidomastoid

Inhalation	Exhalation	Description
1.	2.	The fiber direction of these short muscles between the ribs elevates the ribcage as a whole when they contract.
3.	4.	Contraction causes this muscle to flatten and increase the size of the ribcage.
5.	6.	This muscle's attachment to the sternum and lower ribs make it depress the ribcage.
7.	8.	Contraction of these muscles pulls down on each individual rib, which depresses the ribcage as a whole.
9.	10.	These small muscles elevate the first two pair of ribs when they contract.
11.	12.	Contraction of this muscle expands the ribcage laterally.
13.	14.	Contraction of this muscle helps elevate ribs 3 through 5.
15.	16.	Although it is a prime mover in rotation and flexion of the head, contraction of this muscle assists in ventilation by elevating the sternum and clavicle.

EXERCISE 6 • Respiration

Respiration is the physiologic process of **1.** _____. This gaseous exchange takes place in two locations:

- **2.** _____.
- **3.** _____.

External respiration is the **4.** _____, while **5.** _____ is the gas exchange that occurs between the blood and body tissues. The method of exchange is **6.** _____, and the gases are transported by binding to the **7.** _____ on red blood cells, or as a dissolved substance in **8.** _____. O_2 is transported through the blood as **9.** _____. CO_2 is transported through the blood in three ways: approximately 80% of CO_2 is transported by converting it to **10.** _____, while the other 20% is transported either as **11.** _____ or as a dissolved gas.

Color and label the diagram illustrating respiration and the circulation of blood to supply the body with oxygen and eliminate carbon dioxide. Be sure to draw in the arrows showing what direction the gases are moving. If you need to refresh your memory, refer to Figure 13-11 in the textbook.

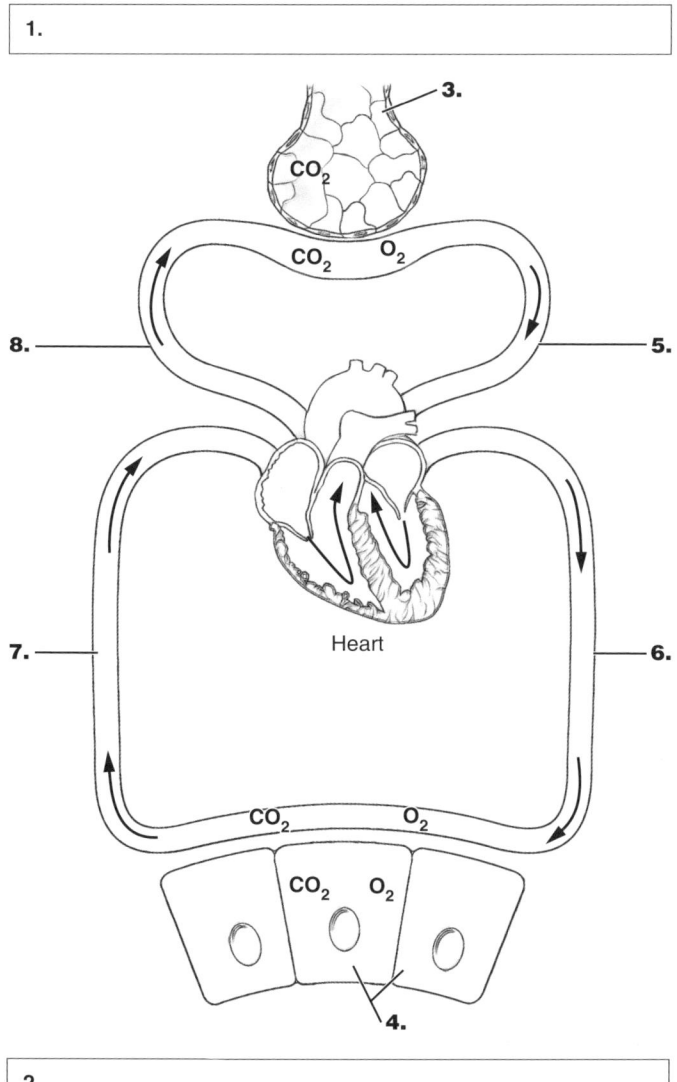

GROUP ACTIVITY 1 • Concept Map

You may recall that a concept map is an organizing tool that goes further than a mind map by asking you to show relationships between linked items. As a group activity, concept maps provide lots of opportunities for discussion and clarification. They allow members of a group to show connections between independent pieces of information in a fun and graphic way. You can develop maps together, or work individually and share your maps to see where your thinking differs. If you need to refresh your memory on how to make a concept map, refer to Chapter 3, Exercise 7.

For the respiratory system, there are lots of terms and concepts you could choose to map. Try making a mind map that explains the control and regulation of respiration by using the following list of terms and phrases:

Stretch receptors

Medulla oblongata

Chemoreceptors

Inspiration center

Pons

Respiratory nerves

Sets basic rhythm of breathing

Walls of bronchioles and alveoli

Carotid and aortic bodies

Pneumotaxic area

Sets the rate of breathing and assists with rhythm

Vagus and glossopharyngeal cranial nerves

GROUP ACTIVITY 2 • Building a Model of a Lung

In order to understand how the changing size of the thoracic cavity impacts the pressure and movement of air into and out of the lungs, build this simple model. For each model you will need the following:

- 1 or 2 L plastic pop bottle
- Rigid plastic straw
- Two balloons
- One rubber band
- Modeling clay
- Scissors

Directions:

1. Cut the bottom off the plastic pop bottle. This will serve as the top and sides of the thoracic cavity.
2. Use the rubber band to fasten one balloon to the bottom of the straw.
3. Position the straw in the neck of the bottle so that the balloon hangs within the bottle. Create an airtight seal around the straw using a clump of modeling clay.
4. Cut off the top of the second balloon and then stretch it across the bottom of the plastic bottle. This flexible bottom will represent the diaphragm.
5. Now, to inflate your "lung," simply pinch the center of the "diaphragm and slowly pull downward. As the "thoracic cavity" expands, notice that the "lung" attached to the end of the straw inflates.

14 The Digestive System

Use this table to identify the study guide exercises and group activities that will help you explore or review each learning objective for this chapter.

No.	Learning Objective	Exercise	Study Group Activity
1	Discuss the importance of the digestive system as it relates to the practice of manual therapy.		See Chapter 1, Activity 1
2	List and explain the functions of the digestive system	1, 5	1
3	List the four layers of the GI tract and describe the functional characteristics of each.	1, 4	1
4	Name and locate the major organs of the GI tract, and describe the functions of each.	1–3, 5, 6	1
5	Name and locate the accessory organs of the digestive system, and describe the general functions of each.	1–3, 5, 6	1
6	Explain the basic metabolic processes of anabolism and catabolism in regard to macronutrients.	1, 7	1
7	Discuss digestive system changes that commonly occur as the body ages.		See Chapter 1, Activity 1

Chapter 14 The Digestive System

EXERCISE 1 • Digestive System Crossword

Use this crossword to review and test your knowledge of the general anatomy and physiology terms from Chapter 14.

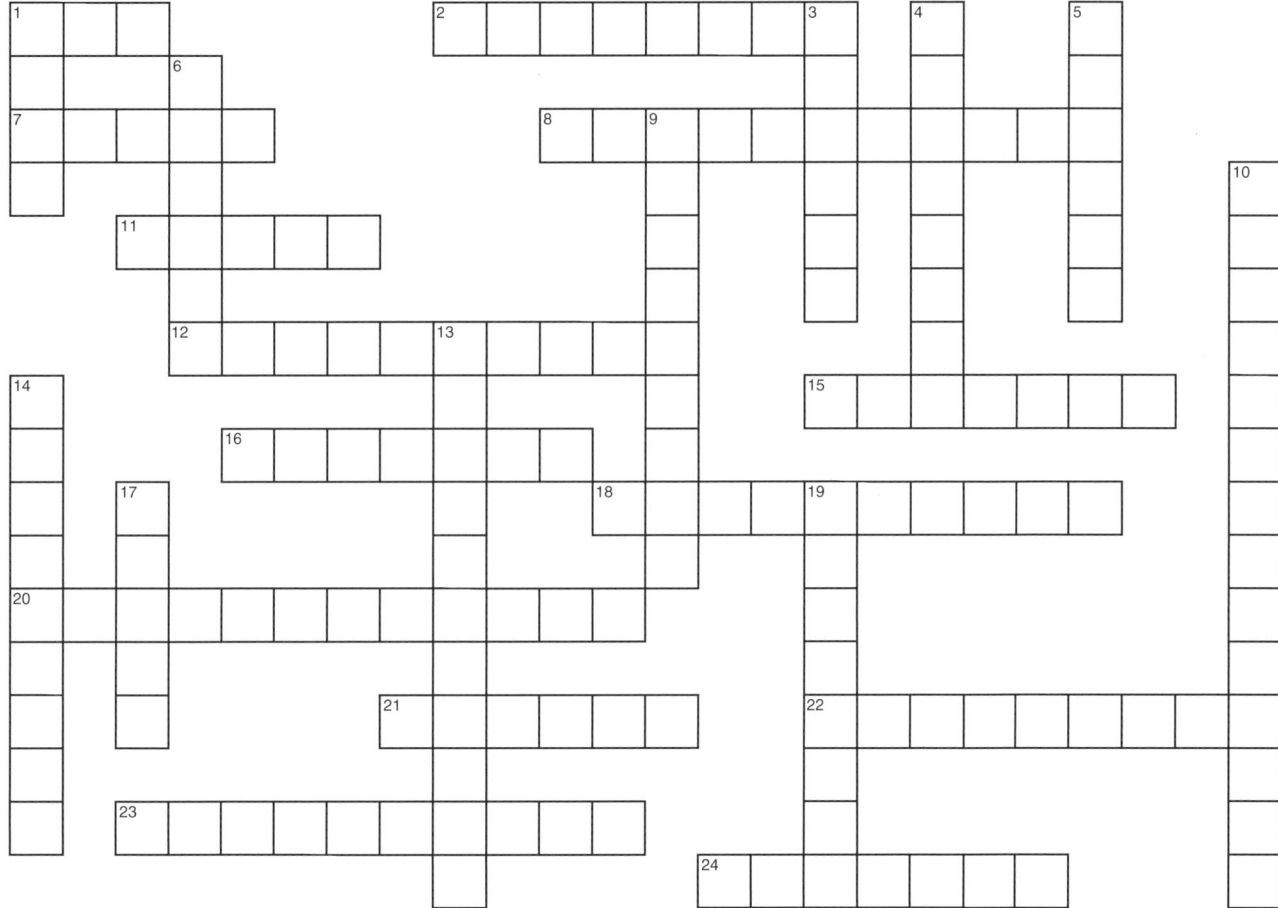

ACROSS

1. Baseline energy needed by the body to support basic life functions.
2. Initial segment of the small intestine.
7. Organ that secretes bile, stores fat and sugar as energy resources, and filters out toxins from blood.
8. The process of chewing.
11. The longest segment of the large intestine.
12. Assimilation of nutrients through the digestive tract into the blood is called _____.
15. Enzyme that digests starch.
16. The complex neuronal network that controls the secretions and smooth muscle contractions of the GI tract is the _____ nervous system.
18. Elimination of feces through the anus.
20. Mechanical digestive process that mixes and churns chyme in the SI.
21. Circular folds in the lining of the small intestine that increase the surface area for absorption.
22. The act of eating or taking in food or liquids.
23. Chewing is an example of this type of digestion.
24. Lower portion of the stomach.

DOWN

1. A fat emulsifier produced by the liver and stored in the gall bladder.
3. Innermost tissue layer of the digestive tract.
4. Movement as a general function is called _____.
5. The upper portion of an organ such as the stomach.
6. Synonym for the visceral peritoneum.
9. Smooth muscle ring that controls the flow of substances through or out of the GI tract.
10. Large fatty extension (apron) of the peritoneum.
13. Wave-like muscular contraction that propels food through the GI tract.
14. The process of breaking down food so that nutrients can be absorbed.
17. Specialized folds in the lining of the stomach that allow it to distend.
19. The action of HCl in the stomach is considered an example of this type of digestion.

EXERCISE 2 • Gastrointestinal Tract Versus Accessory Organs and Functions

Mark each of the items listed as being either an accessory (A) or gastrointestinal (GI) tract organ or function.

_____ 1. Absorption of nutrients

_____ 2. Pancreas

_____ 3. Stomach

_____ 4. Esophagus

_____ 5. Production and secretion of bile

_____ 6. Liver

_____ 7. Peristalsis

_____ 8. Gall bladder

_____ 9. Pharynx

_____ 10. Secretion of amylase, lipase, and trypsin

_____ 11. Absorption of water

_____ 12. Secretion of hydrochloric acid

_____ 13. Remove toxins and most medications from blood

Chapter 14 The Digestive System

EXERCISE 3 • Digestive System Organs

Color and label the diagrams of the digestive system. If you need to refresh your memory, refer to Figures 14-2, 14-8, and 14-11 in the textbook.

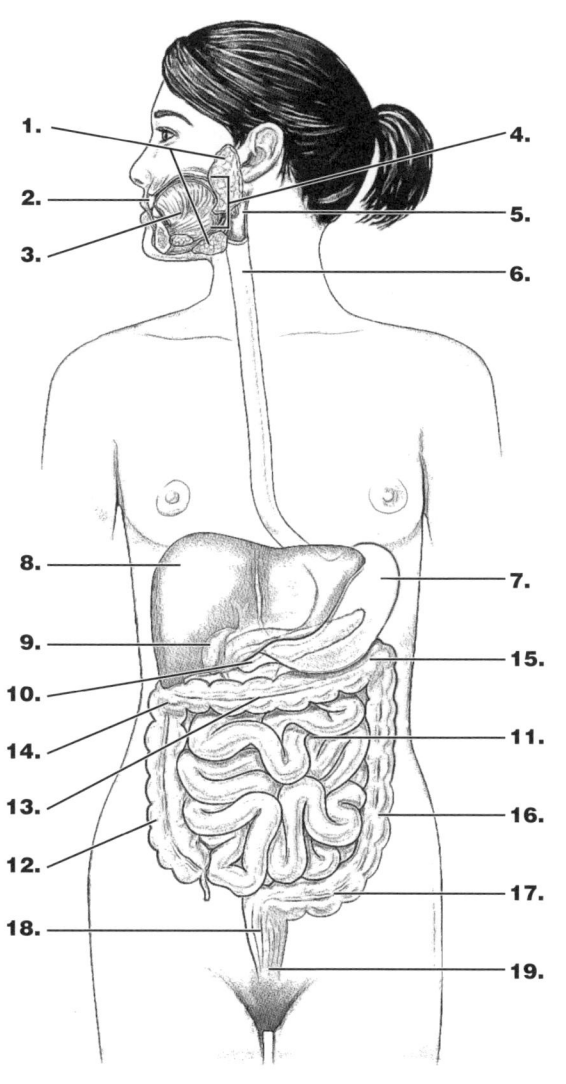
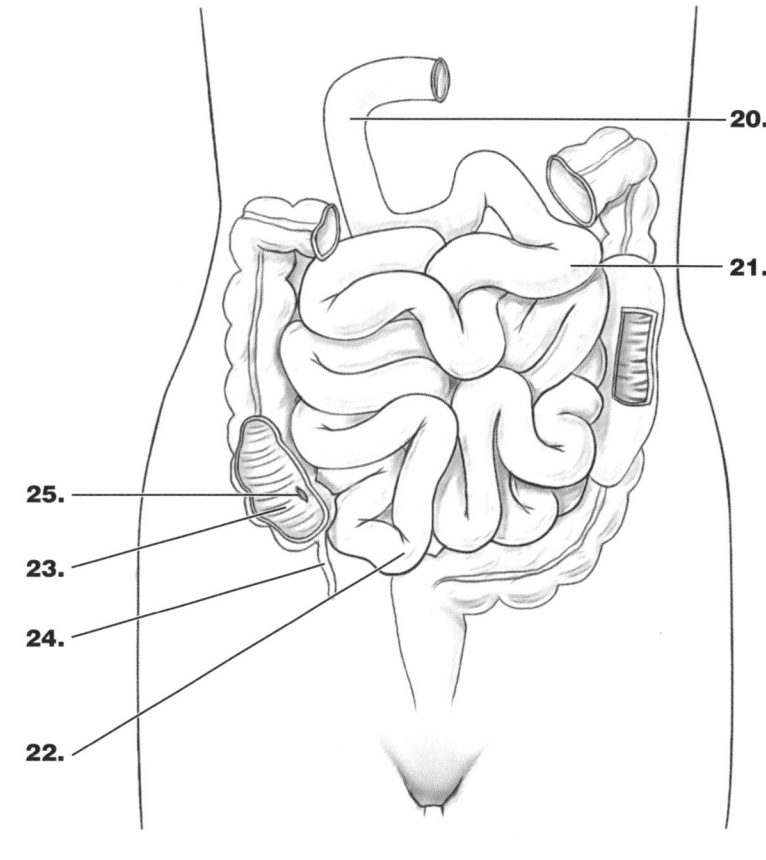

1. _____
2. _____
3. _____
4. _____
5. _____
6. _____
7. _____
8. _____
9. _____
10. _____
11. _____
12. _____
13. _____
14. _____
15. _____
16. _____
17. _____
18. _____
19. _____
20. _____
21. _____
22. _____
23. _____
24. _____
25. _____

EXERCISE 4 • Layers of the GI Tract

Color and label the diagram to identify the layers of the GI tract. Then complete the matching exercise to review or quiz your knowledge about the structure and function of each layer. If you need to refresh your memory, refer to Figure 14-3 in the textbook.

_____ 1. Mucosa A. Propels food forward through the digestive tract

_____ 2. Submucosa B. Visceral peritoneum

_____ 3. Muscularis C. Double fold of peritoneum that supports SI

_____ 4. Serosa D. Includes motor neurons that control muscularis

_____ 5. Myenteric plexus E. Includes motor neurons that control mucosal secretions

_____ 6. Peyer patch F. MALT found in the intestines

_____ 7. Mesentery G. Contains receptors that sense contents and distension of tract

_____ 8. Submucosal plexus H. Causes segmentation in the SI for mechanical digestion

_____ 9. Circular layer I. Includes a third oblique layer in the stomach

_____ 10. Longitudinal layer J. Comprised of areolar connective tissue

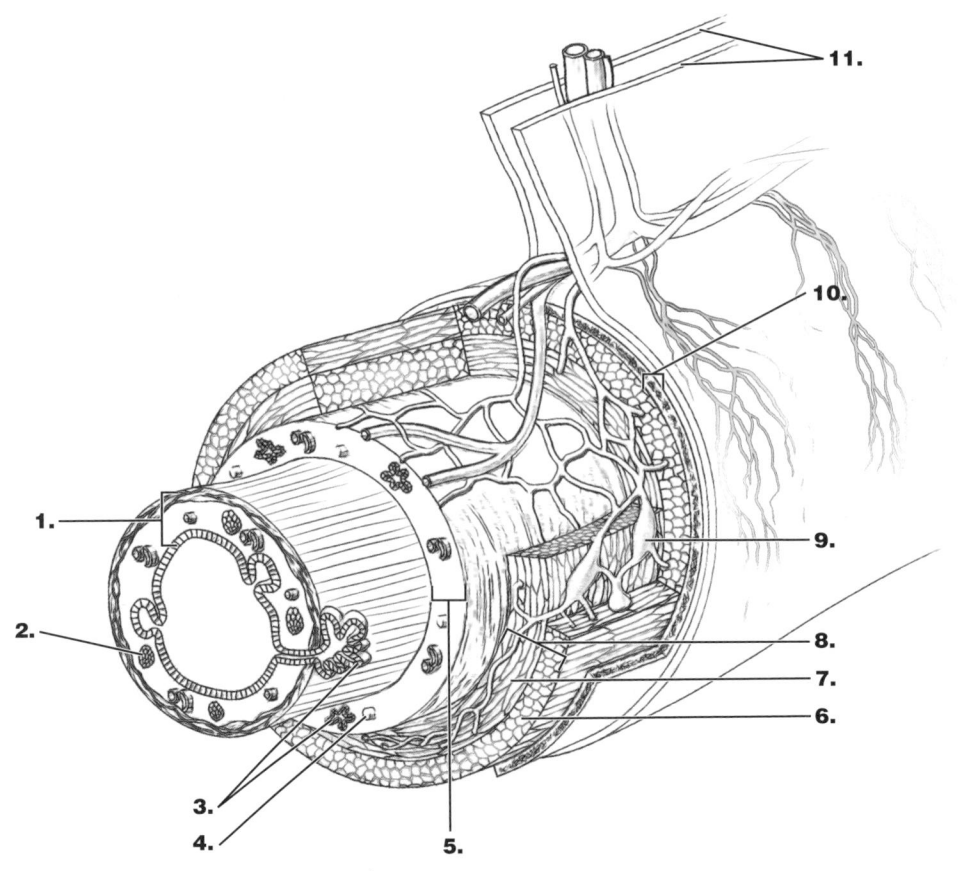

Chapter 14 The Digestive System

EXERCISE 5 • Functions of the Digestive System

Complete the table to summarize the functions of each organ of the digestive system. If you need to refresh your memory, refer back to Table 14-1 in the textbook. Remember that if you do not like tables, this same information can be organized using a mind map.

Organ	Ingestion	Secretion	Digestion M=mechanical C=chemical	Motility	Absorption	Elimination
Mouth and pharynx	Eating	Mucus	M: Chewing C: **1.**	**2.**	Sublingual medications	
Salivary glands		**3.**				
Esophagus		Mucus		**4.**		
Stomach		Mucus, **5.** and **6.**	M: mixing, grinding C: breakdown of all foods via HCl and **7.** via **8.**	Gastric emptying and **9.**	Some medications such as aspirin and **10.**	
Small intestine		Mucus, sucrase, lactase, & maltase plus **11.** Local hormones **12.** and CCK	**13.** M: C: breakdown of all nutrients	**14.** **15.**	**16.** and **17.** and amino acids as well as water and medications	
Large intestine		**18.**		Peristalsis	**19.** and **20.**	Defecation
Liver		**21.**				
Gall bladder		**22.**				
Pancreas		**23.** lipase and trypsin				

EXERCISE 6 • Diagram the Functions of the GI Tract

Sometimes a pictorial representation of information is more helpful than a table or mind map. For example, the schematic provided here can be used to summarize the functions of each organ of the GI tract. First, identify each of the organs labeled with a number on the schematic representation of the GI tract. Next, draw line(s) from each function box to the region(s) of the tract where the function takes place. Finally, complete each function box by placing the number of each organ where the function occurs and provide a brief description. An example has been provided for you under mechanical digestion. Also, consider adding color to further visually organize the information either by coloring each structure a different color and using it to highlight its place in each function box, or by color coding the functions and adding colored squiggles or layers to each organ where the function takes place.

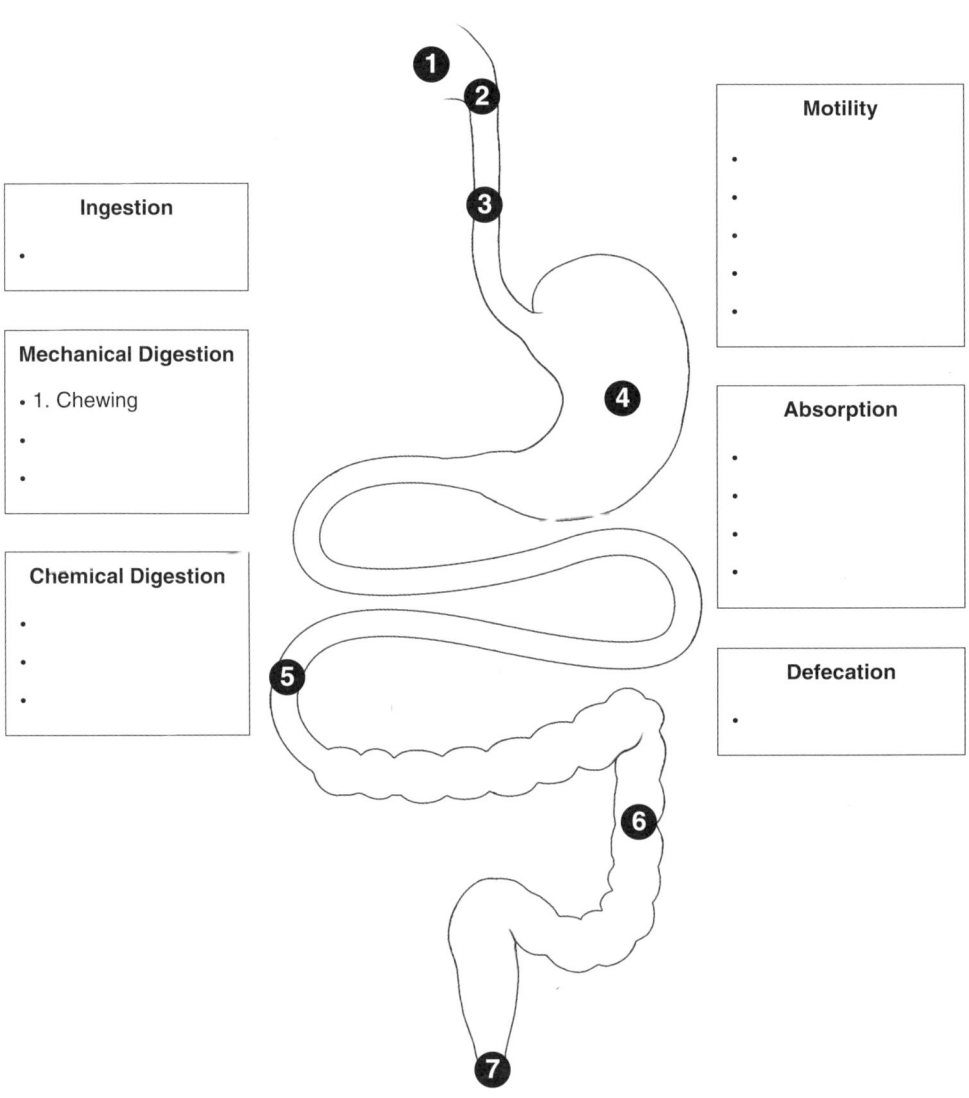

EXERCISE 7 • Metabolism and Nutrients

Metabolism refers to all the 1. _____ _____ that occur within the body. It includes 2. _____ processes, in which complex molecules are formed from simpler ones, tissue is created or 3. _____, and molecules such as hormones, neurotransmitters, and ligands are 4. _____. Metabolism also includes 5. _____ processes such as glycolysis and the Krebs cycle, which break down complex molecules to 6. _____ _____. All of these processes rely on the body's intake and assimilation of two general categories of nutrients through the digestive system.

7. _____ are needed in large quantities to meet the body's tissue building and energy demands. They include

- Carbohydrates that are absorbed as 8. _____ molecules that can be easily catabolized for 9. _____ via glycolysis and the Krebs cycle, or converted into 10. _____ to be stored in skeletal muscle and the liver, or into 11. _____ and stored as adipose tissue.

- 12. _____ are absorbed as triglyceride molecules and broken into 13. _____ and _____ _____, which can be catabolized for energy. They are stored as 14. _____ tissue.

- Proteins absorbed as 15. _____ _____ can be converted in the 16. _____ and catabolized to produce ATP, but they are the body's last choice for energy production. More importantly, these molecules are used for all types of 17. _____ _____ to make and repair tissue, and form 18. _____.

19. _____ are only needed in small amounts by the body to maintain homeostasis and health. These nutrients include

- Vitamins that support normal metabolic function by 20. _____ _____.

- 21. _____ that support homeostatic mechanisms including pH, fluid, and energy balance; are important components of 22. _____ and _____ tissues; and serve as 23. _____.

While not technically a nutrient, 24. _____ is also essential for cellular health and the maintenance of homeostasis.

GROUP ACTIVITY 1 • Pyramid Game

This group activity was introduced back in Chapter 1. If you need to refresh your memory on how to develop and play this game, refer back to Group Activity 3 in that chapter. Some suggested topics for your Digestive System Pyramid Game could include

- Digestive functions
- Layers of the digestive tract
- Digestive secretions
- Organs of the GI tract
- Accessory organs of the digestive system
- Macronutrients
- Micronutrients
- Segments of the large intestine
- Structural characteristics of the small intestine
- Functions of the liver

Have fun brainstorming your own categories!

15 The Urinary System

Use this table to identify the study guide exercises and group activities that will help you explore or review each learning objective for this chapter.

No.	Learning Objective	Exercise	Study Group Activity
1	Explain the function of the urinary system and discuss its relationship and importance to manual therapy practices.		See Chapter 1, Activity 1
2	Name, locate, and explain the general function of urinary system organs.	1, 2	
3	Name the key structural components of the kidneys and describe the general function of each.	1, 3	
4	Describe the role of the urinary system in fluid management.	1	1
5	Name the key structural components of a nephron and describe the processes that occur in each.	1, 4, 5	
6	List and explain the three processes involved in urine formation.	1, 4, 5	
7	Discuss urinary system changes that commonly occur as the body ages.		See Chapter 1, Activity 1

EXERCISE 1 • Urinary System Crossword

Use this crossword to review and test your knowledge of the general anatomy and physiology terms from Chapter 15.

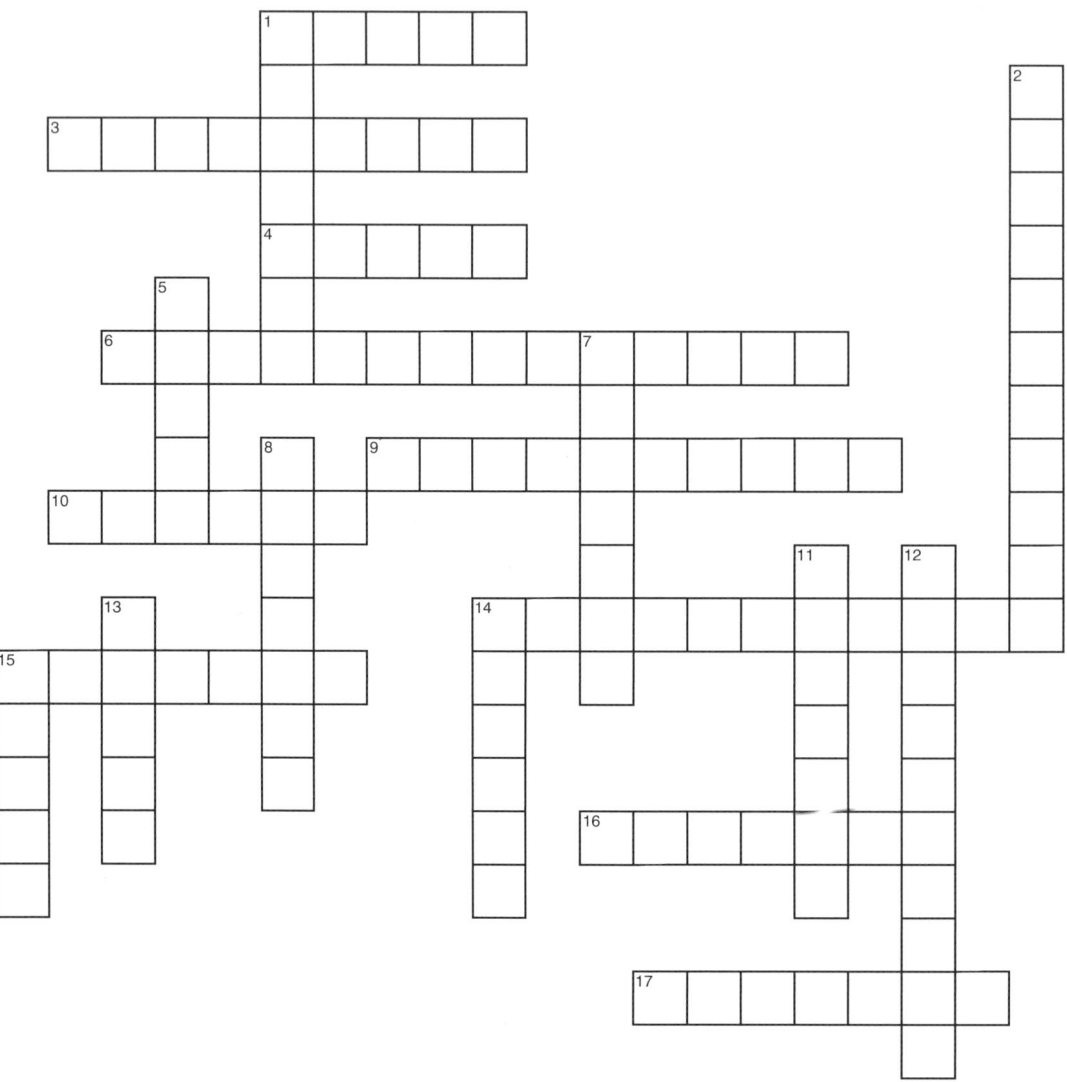

ACROSS

1. Liquid waste formed by the kidneys.
3. In this process, toxins, metabolic wastes, and unused ions and nutrients are moved out of the blood into the renal tubule.
4. Indentation in the kidney where the ureters, blood vessels, and nerves enter and exit the organ.
6. Initial portion of a nephron comprised of the glomerulus and Bowman's capsule.
9. Wad of capillaries found in the nephron.
10. Region of the kidney where urine is collected before being passed into the ureter.
14. Stress initiates the RAA pathway because sympathetic stimulation leads to a decrease in renal _____.
15. Hollow organ that serves as a holding tank for urine.
16. The inner portion of the kidneys is called the renal _____.
17. Microscopic functional unit of the kidney.

DOWN

1. Narrow tube that carries urine from the bladder to the external environment.
2. Urination.
5. Pertaining to the kidneys.
7. These tubes connect the kidneys to the bladder.
8. Blood levels of essential electrolytes are all regulated by the _____.
11. Large fascial envelope that surrounds each kidney and attaches it to the abdominal wall.
12. The specific urine formation process that occurs in the renal corpuscle.
13. Small cup at the bottom of a renal pyramid that collects urine.
14. The renal _____ is the outer portion of the kidney.
15. The kidneys filter and cleanse this fluid through the process of urine formation.

Chapter 15 The Urinary System 201

EXERCISE 2 • Urinary System Organs

Color and label the diagram to identify the organs of the urinary system. Then, for each structural characteristic or function listed, place the letter of the organ described. Note that some organs are described in more than one way, so their letter will be used multiple times. If you need to refresh your memory, refer to Figure 15-1 in the textbook.

_____ 1. This organ carries urine from the kidneys to the bladder.

_____ 2. This organ has rugae for distension.

_____ 3. This organ helps to balance blood pH, electrolytes, and fluid volumes.

_____ 4. This organ is partially situated anterior to 12th rib.

_____ 5. This organ has two muscular sphincters that regulate elimination.

_____ 6. This organ's wall has three layers of smooth muscle.

_____ 7. These mucus-lined tubes are retroperitoneal.

_____ 8. This organ's function is affected by ADH and aldosterone.

_____ 9. This organ secretes the hormone calcitriol.

_____ 10. This organ releases renin in response to stress.

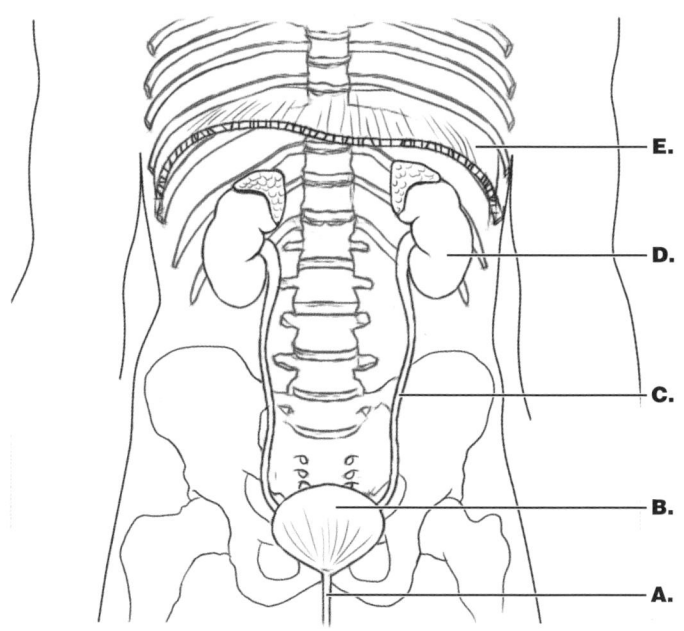

Study & Review Guide for Applied Anatomy and Physiology for Manual Therapists

EXERCISE 3 • Structure of the Kidneys

Color and label the diagram detailing the structure of the kidney. Provide a brief definition of each component identified. If you need to refresh your memory, refer to Figure 15-2 in the textbook.

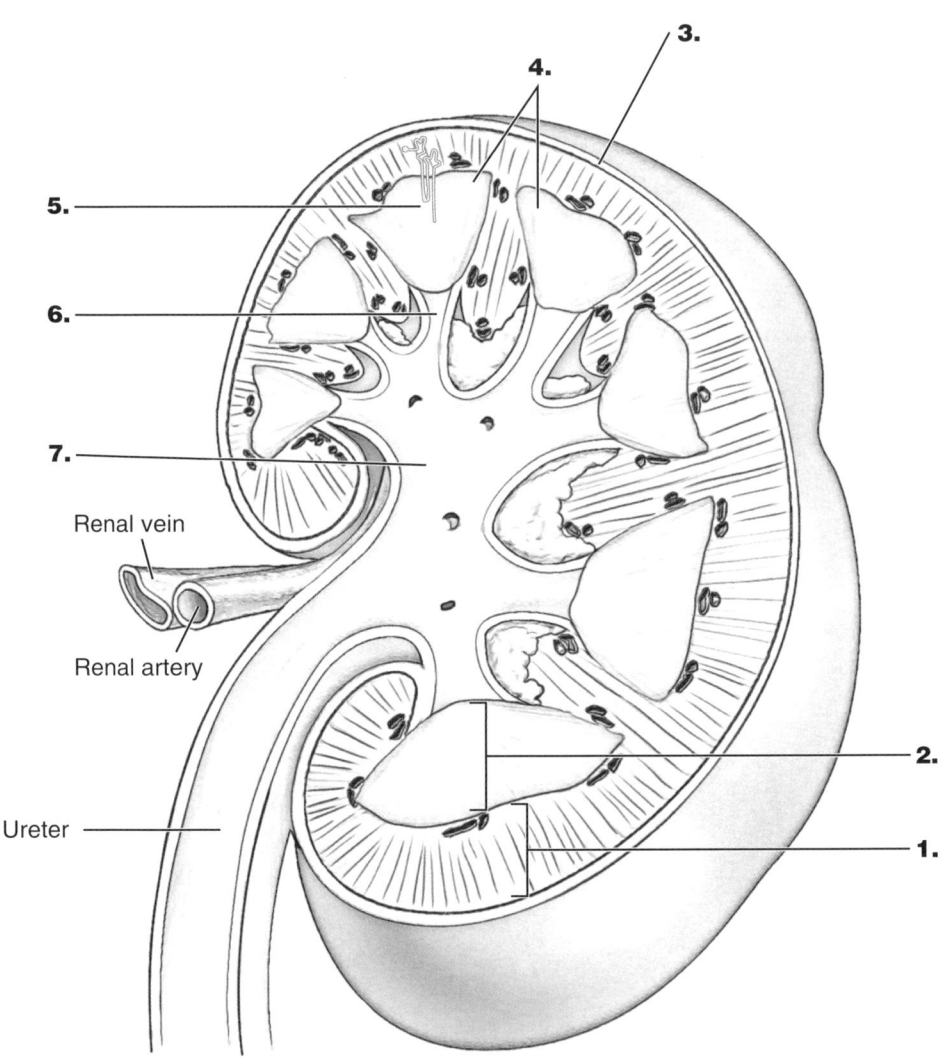

EXERCISE 4 • Parts of a Nephron

Color and label the structural components of the nephron. You may want to look at the next exercise for some of the names of the structures, or if you need to refresh your memory, refer to Figure 15-5 in the textbook.

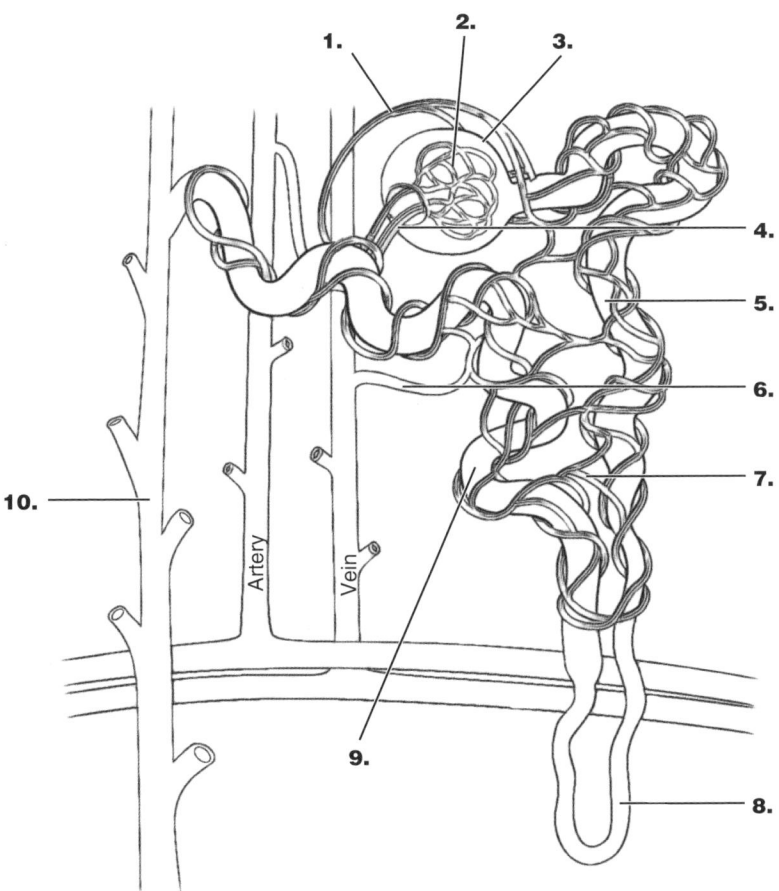

EXERCISE 5 • Structure and Function of a Nephron

Match each of the structures and functions of a nephron to its proper description.

_____ 1. Glomerulus

_____ 2. Distal convoluted tubule

_____ 3. Filtration

_____ 4. Renal corpuscle

_____ 5. Collecting duct

_____ 6. Bowman capsule

_____ 7. Secretion

_____ 8. Proximal convoluted tubule

_____ 9. Reabsorption

_____ 10. Peritubular capillaries

A. The first step in urine formation

B. Nephron segment where filtration occurs

C. The outer portion of the renal corpuscle

D. Where most reabsorption takes place

E. Process in which water, sodium, and other electrolytes move from the renal tubule into blood

F. Ball of capillaries inside the renal corpuscle

G. Network of blood vessels around the renal tubule for the exchange of fluid and substances between blood and urine

H. Elimination of ammonia, urea, and excess hydrogen ions from blood to urine

I. Site where fluid from several nephrons is concentrated into urine

J. Nephron segment where most secretion takes place

GROUP ACTIVITY 1 • The Kidney's Role in Fluid Management

As the kidneys filter and cleanse the blood, they play a central role in managing the volume and composition of the blood. Use the mind map provided to direct a group discussion about the kidney's role in fluid management. Specifically explain how the kidneys perform each regulatory role. As your mind map expands, be sure to also consider the links between the itemized roles. For example, explore the connection between blood pressure and blood volume, or between blood pH and electrolytes.

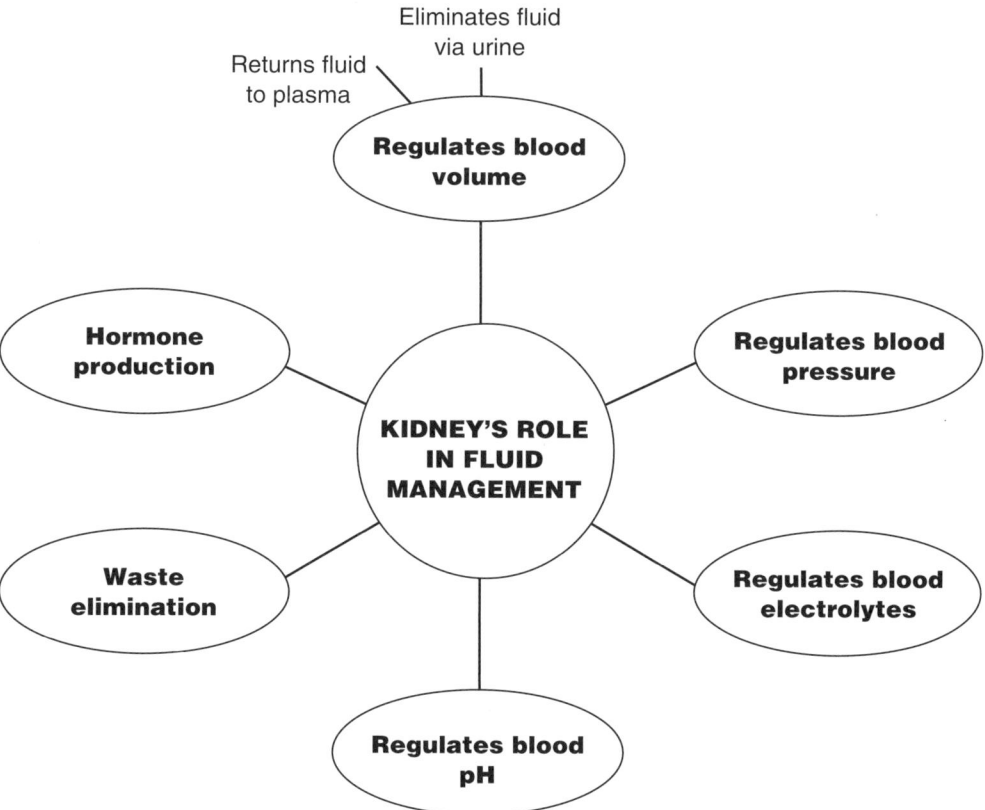

16 The Reproductive System

Use this table to identify the study guide exercises and group activities that will help you explore or review each learning objective for this chapter.

No.	Learning Objective	Exercise	Study Group Activity
1	Explain the function of the male and female reproductive systems and discuss their relationship and importance to manual therapy practices.		See Chapter 1, Activity 1
2	List the structural features and hormonal control processes that the male and female reproductive systems have in common.	1, 2	1
3	Name, locate, and explain the general function of the male genitalia in terms of the primary and accessory reproductive organs.	1–4	1
4	Name, locate, and explain the general function of the female genitalia in terms of the primary and accessory reproductive organs.	1, 2, 5, 6	1
5	Describe the stages and hormonal regulation of the female reproductive cycle.	1, 2	1
6	Explain the key physiologic processes that occur during each stage of pregnancy and childbirth.	1	1, 2
7	Discuss the reproductive system changes that occur as the body ages.		See Chapter 1, Activity 1

EXERCISE 1 • Reproductive System Crossword

Use this crossword to review and test your knowledge of the general anatomy and physiology terms from Chapter 16.

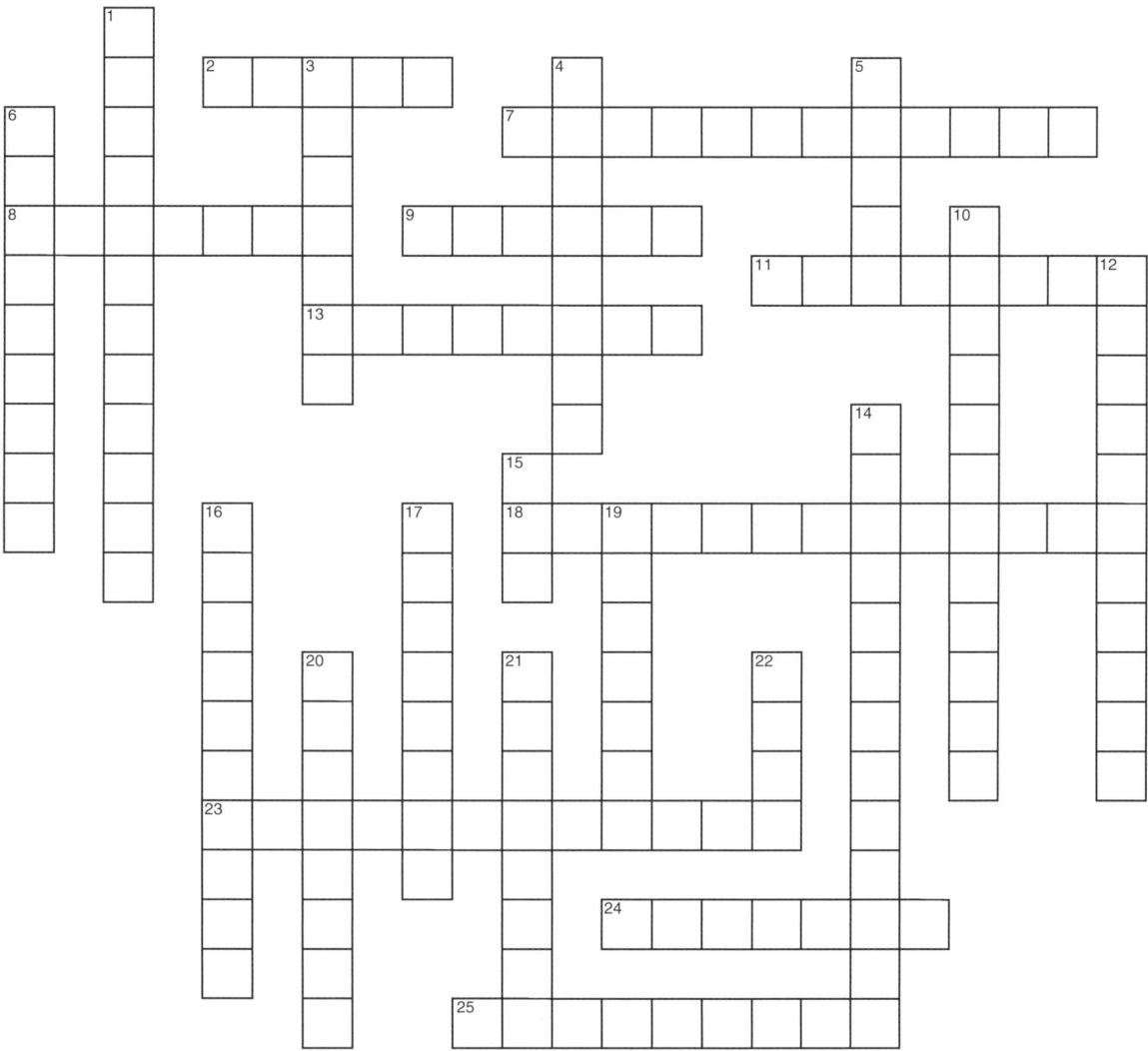

ACROSS

2 Male gamete.
7 Hormone produced by Leydig cells.
8 Passageway for both sperm and urine in males.
9 Fertilized egg.
11 The first menstrual period and beginning of the reproductive cycle.
13 Embryonic layer that differentiates to form the epidermis, nervous tissue, and sense organs.
18 Days 6 through 14 of the female reproductive cycle when the endometrium thickens is called the _____ phase.
23 Glandular mass formed from the follicle once the ovum has been discharged.
24 Gametes are produced through this cell division process.
25 Period of fetal development from conception until birth.

DOWN

1 Painful or difficult menstruation.
3 In the first stage of labor, the cervix dilates and _____.
4 Middle embryonic layer that differentiates to form muscle and connective tissues.
5 Thick, whitish fluid consisting of sperm and secretions from several accessory reproductive organs.
6 The expelling of an egg from the ovary.
10 Female steroid hormone that stimulates the development and maintenance of the endometrium.
12 Inner lining of the uterus that thickens and sloughs off with each menstrual cycle.
14 A synonym for conception.
15 A common condition for men over 50.
16 Multi-celled mass of tissue that develops into an embryo.
17 The region between the mons pubis and anus in females, or the scrotum and anus in males.
19 Synonym for fallopian tube.
20 Hormone that stimulates the maturation of ova within the ovaries.
21 Specialized ring of cells surrounding an ovum.
22 Female gamete.

EXERCISE 2 • Mind Map of Common Characteristics

Complete the mind map by specifying the male and female reproductive features for each of the common characteristics identified. If you need to refresh your memory, refer to Table 16-1 in the textbook.

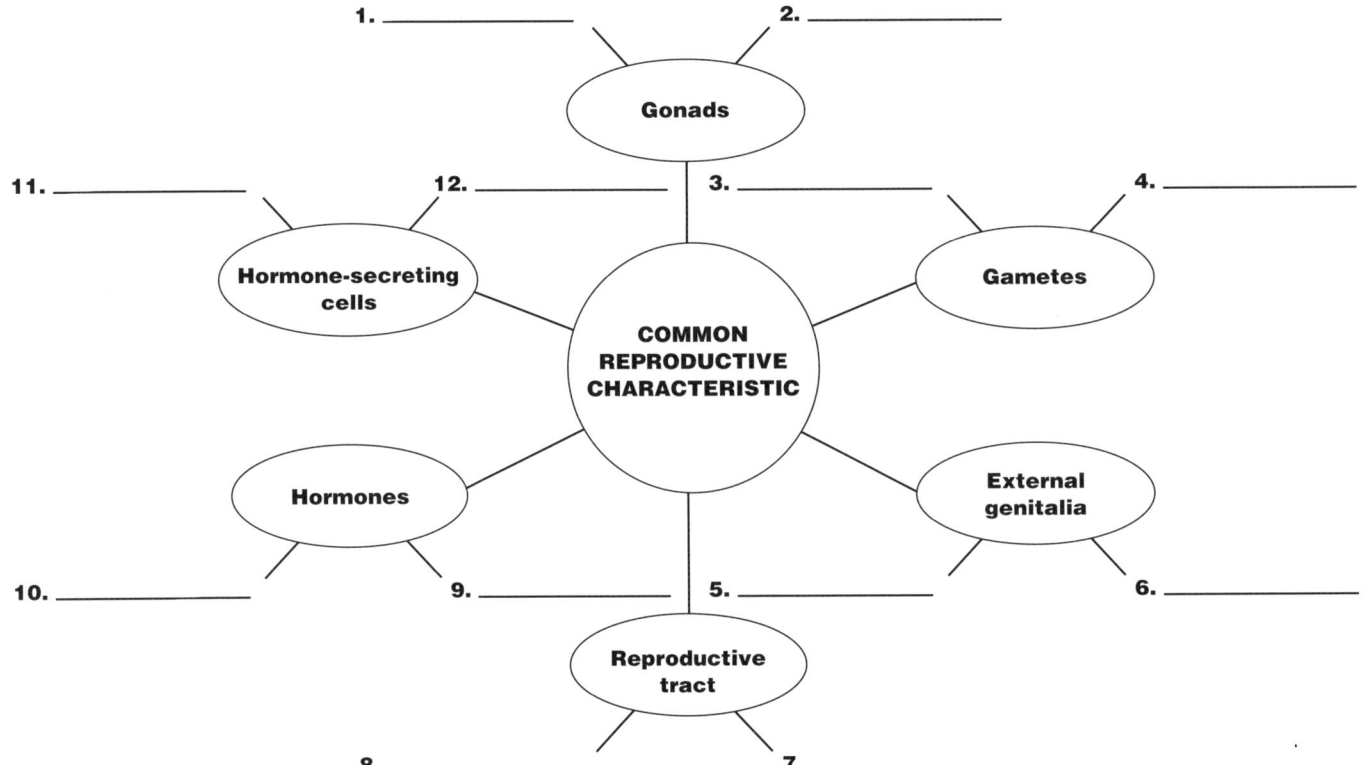

Chapter 16 The Reproductive System

EXERCISE 3 • Male Pelvic Anatomy

Color and label the sagittal section to identify the structures of the male pelvic cavity. Highlight the labels of the reproductive components to help differentiate them from other pelvic structures. If you need to refresh your memory, refer to Figure 16-1 in the textbook.

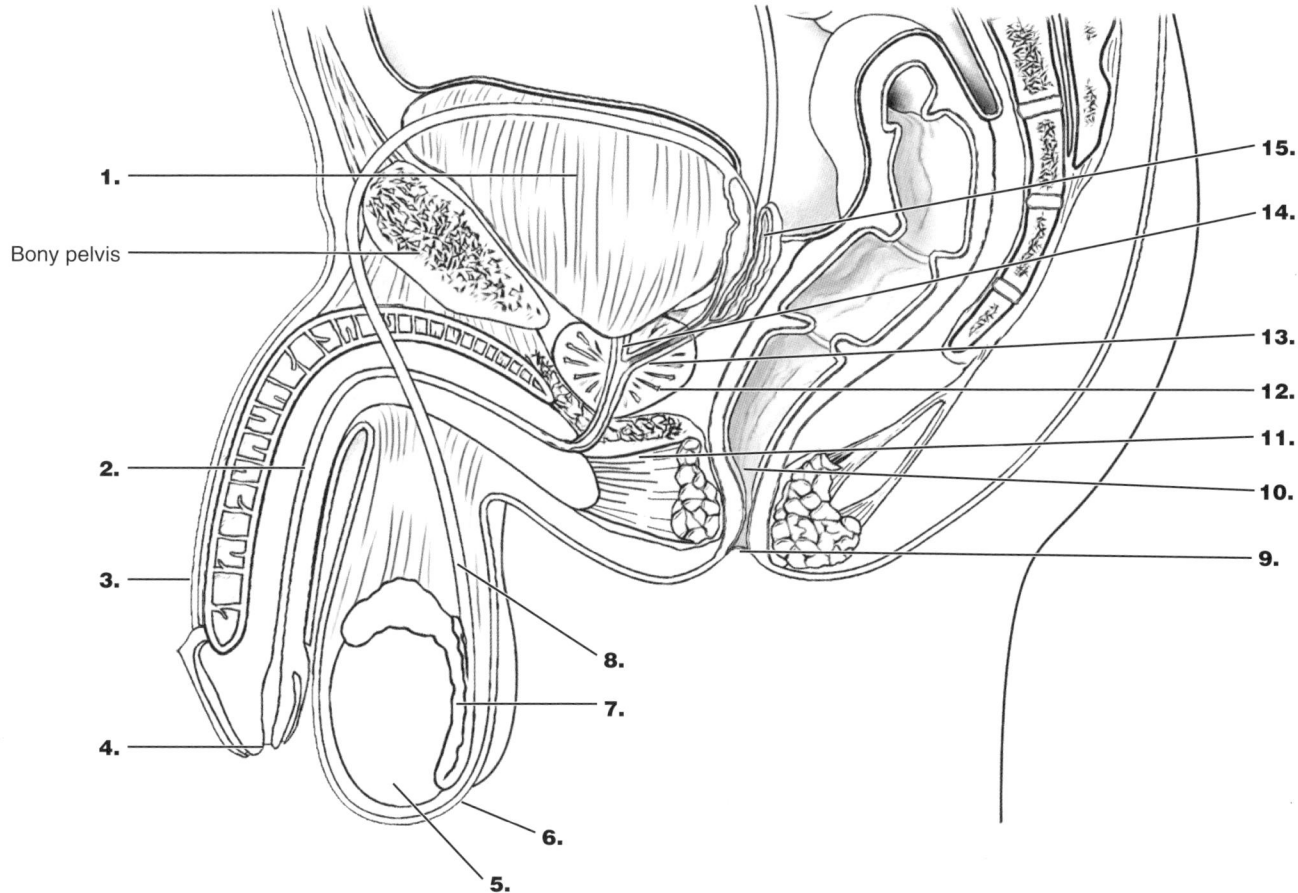

EXERCISE 4 • Male Reproductive Structures and Functions

Match each of the structures in the male reproductive system with its function or key structural characteristic.

_____ 1. Seminal vesicle

_____ 2. Testes

_____ 3. Vas deferens

_____ 4. Seminiferous tubule

_____ 5. Epididymis

_____ 6. Ejaculatory duct

_____ 7. Leydig cells

_____ 8. Prostate gland

_____ 9. Bulbourethral glands

A. Sperm mature, develop their motility and ability to fertilize in this structure

B. Sperm production and secretion of testosterone

C. Duct that carries sperm from the prostate to the urethra

D. Produces testosterone

E. Produces 60% of the fluid portion of semen

F. Secretes a milky fluid directly into the urethra to support sperm motility

G. Stores sperm for several months, and carries it out of the scrotum to the spermatic cord

H. Produces mucus-like substance that lubricates the lining of the urethra to protect sperm during ejaculation

I. Male gonads that produce male gametes

EXERCISE 5 • Female Pelvic Anatomy

Color and label the sagittal section to identify the structures of the female pelvic cavity. Highlight the labels of the reproductive components to help differentiate them from other pelvic structures. If you need to refresh your memory, refer to Figure 16-3 in the textbook.

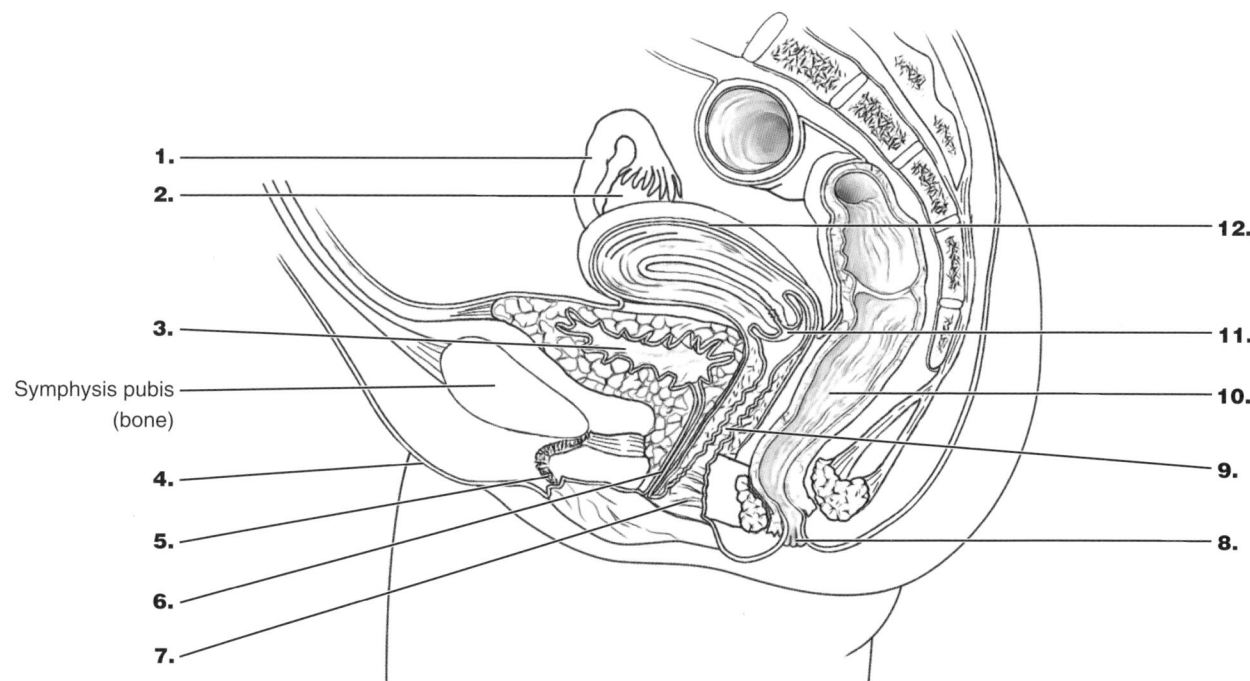

EXERCISE 6 • Female Reproductive Structures and Functions

Match each of the structures in the Female reproductive system with its function or key structural characteristic.

_____ 1. Follicle

_____ 2. Corpus luteum

_____ 3. Endometrium

_____ 4. Fallopian tube

_____ 5. Fimbriae

_____ 6. Vagina

_____ 7. Uterus

_____ 8. Ovary

_____ 9. Placenta

_____ 10. Labia

A. Short muscular tube that carries eggs from the ovary to the uterus

B. Produces ova, estrogen, and progesterone

C. Blood-rich, protective membrane for the fetus

E. Canal between the cervix and exterior environment

F. Inner lining of the uterus that thickens and sloughs off with each menstrual cycle

G. Hormone-secreting, glandular mass formed from the follicle once the ovum has been discharged

H. Lateral tissue folds that surround the vaginal and urethral openings

I. Specialized ring of cells surrounding an ovum inside the ovaries

J. Finger-like projections off the fallopian tube that surround the ovaries to help "catch" the egg

K. Hollow, muscular organ that houses the developing fetus

GROUP ACTIVITY 1 • Pyramid Game

This group activity was introduced back in Chapter 1. If you need to refresh your memory on how to develop and play this game, refer back to Group Activity 3 in that chapter. Some suggested topics for your Reproductive System Pyramid Game could include

- Reproductive hormones
- Common characteristics of the male and female reproductive systems
- Structures of the male reproductive tract
- Structures of the female reproductive tract
- Phases of the female reproductive cycle
- Stages of labor
- Body changes due to pregnancy
- Signs of menopause
- Gonads and gametes
- Signs of puberty

Have fun brainstorming your own categories.

GROUP ACTIVITY 2 • Discussing Pregnancy and Childbirth

Mind map a discussion about pregnancy and childbirth. Explain the changes that occur both for the mother and growing baby as you map out each stage of gestation and labor. Also, discuss how manual therapy can be used to support a mother through each of these processes and any specialty training that may be required.

PRACTICE EXAM UNIT 6 • Chapters 13–16

1. The primary functions of the urinary system are to filter blood to help regulate fluid volume, blood pressure, pH;

   A. recycle old RBCs; and enrich blood with more WBCs.
   B. balance hormone levels; and purify blood plasma.
   C. balance electrolytes; and eliminate liquid waste products via excretion of urine.
   D. balance vitamins and electrolytes; and enrich blood with recycled nutrients.

2. Which of these statements best summarizes the functions of the digestive system?

   A. Nutrient–waste exchange between blood and tissues, helps balance fluid and pH levels, excretion of liquid waste products
   B. Provides nutrients for cellular metabolism, assists in regulating body temperature, elimination of solid wastes
   C. Assists in balancing fluid, pH, blood pressure, and purifying blood.
   D. Generates heat via digestion; balances hormone, electrolyte, and pH levels in blood; and excretion of all metabolic by-products.

3. How does the respiratory system help the body regulate temperature, pH, and fluid balance?

   A. Each exhale expels carbon dioxide to help balance pH and eliminates heat and water.
   B. Inhalation brings in oxygen and moisture to help balance pH and fluids, and exhalation eliminates heat.
   C. The exchange of gases in the lungs balances pH and temperature, and moisture is added to blood by the respiratory membrane.
   D. Each exhale eliminates toxins and fluid, and inhales bring in "buffer" chemicals like nitrogen.

4. The functions of the reproductive system are to produce offspring and

   A. stimulate emotional development.
   B. maintain the purity of the genetic code from parents.
   C. trigger the stress response when reproduction is threatened.
   D. produce hormones for development of sex cells and secondary sex traits at puberty.

5. Which respiratory structure serves as a passageway for air and houses the voice box?

   A. Trachea
   B. Pharynx
   C. Palatine tonsils
   D. Larynx

6. What is the positional relationship between the esophagus and trachea?

   A. The esophagus is anterior to the trachea.
   B. The trachea is on the right side and parallel to the esophagus.
   C. The esophagus is on the right side and parallel to the trachea.
   D. The trachea is anterior to the esophagus.

7. Swallowing, segmentation, and peristalsis are all different types of which digestive process?

    A. Chemical digestion
    B. Mechanical digestion
    C. Motility
    D. Ingestion

8. The successful fertilization of an egg is dependent on sexual intercourse occurring within a window of 24 hours before ovulation, and no more than _____ after.

    A. 48 hours
    B. 3–4 days
    C. 24 hours
    D. 1 week

9. What is the name of the indentation along the medial border of each kidney where the ureters, blood vessels, and nerves enter and exit the organ?

    A. Hilus
    B. Medial indentation
    C. Renal neurovasal fossa
    D. Renal–ureter junction

10. What simultaneous action occurs when the micturition reflex signals the internal urethral sphincter to relax?

    A. The external urethral sphincter is also relaxed.
    B. A motor signal is sent to the muscles in the pelvic floor to relax.
    C. A motor signal is sent to the external urethral sphincter to contract.
    D. Smooth muscles in the bladder and prostate of males are signaled to contract.

11. What hormone produced by the kidneys plays a vital role in calcium absorption as the active form of vitamin D?

    A. Calcitonin
    B. Erythropoietin
    C. Precursor D
    D. Calcitriol

12. The six individual processes of the digestive system are ingestion, digestion, motility, elimination, _____, and _____.

    A. energy storage and defecation
    B. secretion and absorption
    C. anabolism and micturition
    D. segmentation and peristalsis

13. What is the difference between digestion and metabolism?

    A. Digestion is carried out by organs in the GI tract, and metabolism by the accessory organs.
    B. Digestion is breaking down food into usable components, and metabolism is the use of these.
    C. Metabolism is the chemical processing of food, and digestion is the mechanical processing.
    D. Proteins and fats are digested, and carbohydrates are metabolized.

14. Oxyhemaglobin is formed during what respiratory system process?

    A. External respiration
    B. Internal respiration
    C. Ventilation
    D. Pulmonary absorption

15. The two primary nerves for muscles of ventilation are the phrenic and

    A. vagus.
    B. splenic.
    C. intercostal.
    D. abdominal oblique.

16. In males, the fluids that provide nourishment to sperm and assist its movement through the duct system are produced and secreted by the bulbourethral glands, _____ and _____.

    A. urethral lining and Leydig cells
    B. epididymis and prostate.
    C. vas deferens and epididymis.
    D. seminal vesicles and prostate.

17. What is the function of progesterone?

    A. Building and maintaining the uterine lining
    B. Production of female gametes
    C. Development of secondary gender characteristics in females
    D. Signaling the release of ova from the ovaries

18. In the male reproductive system, where are the Leydig cells that produce testosterone located?

    A. Epididymis
    B. Vas deferens
    C. Seminiferous tubules
    D. Prostate

19. The proper sequence for the kidney's physiologic processing of blood to form urine is

    A. secretion, absorption, filtration, and excretion.
    B. secretion, excretion, and filtration.
    C. filtration, resorption, secretion, and excretion.
    D. filtration, diffusion, osmosis, and excretion.

20. What structure in the digestive system functions to insulate and cushion the abdominopelvic cavity?

    A. Greater omentum
    B. Lesser omentum
    C. Mesenteric peritoneum
    D. Visceral peritoneum

21. Which of these organs is an accessory digestive organ?

    A. Esophagus
    B. Salivary glands
    C. Small intestines
    D. Colon

22. Which of these skeletal muscles are considered the primary muscles of ventilation?

    A. Sternocleidomastoid and scalenes
    B. Diaphragm and intercostals
    C. Intercostals and abdominal obliques
    D. Diaphragm and serratus anterior

23. What is the anatomic term for the respiratory process that is the exchange of gases between the lungs and blood?

    A. Inhalation
    B. Exhalation
    C. External respiration
    D. Internal respiration

24. What is the anatomic name for the lining of the uterus?

    A. Intrauterine mucosal layer
    B. Reproductive membrane
    C. Endoperitonium
    D. Endometrium

25. The functions of the liver include filtration and detoxification of blood, storage of glycogen, conversion of ammonia to urea, storage of fat soluble vitamins and minerals, and

    A. destruction of old RBCs, plus production and secretion of bile.
    B. secretion of bile, plus absorption of amino acids.
    C. secretion of proteases for protein digestion, plus production of bilirubin.
    D. production of hemoglobin, plus storage of bile.

26. Which organ secretes the digestive enzymes amylase, lipase, and trypsin?

    A. Stomach
    B. Small intestine
    C. Liver
    D. Pancreas

27. What are the functions of the large intestine?

    A. Completion of protein digestion and absorption of amino acids
    B. Secretion of bicarbonates and absorption of water
    C. Absorption of water and elimination
    D. Segmentation and elimination

28. Which of these is the best description of the respiratory mucosa?
    A. The membrane that covers the lungs and lines the thoracic cavity
    B. The highly vascular membrane that lines the upper and lower respiratory tracts
    C. The combination of capillary and alveolar walls through which gases are exchanged
    D. The fluid-producing membrane between the visceral and parietal layers of pleura

29. When the pulmonary stretch receptors are activated, they send a signal to the brain that does what?
    A. Inhibits the inspiration areas of the brain
    B. Contracts the lungs for exhalation
    C. Speeds up the ventilation rate
    D. Alters the rhythm and depth of breathing

30. Which of these exert the strongest influence over the respiratory centers of the brainstem?
    A. Pulmonary stretch receptors
    B. Phrenic nerve
    C. Chemoreceptors
    D. Vagus nerve

31. How are amino acids most often used in the digestive system?
    A. To emulsify fats in the small intestine
    B. Production of hormones, enzymes, and plasma proteins
    C. In anabolic processes like repairing tissue and forming ligands
    D. Stored in the liver as glycogen

32. Which digestive organ carries out segmentation, peristalsis, and absorption?
    A. Stomach
    B. Esophagus
    C. Large intestine
    D. Small intestine

33. What is the name for the tube that carries urine from the kidneys to the bladder?
    A. Urethra
    B. Ureter
    C. Upper urinary tract
    D. Perirenal tubule

34. What portion of the nephron carries out filtration of blood?
    A. Proximal tubule
    B. Renal corpuscle
    C. Distal tubule
    D. Loop of Henle

35. In which step of nephron processing does hydrogen, potassium, ammonia, and urea get removed from blood?
    A. Filtration
    B. Reabsorption
    C. Secretion
    D. Excretion

Answer Key

CHAPTER 1

EXERCISE 1 • Key Terminology Crossword

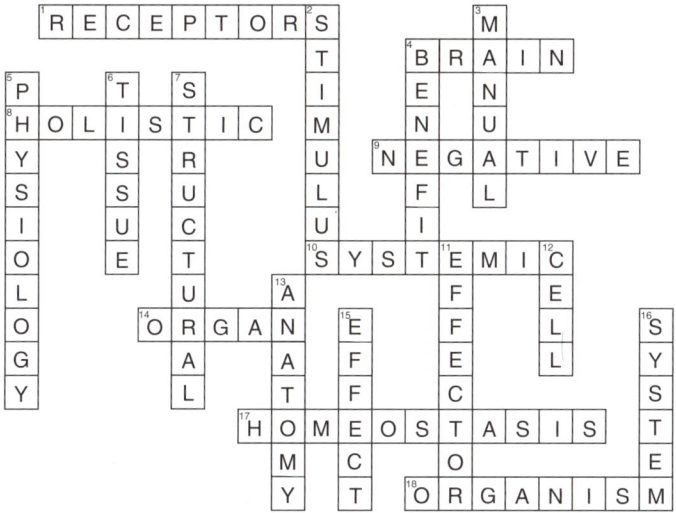

EXERCISE 2 • Levels of Organization

1. Organism or Whole body
2. System = a group of organs working together
3. Organ = a group of tissues working together
4. Tissue = a group of like cells working together
5. Cell = basic building block of life; smallest functional unit of the body

EXERCISE 4 • Homeostasis Flow Chart

Integration center (bow tie shape) receives input from receptor, interprets information, and passes command to the effector

Stimulus (sun burst shape) change in the environment

Effector (rectangle) cells, tissue, or organs that respond to change

Receptor (oval) sense organ sensitive to specific type of stimulus

EXERCISE 5 • Charting Negative and Positive Feedback

1. Counteracts or reverses
2. Reinforces or sustains
3. Increased urination
4. Increased heart rate and blood pressure
5. Negative
6. Low level of calcium in blood

EXERCISE 6 • Linking Body, Mind, and Spirit

Following are just examples. Your answers should reflect your own ideas, thoughts, and feelings.

TENSE:
Body: tight and head aches
Mind: scattered but alert
Spirit: uptight and constricted

FEAR:
Body: uptight and on alert
Mind: worried and concerned
Spirit: nervous and suspicious

JOY:
Body: loose and energetic
Mind: alert and creative
Spirit: happy and content

EXERCISE 7 • Benefits and Effects of Manual Therapy

1. B
2. E — STRUCTURAL
3. E — SYSTEMIC
4. B
5. E — SYSTEMIC
6. B
7. B
8. E — STRUCTURAL
9. E — STRUCTURAL
10. E — SYSTEMIC

EXERCISE 8 • Manual Therapy Categories

1. Sliding/gliding style of work that uses a lubricant for a full-body session
2 & 3. Traditional massage, Wellness/health maintenance massage
4. Loosening
5. Broadening
6–8. Improve structural alignment; improve range of motion (ROM); decrease pain
9–12. Any four of the following: Active Release Technique (ART™), Aston Patterning®, Cranio-sacral, Hellerwork®, Joint mobilization, Myofascial Release (MFR), Rolfing®, Soft tissue release (STR), or Structural integration
13. Neuromuscular
14 & 15. Decrease pain; loosen myofascial components
16–18. Any three of the following: Myotherapy, Neurokinetics, Neuromuscular Technique (NMT), Positional release, Proprioceptive Neuromuscular Facilitation (PNF), Strain Counterstrain®, Tender point or Trigger point
19. Lymph flow
20 & 21. Any two of the following: Lymphatic massage, Lymphatic facilitation, Lymphatic techniques, Lymphedema techniques, or Manual Lymphatic Drainage (MLD)®
22. Movement Therapies
23–25. Any three of the following: Achieve pain-free movement; general relaxation and body awareness; decrease muscle tension; or release holding patterns (emotional or physical)
26–28. Any three of the following: Feldenkrais®, Hakomi, Qi gong, Rosenwork, Tai Chi, or Trager®
29. The use of light or deep pressure to stimulate defined energy zones, dermatomes, or points
30 & 31. Any two of the following: Bindegewebs (CTM), Reflexology, Shiatsu, or Therapeutic Touch®
32. Energy Techniques
33. Decongest
34. Balance
35 & 36. Any two of the following: Polarity®, Qi Gong, Reiki®, or Therapeutic Touch®

EXERCISE 9 • Creating a Body Systems Table

Remember, your answers do not need to be exactly the same as the ones offered here.

1. Protective outer covering; sensory organ; regulation of body temperature
2. Bone, cartilage, and joints
3. Bone landmarks for postural assessment; structural effects on the joint receptors and connective tissues
4. Skeletal muscle and tendon
5. Maintain posture; create movement; generation of heat
6. Brain, spinal cord, nerves, special and general sensory receptors
7. Mediates benefits and physiologic effects of manual therapy
8. Hypothalamus, pituitary, thyroid, parathyroids, thymus, adrenals, pancreas, gonads
9. Benefits such as stress reduction, improved mental focus, and restorative sleep involve changes in endocrine function
10. Transportation of nutrients, wastes, and hormones
11. Manual therapies can improve local blood flow and decrease blood pressure
12. Tonsils, thymus, spleen, white blood cells, lymph nodes, and vessels
13. Fluid and protein return; resistance to disease
14. Regulation and exchange of oxygen and carbon dioxide; vocalization
15. Manual therapies can improve the efficiency and ease of breathing
16. Mouth, salivary glands, esophagus, stomach, small and large intestines, anus, liver, gall bladder, pancreas
17. Break down of food; absorption of nutrients; elimination of solid waste
18. Kidneys, ureters, bladder, and urethra
19. Female: ovaries, fallopian tubes, uterus, vagina, and vulva. Male: testes, seminal vesicles, vas deferens, prostate, penis
20. Manual therapies can impact fertility and the reproductive cycle. They can also be used to support women during pregnancy, labor, and childbirth.

EXERCISE 10 • Body Systems Anatomy Mind Map

Integumentary: skin, glands, hair, nails, sensory receptors

Nervous: brain, spinal cord, nerves, special sensory receptors, general sensory receptors

Endocrine: thyroid, thymus, gonads, parathyroids, adrenals, pancreas, pituitary, hypothalamus

Reproductive: vulva, uterus, vagina, penis, prostate, tubes, gonads

Urinary: kidneys, ureters, bladder, urethra

Digestive: pancreas, anus, liver, stomach, intestines, esophagus, mouth, gall bladder

Respiratory: bronchi, lungs, trachea, nose, sinuses

Cardiovascular: blood vessels, heart, blood

Lymphatic: lymph nodes, white blood cells, thymus, tonsils, spleen, lymphatic vessels

Skeletal muscular: muscle, tendon

Skeletal: bone, joints, cartilage

EXERCISE 11 • Body Systems Physiology Mind Map

Integumentary: protection, covering, sensory, regulation of body temperature

Nervous: coordination, communication, control

Endocrine: coordination, communication, control

Reproductive: reproduction

Urinary: cleanse blood, eliminate waste

Digestive: absorb nutrients, eliminate solid wastes, break down food into useable nutrients

Respiratory: oxygen and carbon dioxide exchange

Cardiovascular: transportation

Lymphatic: resistance to disease, fluid and protein return

Skeletal muscular: heat, movement, posture

Skeletal: structure, protection, levers, blood cell production, mineral storage

CHAPTER 2

EXERCISE 2 • Planes of the Body

1. Frontal or coronal
2. Sagittal or median
3. Transverse or horizontal
4. Frontal or coronal
5. Transverse or horizontal
6. Sagittal or median

EXERCISE 3 • Location and Movement Terms Crossword

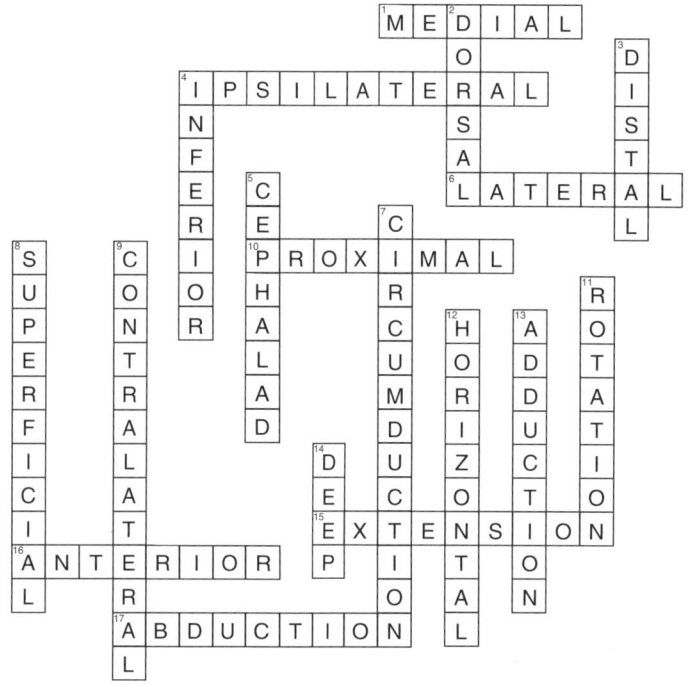

EXERCISE 4 • Mix-and-Match Word Parts

1. C
2. D
3. H
4. G
5. A
6. I
7. J
8. B
9. F
10. E

EXERCISE 5 • Body Cavities Color and Label

1. Cranial
2. Spinal
3. Thoracic
4. Abdominopelvic
5. Diaphragm
6. Abdominal
7. Pelvic

EXERCISE 6 • Body Regions Matching

1. J
2. D
3. G
4. K
5. B
6. M
7. A
8. N
9. E
10. F
11. H
12. Q
13. T
14. C
15. S
16. I
17. L
18. O
19. P
20. R

EXERCISE 7 • Body Regions Labeling

1. Frontal
2. Orbital
3. Sternal
4. Pectoral
5. Brachial
6. Antecubital
7. Antebrachial
8. Digital
9. Inguinal
10. Patellar
11. Tarsal
12. Acromial
13. Cervical
14. Scapular
15. Vertebral or spinal
16. Sacral
17. Popliteal
18. Sural
19. Calcaneal
20. Plantar

EXERCISE 8 • Abdominal Regions Labeling

1. Right hypochondriac
2. Epigastric
3. Left hypochondriac
4. Right lumbar
5. Umbilical
6. Left lumbar
7. Right iliac
8. Hypogastric
9. Left iliac

EXERCISE 9 • Pathology Terms Case Study

1. Etiology is infected tonsils.
2. Diagnosis is tonsillitis.
3. Symptoms include headache; feeling tired and generally run down; a throat that feels scratchy and swollen; painful swallowing; trouble sleeping.
4. Signs include swollen lymph nodes in his neck, a fever of 102°, as well as red and pus-marked tonsils causing severe sore throat.
5. Prognosis is for a complete recovery within 2 or 3 days after surgery with a prescription of antibiotics.

EXERCISE 10 • Classes of Disease Table

1. Disease caused by a specific pathogen such as a bacteria, virus, fungus, or parasite, which creates a physiologic disruption.
2. Examples include the common cold, influenza, tuberculosis, malaria, dysentery, tape worms, lice, and many more.
3. Environmental.
4. Disease caused by exposure to harmful substances in surroundings.
5. Hereditary.
6. Examples include hemophilia, sickle cell anemia, Down syndrome, polycystic kidney disease, muscular dystrophy, and many more.
7. Disease related to poor nutrition or unhealthy lifestyle.
8. Examples include scurvy, anemia, type 2 diabetes, osteoporosis, atherosclerosis, and some types of cancer.

EXERCISE 11 • A&P Terminology Crossword

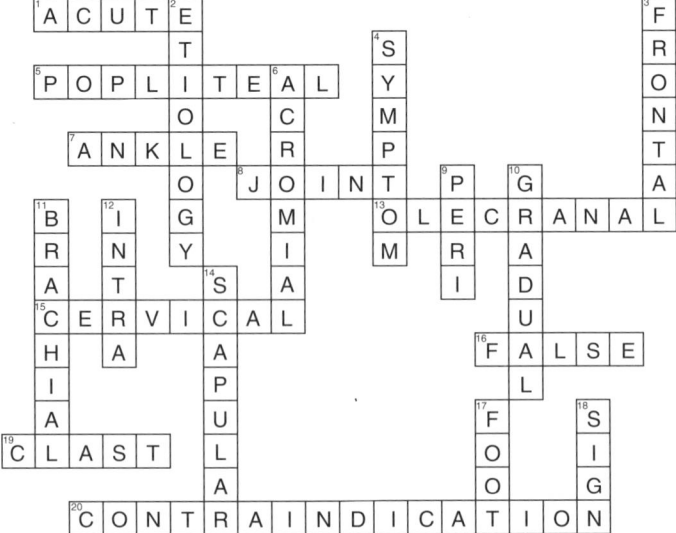

CHAPTER 3

EXERCISE 1 • Chemistry Crossword

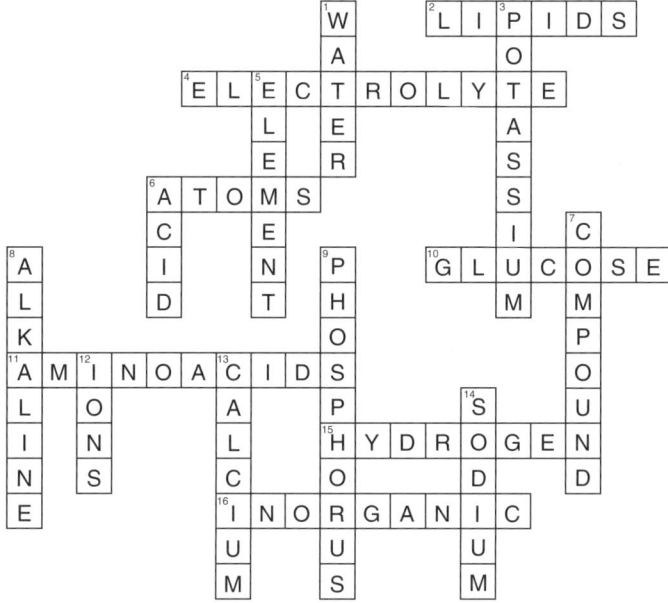

EXERCISE 2 • Cellular Components Flow Chart

1. Plasma membrane
2. Phospholipid
3. Cytoplasm
4. Nucleus
5. Genetic blueprint
6. IMPs
7. Cytosol
8. Water
9. Organic compounds
10. Organelles
11. Nuclear envelope
12. Nucleolus
13. DNA
14. Genes
15. Receptor proteins
16. Effector proteins
17–19. Channel proteins, transport proteins, linker proteins
20–25. Mitochondria, lysosomes, Golgi apparatus, vesicle, cytoskeleton, centrosome
26. Endoplasmic reticulum
27. Ribosomes

EXERCISE 3 • Color and Label a Cell

1. Ribosome
2. Rough ER
3. Smooth ER
4. Cytoskeleton
5. Centrosome
6. Protein
7. Lysosome
8. Mitochondrion
9. Plasma membrane
10. Cytosol
11. Golgi apparatus
12. Nuclear envelope
13. Nucleolus
14. Nucleus

EXERCISE 4 • A Cell Analogy

1. Plasma membrane
2. Nucleus
3. DNA
4. Mitochondria
5. Ribosomes
6. Golgi apparatus
7. Lysosomes
8. Endoplasmic reticulum
9. Rough
10. Smooth

EXERCISE 5 • Cellular Transport

1. Intracellular fluid
2. Extracellular fluid
3. Interstitial fluid
4. Passive
5. Active
A. Diffusion
B. Osmosis
C. Phagocytosis

EXERCISE 6 • Cellular Processes Matching

1. D
2. I
3. F
4. L
5. A
6. N
7. B
8. H
9. O
10. C
11. K
12. M
13. G
14. E
15. J

CHAPTER 4

EXERCISE 1 • Terminology Crossword

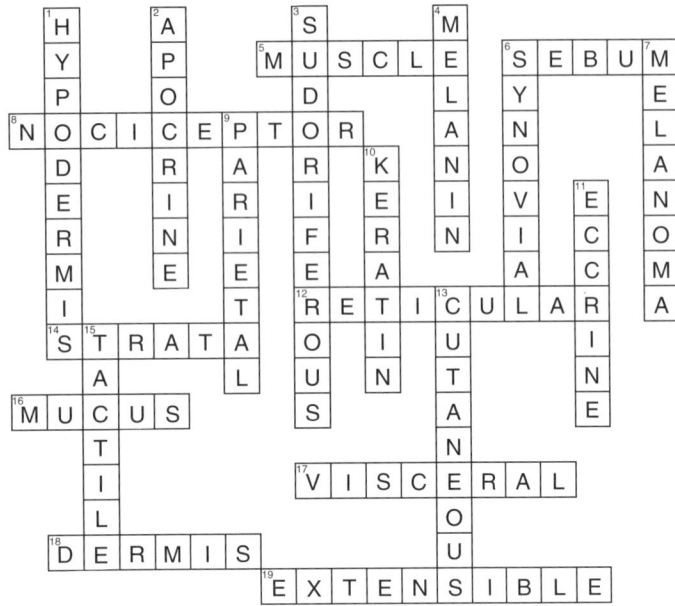

EXERCISE 2 • Membranes Organizational Chart

1. A broad flat sheet of at least two layers of tissue
2. Connective tissue membranes
3. Epithelial membranes
4. Synovial membranes; structure—thick fibrous connective tissue layer with a thin internal layer of simple epithelium; function—line synovial joint cavities and secrete synovial fluid; examples—knee, ankle, elbow, shoulder, hip
5. Mucous membranes; structure—simple columnar epithelium attached to a thin basement membrane; function—line cavities with openings to the external environment and secrete mucus; examples—lining respiratory, digestive, urinary, and reproductive tracts
6. Serous membranes; structure—thin simple epithelial layer attached to a basement membrane. Fold into two layers; parietal and visceral layers; function—parietal layer lines cavities without openings to the external environment and visceral layer covers internal organs; examples—pleura in the thoracic cavity, peritoneum of the abdominopelvic cavity
7. Cutaneous membrane; structure—epidermis and dermis; function—protection, temperature regulation, excretion, absorption, general sensory organ, and synthesis of vitamin D; example—the skin

EXERCISE 3 • Functional Mnemonic

The mnemonic will differ; however, here is a summary of the functions:

Protection—Serves as a physical barrier to pathogens and contaminants.

Temperature regulation—Sweat helps to cool us and the hypodermis insulates to help us retain body heat.

Excretion—Sweating eliminates trace amounts of metabolic waste products.

Absorption—Pores allow oils, herbal extracts, or medications to be absorbed.

General sensory organ—Numerous cutaneous receptors collect information about what is happening to the surface of the body.

Synthesis of vitamin D—Ultraviolet light absorbed by the skin stimulates the synthesis of vitamin D.

EXERCISE 4 • Label and Color the Skin Diagram

1. Epidermis
2. Dermis
3. Hypodermis
4. Hair shaft
5. Hair root
6. Sebaceous gland
7. Arrector pili muscle
8. Hair follicle
9. Apocrine sweat gland
10. Blood vessels
11. Fat/adipose tissue
12. Sensory receptors
13. Nerve
14. Pore
15. Eccrine sweat gland

EXERCISE 6 • Matching Structures and Functions

1. E
2. I
3. D
4. L
5. C
6. H
7. M
8. B
9. K
10. F
11. N
12. G
13. J
14. O
15. A

EXERCISE 7 • Pathology Mind Map

1-4. Fungal infections, Bacterial infections, Viral infections, Parasitic infections

5-9. Acne, Eczema, Hives, Psoriasis, Vitiligo

CHAPTER 5

EXERCISE 1 • Bony Terms Crossword

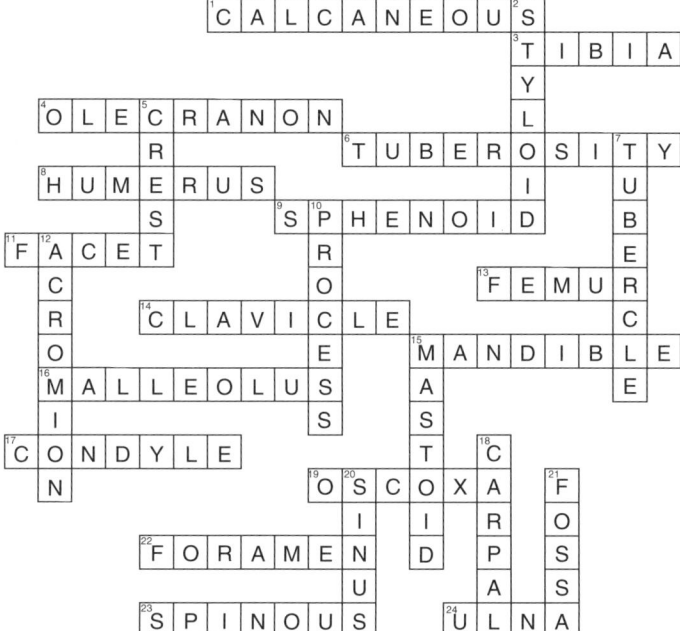

EXERCISE 3 • Label the Skeleton

1. Cranium
2. Facial bones
3. Hyoid
4. Clavicle
5. Scapula
6. Sternum
7. Ribs (costal bones)
8. Humerus
9. Radius
10. Ulna
11. Carpals
12. Metacarpals
13. Phalanges
14. Femur
15. Patella
16. Tibia
17. Fibula
18. Tarsals
19. Metatarsals
20. Phalanges
21. Ilium
22. Pubic
23. Ischium
24. Vertebra
25. Sacrum
26. Coccyx
27. Coxal bone

EXERCISE 4 • Draw Me a Bone

Short bone—carpals and tarsals
Long bones—humerus, radius, ulna, femur, tibia, fibula
Flat bones—cranial bones, mandible, ribs, sternum
Irregular—scapula, vertebra, pelvic bones

EXERCISE 5 • Parts of a Long Bone

Matching portion:

1. C
2. I
3. F
4. A
5. K
6. E
7. J
8. B
9. L
10. H
11. D
12. G

Labeling portion:

1. Epiphysis
2. Metaphysis
3. Diaphysis
4. Articular cartilage (hyaline)
5. Red marrow
6. Epiphyseal line
7. Spongy bone
8. Endosteum
9. Medullary cavity
10. Yellow marrow
11. Compact bone
12. Periosteum

EXERCISE 6 • Build a Long Bone

1. Diaphysis
2. Medullary cavity
3. Yellow bone marrow
4. Epiphyses
5. Red bone marrow
6. Articular cartilage
7. Periosteum

EXERCISE 7 • Skeletal Landmarks Labeling

1. H
2. N
3. K
4. A
5. F
6. O
7. L
8. E
9. C
10. D
11. B
12. M
13. G
14. I
15. J
16. P
17. S
18. T
19. Q
20. R

EXERCISE 8 • Color and Label a Synovial Joint

1. Synovial membrane
2. Ligament
3. Joint capsule
4. Menisci
5. Bursa
6. Articular cartilage
7. Synovial fluid in the synovial space

EXERCISE 9 • Diarthrotic Joint Movements

1. Pivot
2. Rotation
3. Ball and socket
4. Flexion, extension, ABduction, adduction, rotation, circumduction
5. Pivot
6. Rotation
7. Hinge
8. Flexion, extension
9. Condyloid
10. Flexion, extension, ABduction, adduction
11. Saddle
12. Flexion, extension, ABduction, adduction
13. Condyloid
14. Flexion, extension, ABduction, adduction
15. Hinge
16. Flexion, extension
17. Ball and socket
18. Flexion, extension, ABduction, adduction, rotation, circumduction
19. Hinge
20. Flexion, extension
21. Hinge
22. Dorsiflexion, plantar flexion
23. Gliding
24. Sliding, shifting for inversion, eversion

EXERCISE 10 • Joint Crossword

Across/Down answers: GLENOHUMERAL, CIRCUMDUCTION, STERNOCLAVICULAR, CONDYLOID, PIVOT, RETRACTION, SADDLE, PLANTARFLEXION, TEMPOROMANDIBULAR, SYNARTHROSIS, SUPINATION, ANKLE

GROUP ACTIVITY 1 • Quiz Show

Level 1	Dem Bones	Tissue? I Hardly Know You!	Joint Classification	Landmark Terminology	Specific Landmarks
100	What is the patella?	What is dense/hard or cortical bone?	What is an amphiarthrosis?	What is a foramen?	What is the ischial tuberosity?
200	What is a long bone?	What is yellow marrow or fat/adipose?	What are fibrous joints?	What is a shallow dish-like depression?	What is the mastoid process?
300	What are the parietal bones?	What is spongy bone?	What is a pivot joint?	What is a tuberosity?	What is the base?
400	What are the cuneiforms?	What are trabeculae?	What is a ball and socket joint?	What is a crest or ridge?	What is the linea aspera?
500	What is the mandible?	What is cortical bone?	What is the first carpometacarpal joint?	What is a fovea?	What is the medial femoral epicondyle?

Level 2	More Landmarks	Synovial Joint Structures	Special Movements	Common Names	What's Wrong?
200	What is the radial notch?	What is the joint capsule?	What is supination?	What is the shoulder?	What is osteoporosis?
400	What is the coracoid process?	What is the synovial membrane?	What is horizontal ABduction?	What is the knee?	What is osteoarthritis (OA)?
600	What is the tibial plateau?	What is a ligament?	What is elevation?	What is the elbow?	What is rheumatoid arthritis (RA)?
800	What are the malleoli?	What is articular or hyaline cartilage?	What is inversion?	What is the hip?	What is gout?
1000	What is the temporal styloid process?	What is a bursa?	What is plantar flexion?	What is the ankle?	What is scoliosis?

CHAPTER 6

EXERCISE 1 • Muscle Terminology Crossword

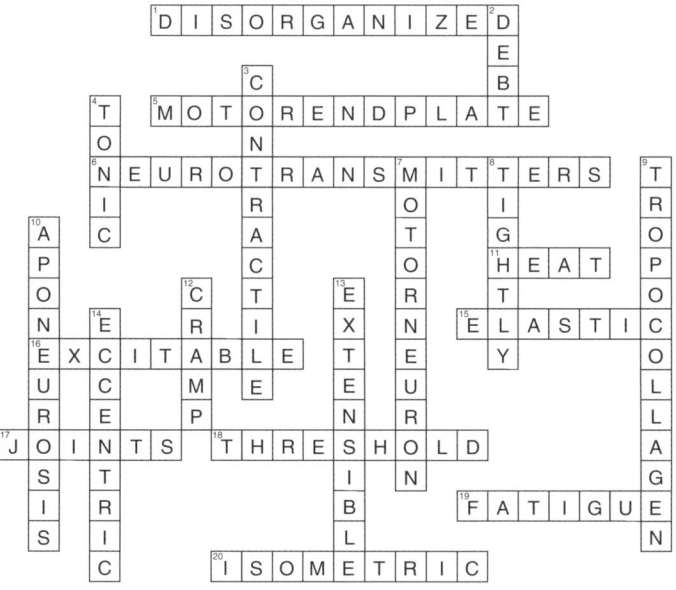

EXERCISE 2 • Major Parts of a Skeletal Muscle

1. Bone
2. Tendon
3. Tenoperiosteal junction
4. Musculotendinous junction
5. Epimysium
6. perimysium
7. Fascicle
8. Endomysium
9. Fiber (muscle cell)
10. Sarcolemma

EXERCISE 3 • Comparing Fascia and Tendons

There are many possible answers for this exercise. Some examples include the ones listed in the chart below:

Fascia characteristics	Shared characteristics	Tendon characteristics
Disorganized fibers	Comprised of fibrous connective tissue	Organized fibers
More ground substance	Component of skeletal muscles	Little ground substance
Includes lots of elastic and reticular fibers	Focus and transfer muscle contraction to bone	Thickly packed collagen fibers

EXERCISE 4 • Skeletal Muscle Fiber Organization

Matching:

1. F
2. D
3. J
4. A
5. K
6. E
7. I
8. B
9. L
10. H
11. C
12. G

Labeling:

1. Sarcomere
2. Myosin
3. Actin
4. Z lines
5. A band
6. I bands
7. Myofilaments (actin and myosin)
8. Myofibril
9. Mitochondrion
10. Nucleus
11. Sarcoplasmic reticulum
12. Sarcolemma

EXERCISE 5 • Skeletal Muscle Contraction

1. Sliding filament mechanism
2. Sarcomeres
3. Motor unit
4. Motor neuron
5. Fibers
6. Neuromuscular junction
7. Neurotransmitters
8. Motor neuron
9. Motor end plates
10. Threshold stimulus
11. All-or-none response
12. Threshold
13. All
14. None

15–16. Graded response; motor unit recruitment

17. Calcium
18. Sarcoplasmic reticulum
19. Actin filaments
20. Myosin heads
21. Pull the two myofilaments across one another
22. Myosin heads
23. Continued sliding of the filaments across one another
24. Calcium
25. Sarcoplasmic reticulum

EXERCISE 6 • Picturing Energy for Muscle Contraction

1. Creatine phosphate
2. ADP
3. ATP
4. Creatine
5. Glucose
6. 2 ATP
7. Lactic acid
8. Anaerobic
9. Pyruvic acid
10. Krebs
11. 30–32 ATP

12–14. H_2O, CO_2, and heat

15. Aerobic

EXERCISE 7 • Organizing Methods of ATP Production

1. Direct phosphorylation
2. ATP + creatine
3. Glucose is converted into pyruvic acid to release ATP
4. No, anaerobic process
5. Aerobic cellular metabolism or Krebs cycle
6. Pyruvic acid is converted into H_2O and CO_2 releasing heat and providing ATP (can also convert fatty acids and amino acids into energy)
7. H_2O, CO_2, and heat plus lots of ATP

EXERCISE 8 • Types of Fiber Arrangements

Specific muscle examples may differ. Check with your instructor.

1. Infrahyoids, rectus abdominis
2. Fusiform
3. Circular
4. Pectoralis major, latissimus dorsi
5. Extensor digitorum longus, peroneus longus
6. Bipennate
7. Multipennate

EXERCISE 9 • Muscle Assignments

Agonist—This muscle is generally the largest and the strongest or has the best angle of pull across a joint to its attachment point; the prime mover.

Antagonist—A muscle that opposes the agonist.

Synergist—A muscle that helps or assists the prime mover.

Stabilizer—A muscle that stabilizes the prime mover's bone of origin to make the movement created by the agonist more efficient.

Answers for the table may differ. If you have questions or your answer does not appear below, check with your fellow classmates or instructor.

1. Biceps femoris, semimembranosus, or semitendinosus
2. Vastus medialis, vastus intermedius, or vastus lateralis

3. Biceps femoris
4. Rectus femoris, vastus medialis, vastus intermedius, or vastus lateralis
5. Latissimus dorsi or posterior deltoid
6. Pectoralis major, coracobrachialis, or anterior deltoid
7. Latissimus dorsi, teres major, or posterior deltoid
8. Depending on specific answer to No. 6, could be pectoralis major, coracobrachialis, anterior deltoid, or biceps brachii
9. Deltoid
10. Pectoralis major, coracobrachialis, latissimus dorsi, or teres major
11. Deltoid
12. Coracobrachialis, latissimus dorsi, or teres major
13. Infraspinatus, teres minor, posterior deltoid
14. Subscapularis, pectoralis major, latissimus dorsi, teres major, or anterior deltoid
15. Teres minor, posterior deltoid

EXERCISE 10 • Naming Muscles

While your specific muscle examples may differ, the naming themes and some examples include

Shape—Deltoid, rhomboids, quadratus lumborum

Function—Supinator, pronator teres, extensor digitorum, flexor digitorum, flexor hallucis

Fiber direction—Rectus abdominis, external obliques, internal obliques, transverse abdominis

General location—Tibialis anterior, tibialis posterior, brachialis

Origin or insertion—Sternocleidomastoid, coracobrachialis, palmaris longus, brachoradialis

Number of origins—Biceps brachii, triceps brachii, biceps femoris

EXERCISE 11 • Locating Major Muscles

Anterior view:
1. Temporalis
2. Orbicularis oculi
3. Masseter
4. Sternocleidomastoid
5. Trapezius
6. Deltoid
7. Pectoralis major
8. Serratus anterior
9. Biceps brachii
10. Brachialis
11. Brachioradialis
12. Flexor carpi radialis
13. Palmaris longus
14. Peroneus longus
15. Tibialis anterior
16. Vastus medialis
17. Rectus femoris
18. Vastus lateralis
19. Gracilis
20. Sartorius
21. Adductor longus
22. Pectineus
23. Iliopsoas
24. Tensor fascia latae
25. Extensor digitorum superficialis
26. Extensor carpi radialis
27. External obliques
28. Rectus abdominis
29. Internal obliques
30. Orbicularis oris
31. Zygomaticus
32. Frontalis

Posterior view:
1. Temporalis
2. Masseter
3. Infraspinatus
4. Teres minor
5. Teres major
6. Latissimus dorsi
7. External obliques
8. Flexor carpi ulnaris
9. Extensor carpi ulnaris
10. Gluteus medius
11. Gluteus maximus
12. Adductor magnus
13. Iliotibial tract or band
14. Gracilis
15. Gastrocnemius
16. Peroneus longus
17. Soleus
18. Soleus
19. Semimembranosus
20. Semitendinosus
21. Biceps femoris
22. Flexor carpi ulnaris
23. Extensor carpi ulnaris
24. Extensor digitorum superficialis
25. Extensor carpi radialis
26. Brachioradialis
27. Triceps brachii
28. Deltoid
29. Trapezius
30. Occipitalis

GROUP ACTIVITY 1 • Quiz Show

Level 1	Functions and Junctions	Let's Get Connected	Under the Microscope	Movement Roles	Prime Functions
100	What is movement?	What is disorganized?	What is the sarcolemma?	What is the agonist or prime mover?	What is the biceps brachii?
200	What is posture?	What is a tendon?	What is the sarcoplasmic reticulum?	What are synergists?	What is wrist flexion?
300	What is heat?	What is the perimysium?	What is myosin?	What are antagonists?	What is plantar flexion?
400	What is the musculotendinous junction?	What is tropocollagen?	What is the Z line?	What are fixators or stabilizers?	What is the deltoid?
500	What is the tenoperiosteal junction?	What is an aponeurosis?	What is the A band?	What is an eccentric contraction?	What is the iliopsoas?

Level 2	Not all Contractions Are the same	Origins	Insertions	Muscle Groups	I Am What I Do
200	What is an isometric contraction?	What is the sternocleido-mastoid?	What is the Achilles tendon?	What is 5?	What is the tibialis anterior?
400	What is an isotonic contraction?	What is the coracoid?	What is the tibial tuberosity?	What are the hamstrings?	What is the gracilis?
600	What is a twitch?	What is the ischial tuberosity?	What is the IT tract or band?	What is the erector spinae group?	What is the subscapularis?
800	What are tonic contractions?	What is the lateral humeral epicondyle?	What is the greater tubercle of the humerus?	What is the transverse abdominis?	What is the rectus femoris?
1000	What is motor tone?	What is the common origin of the wrist flexors?	What is the olecranon of the ulna?	What is the deepest group of the paraspinals?	What is the external obliques?

CHAPTER 7

EXERCISE 1 • Nervous System Crossword

(Crossword solution with answers including: MEDULLA OBLONGATA, VAGUS, PIA MATER, SCIENCE, DURA MATER, CERVICAL, LUMBAR, BASAL GANGLIA, BLOOD BRAIN BARRIER, MYOTOME, ARACHNOID, CEREBROSPINAL, FACIAL, etc.)

EXERCISE 2 • Functional Organization of the Nervous System

1. Central nervous system (green)
2. Peripheral nervous system (blue and red)
3. Spinal cord (green)
4–7. Cerebrum, Diencephalon, Brain Stem, Cerebellum (green)
8. Somatic division (blue and red)
9. Sympathetic division (red)
10. Parasympathetic division (red)

EXERCISE 3 • Neuroglia Mind Map

1. Microglia (green)
2. Satellite cells (purple)
3. Oligodendrocytes (green)
4–5. Maintenance of chemical environment for impulse conduction, scar tissue formation
6. Form CSF
7. Make and maintain myelin in the PNS

Astrocytes and ependymal cells (green)
Schwann cells (purple)

EXERCISE 4 • Neurons: Matching Parts

Diagram:
1. Dendrites
2. Cell body
3. Nucleus
4. Axon hillock
5. Axon
6. Myelin
7. Axon terminal with synaptic bulb

Matching:
1. D
2. J
3. A
4. N
5. G
6. E
7. L
8. B
9. O
10. C
11. M
12. K
13. H
14. F
15. I

EXERCISE 5 • Structure of a Nerve

12 pairs of cranial nerves
31 pairs of spinal nerves

Diagram:
1. Epineurium
2. Fascicle
3. Perineurium
4. Nerve fibers (axons)
5. Endoneurium
6. Schwann cells
7. Myelin
8. Axon
9. Artery and vein (blood vessels)

EXERCISE 7 • Diagram a Reflex Arc

1. Motor outcome or response
2. Sensory stimulus
3. Deep tendon
4. Withdrawal
5. Spinal cord (green)
6. Sensory receptors (stretch receptors in skeletal muscle) (blue)
7. Sensory neuron (blue)

8. Sensory receptors (pain receptors in skin) (blue)
9. Sensory neuron (blue)
10. Synapse (green)
11. Interneuron (green)
12. Motor neuron (red)
13. Skeletal muscle effector or quadriceps (red)
14. Skeletal muscle effector or biceps (red)

EXERCISE 8 • Sensory Receptors Table

1. Photoreceptors
2. Retina of the eye
3. Tissue damage (pain)
4. Skin, joint capsules, fascia, periosteum, walls of blood vessels
5. Proprioceptors
6. Movement, muscle tension, and length of muscles
7. Touch, pressure, and movement stimulus such as stretch, compression, and torsion
8. Skin, hollow organs, cochlea, and bony labyrinth of the ear
9. Chemoreceptors
10. Nose, tongue, and blood vessels
11. Temperature changes
12. Skin

EXERCISE 9 • Meninges Diagram

1. Dura mater
2. Arachnoid mater
3. Subarachnoid space
4. Arachnoid villus
5. Pia mater

EXERCISE 10 • Nervous Terminology: Reviewing Synonyms

1. Afferent
2. Motor
3. Ascending tracts. Synonyms include sensory, afferent, posterior, and dorsal
4. Descending tracts. Synonyms include motor, efferent, afferent, and ventral
5. Dorsal root. Synonyms include sensory, afferent, and posterior
6. Ventral root. Synonyms include motor, efferent, and anterior

EXERCISE 11 • Spinal Cord Gray Matter Organization

1. Posterior
2. Lateral
3. Anterior
4. Somatic sensory
5. Visceral sensory
6. Visceral motor
7. Somatic motor

EXERCISE 12 • Matching Brain Parts and Their Functions

1. Cerebrum, G
2. Corpus callosum, C
3. Thalamus, A
4. Hypothalamus, F
5. Pituitary gland, D
6. Pineal gland, K
7. Midbrain, I
8. Pons, H
9. Medulla oblongata, B
10. Reticular formation, J
11. Cerebellum, E

EXERCISE 13 • Cerebral Structures

Fill in the blank:
1. Gyri (singular gyrus)
2. Fissures
3. Hemispheres
4. Sulci (singular sulcus)
5. Lobes

Diagram labels:
1. Longitudinal fissure
2. Transverse fissure
3. Right cerebral hemisphere
4. Left cerebral hemisphere
5. Central sulcus
6. Lateral sulcus
7. Frontal lobe
8. Parietal lobe
9. Temporal lobe
10. Occipital lobe

EXERCISE 14 • Pathways of the Nervous System

Sensory neurons, a (blue)
Somatic motor neurons, b (red)
Sympathetic motor neurons, d (red)
Parasympathetic motor neurons, c (red)
Spinal cord, 5
Cauda equina, 8
Ascending tracts, 7 (blue)
Descending tracts, 6 (red)
Cerebrum, 1
Diencephalon, 2
Brain stem, 3
Cerebellum, 4

EXERCISE 16 • Structural Features of the ANS

1. Fight or flight
2. Feed and breed
3. Thoracolumbar
4. Craniosacral
5. 2
6. 2
7. Paravertebral chain
8. In or near effector
9. Widespread
10. Targeted
11. Norepinephrine
12. Acetylcholine

GROUP ACTIVITY 2 • Quiz Show

Level 1	Neurons or Neuroglia	In the Periphery	Impulse Conduction	Parts of the Brain	Cranial Nerves
100	What is unipolar?	What is a nerve?	What is threshold?	What is the cerebellum?	What is 12?
200	What is a Schwann cell?	What is 31 pairs?	What is negative inside and positive outside?	What is the parietal lobe?	What is the vagus nerve?
300	What is forming CSF?	What is the posterior or dorsal root?	What is sodium?	What is the diencephalon?	What is tic douloureux?
400	What is neurilemma?	What is efferent?	What is dendrite-cell body-axon?	What is the corpus callosum?	What is the facial or cranial nerve VII?
500	What are integrative or interneurons?	What are skeletal muscles?	What is the axon hillock?	What is the medulla oblongata?	What are the olfactory and optic nerves?

Level 2	The ANS	Nerves and Plexuses	More Brain	The Spinal Cord	Sensory Receptors
200	What is 2?	What is the brachial plexus?	What is the occipital lobe?	What is ascending?	What are general sense receptors?
400	What is the parasympathetic division?	What is the phrenic nerve?	What is the limbic system?	What is anterior or ventral?	What are baroreceptors, tactile receptors, and mechanoreceptors of the ear?
600	What is parallel and slightly anterior to the spine?	What is the sacral plexus?	What is the sensory clearing house; prioritize and route sensory info?	What is the central canal?	What are joint receptors, muscle spindles, and Golgi tendon organs?
800	What is the lateral horn?	What are the axillary, musculocutaneous, radial, ulnar, and median nerves?	What are consciousness, cognition, and motor commands?	What is the pia mater?	What is a muscle spindle?
1000	What are the adrenals, sweat glands, and smooth muscle of blood vessels (vasomotor)?	What is the accessory nerve?	What is the amygdala?	What is the primary reflex center and information relay to and from the brain?	What are baroreceptors?

CHAPTER 8

EXERCISE 1 • Neuromuscular and Myofascial Terminology Crossword

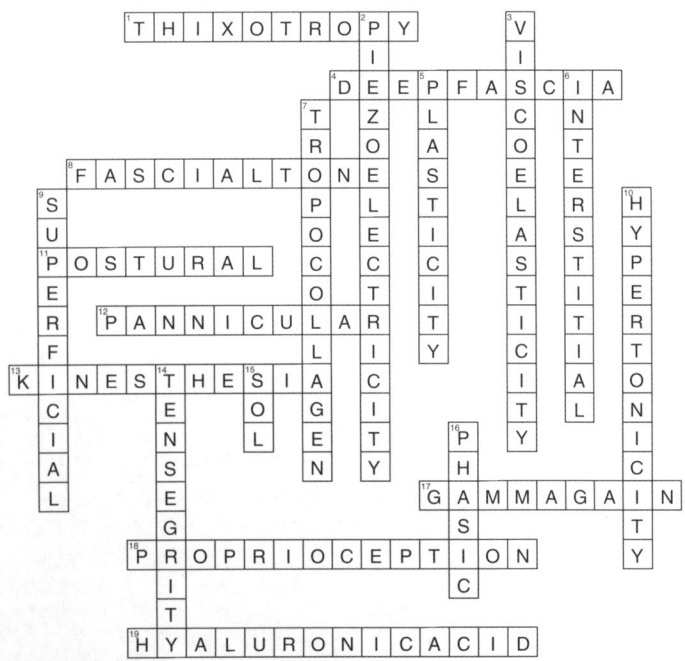

EXERCISE 2 • Neuromuscular Reflexes Table

1. A
2. G
3. C
4. D
5. E
6. F

EXERCISE 3 • Neuronal Loops

Fill in the blank:

1. Lengthening or stretching
2. Contraction
3. Stretch reflex
4. Alpha sensory
5. Alpha motor
6. Extrafusal
7. Stretch reflex
8. Control and coordinate voluntary movement
9. Gamma loop
10. Gamma sensory
11. Gamma motor
12. Intrafusal
13. Sensitivity
14. Length and tension
15. Tension
16. Sensitivity
17. Gamma gain or loading

EXERCISE 4 • Trigger Versus Tender Points

1. TeP
2. B
3. TeP
4. TrP
5. TrP
6. TrP
7. TrP
8. TeP
9. TeP
10. TrP
11. TeP
12. TeP

EXERCISE 5 • Tensegrity

1. Tension
2. Integrity
3. Compression
4. Tension
5. Upright posture

All homeostatic mechanisms are basically functional tensegrity systems.

EXERCISE 6 • Fascial Layers, Bands, and Planes

1. Tube
2. Sleeve
3. Lumbosacral aponeurosis
4. Flattened horizontal straps
5. Spinal junction
6. Curve
7. Deep fascia
8. Body cavities
9. Strength
10. Blood vessels, nerves, and organs

EXERCISE 7 • Mechanical Properties of Fascia

1. The ability of tissues to extend and rebound rather than stretch and recoil
2. The ability to vacillate between a more viscous (gel) state and more liquid (sol) state in response to temperature or movement
3. The ability to produce a small electrical charge in response to mechanical pressure
4. Slow steady pace; gradual application of superficial to deep pressure to assist in warming; constant movement of tissue with hands (instrument) to maintain warming and increase soluble change; increased duration to fully affect change
5. Sustained, moderate pressure and movement to affect fascial components

EXERCISE 8 • Fascial Receptors

1. P
2. R
3. GO
4. IMF
5. P
6. IMF
7. R
8. P
9. IMF
10. GO

EXERCISE 9 • Concepts in Posture, Balance, and Coordinated Movement

1. G
2. B
3. A
4. F
5. H
6. E
7. D
8. C

GROUP ACTIVITY 1 • Making Manual Therapy Choices

1. RI
2. RI
3. Engage quadriceps in isometric contraction
4. PR and/or CR
5. GG and ISR
6. PR for suboccipitals and pectorals; Contract relax for all neck flexors (stretch into extension); Contract relax is also appropriate for pectorals and interscapular muscles.
7. RI, CR, and/or SS
8. RI, ISR, and SR
9. Reciprocal inhibition is the best choice for the calf muscles of the injured leg to avoid irritating the strain. CR can be effective in all other muscles; and static stretch is good homework/self-care.

CHAPTER 9

EXERCISE 1 • Endocrine System Crossword

Across/Down answers filled in crossword grid:
MINERALCORTICOIDS, SOMATOTROPIN, NEGATIVE, BMR, RESISTANCEREACTION, STEROID, LANGERHANS, WATERSOLUBLE, PITUITARY, SYNDES(?), ADRENAL, CONGRISTS(?), PEPTIDE, HORMONE, etc.

EXERCISE 2 • Locating Endocrine Glands

1. Hypothalamus
2. Pituitary
3. Pineal
4. Thyroid
5. Parathyroids
6. Thymus
7. Adrenal
8. Pancreas
9. Gonads

EXERCISE 3 • Comparing the Communication Systems

1. No
2. Yes
3. Slow
4. Immediate
5. Long-term change like growth and maturation
6. Short-term, instantaneous changes like movement, breathing, and heart rate
7. Pituitary (endocrine gland connected to the hypothalamus)
8. Hypothalamus (brain region connected to the pituitary)
9. Hormones through the blood stream
10. Nerve impulses along neurons

EXERCISE 4 • Mechanisms of Hormone Action

1. Water-soluble
2. Lipid-soluble
3. Water-soluble
4. Plasma membrane
5. G-protein
6. Cyclic AMP (cAMP)
7. Physiologic change or cellular response
8. Second-messenger mechanism
9. Lipid-soluble
10. Plasma or cell membrane
11. Cytoplasm
12. Nuclear membrane
13. DNA
14. mRNA
15. Protein

EXERCISE 5 • Stimulating and Regulating Hormone Activity

1. Hormonal stimulus—Hypothalamus stimulates the anterior pituitary; anterior pituitary stimulates the gonads, thyroid, and a portion of the adrenal cortex.
2. Changes in blood concentrations—Calcitonin release from the thyroid gland; PTH from the parathyroid; glucagon and insulin from the pancreas.
3. Neurologic stimulus—Hypothalamus and posterior pituitary, and the sympathetic stimulation of the adrenal glands.

EXERCISE 6 • Glands and Their Hormones

Pineal—melatonin
Pituitary—TSH, ACTH, FSH, LH, prolactin, and GH from the anterior pituitary; ADH and oxytocin from the posterior pituitary
Thyroid—T_3, T_4, and calcitonin
Parathyroids—PTH
Thymus—thymosin
Adrenals—mineralocorticoids (aldosterone), glucocorticoids (cortisol), and androgens (DHEA) from the cortex; adrenaline and noradrenaline (catecholamines) from the medulla
Ovaries—estrogens and progesterone
Testes—testosterone (androgens)

EXERCISE 7 • Matching Hormones and Physiologic Responses

1. R
2. G
3. J
4. E
5. I
6. Q
7. B
8. O
9. P
10. C
11. N
12. D
13. K
14. F
15. L
16. H
17. A
18. M

EXERCISE 8 • Diagramming Stress

1. Hypothalamus
2. Alarm Response
3. Resistance Reaction
4. Sympathetic nervous system
5. Endocrine system (pituitary)
6. Release of catecholamines from the medulla, which support and prolong
7. ↑ HR, ↑ breathing, dilate bronchioles, dilate pupils, changes in blood flow patterns, ↓ digestion, etc.
8. Adrenals
9. Liver
10. Thyroid
11. Aldosterone ↑ sodium retention to ↑ BP; Cortisol to ↓ inflammatory response
12. Exhaustion

CHAPTER 10

EXERCISE 1 • Cardiovascular Crossword

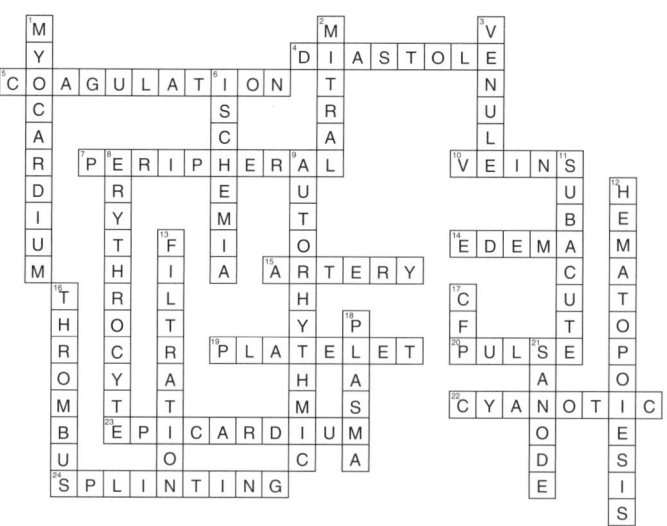

EXERCISE 2 • Matching Blood Components

1. C
2. I
3. E
4. H
5. B
6. F
7. A
8. J
9. D
10. G

EXERCISE 3 • Blood Vessel Structure

1. Artery
2. Arteriole
3. Capillary
4. Venule
5. Vein
A. Inner layer (tunica interna)
A_1. Endothelium
A_2. Basement membrane
B. Middle layer (tunica media)
B_1. Elastic fiber
B_2. Smooth muscle
C. Outer layer (tunica externa)
D. Valve

EXERCISE 5 • Primary Arteries of the Body

1. I (pulse point)
2. E (pulse point)
3. R (pulse point)
4. N
5. H (pulse point)
6. O (pulse point)
7. M
8. A (pulse point)
9. B
10. G
11. L
12. J (pulse point)
13. P (pulse point)
14. C
15. F (pulse point)
16. K
17. D
18. Q (pulse point)

EXERCISE 6 • Primary Veins of the Body

1. R
2. N
3. A
4. O
5. G
6. H
7. P
11. I
12. J
13. C
14. L
15. K
16. B
17. F

8. T
9. M
10. D
18. E
19. Q
20. S

3. B
4. C
5. A

Diagram:
1. SA node initiate signal
2. Signal passes through atria stimulating contraction
3. Signal is delayed at AV node
4. AV bundle passes signal through to the interventricular septum
5. Bundle branches pass signal down to the apex
6. Purkinje fibers carry signal through the ventricles creating a wringing action

EXERCISE 7 • The Layers of the Heart

1. Fibrous pericardium
2. Serous pericardium (parietal layer)
3. Pericardial cavity or space
4. Serous pericardium (visceral layer) or epicardium (actual heart wall)
5. Myocardium (actual heart wall)
6. Endocardium (actual heart wall)

EXERCISE 8 • Blood Flow through the Heart

Diagram structures:
1. Ascending aorta
2. Superior vena cava
3. Right atrium
4. Fossa ovalis
5. Coronary sinus
6. Inferior vena cava
7. Tricuspid valve
8. Right ventricle
9. Intraventricular septum
10. Left ventricle
11. Bicuspid or mitral valve
12. Aortic valve
13. Left atrium
14. Pulmonary veins
15. Pulmonary valve
16. Pulmonary trunk (arterial)

Blood flow:
1—Right atrium
8—Left atrium
3—Right ventricle
10—Left ventricle
9—Bicuspid valve
2—Tricuspid valve
11—Aortic valve
4—Pulmonary valve
12—Aorta
14—Vena cavae
7—Pulmonary veins
5—Pulmonary arteries
13—Systemic capillaries
6—Lung capillaries

EXERCISE 9 • The Conduction System of the Heart

Matching:
1. D
2. E

EXERCISE 10 • The Cardiac Cycle

Relaxation Phase
Atria are relaxed
Ventricles are relaxed
Semilunar valves are closed
AV valves are open
Blood flows from atria to ventricles

Atrial Systole
Atria are contracted
Ventricles are relaxed
Semilunar valves are closed
AV valves are open
Blood flows from atria to ventricles

Ventricular Systole
Atria are relaxed
Ventricles are contracted
Semilunar valves are open
AV valves are closed
Blood flows from ventricles to great vessels

EXERCISE 11 • Cardiovascular Circulation

1. Pulmonary circuit
2. Systemic circuit
3. Aorta (red)
4. Systemic arterioles (red)
5. Systemic capillaries (red to blue)
6. Systemic venules (blue)
7. Superior and inferior vena cavae (blue)

8. Pulmonary arteries (blue)
9. Pulmonary arterioles (blue)
10. Pulmonary capillaries (blue to red)
11. Pulmonary venules (red)
12. Pulmonary veins (red)

Right side of heart is blue, while left side is red

EXERCISE 12 • Blood Flow

1. Ventricular contraction
2. Arterial recoil
3. Precapillary sphincters
4. Volume
5. Rate
6. Skeletal muscle contractions
7. One-way valves
8. Respiratory pump

EXERCISE 13 • Blood Pressure Regulation

1. Hydrostatic force generated by blood against the vascular wall
2. Systolic
3. Ventricular contraction
4. Diastolic
5. Ventricle relaxes
6. ↑
7. ↑
8. ↓
9. ↑
10. ↓
11. ↑
12. ↓

EXERCISE 14 • Capillary Flow

1. Diffusion
2. Glucose, oxygen, carbon dioxide
3. Starling forces
4. Hydrostatic
5. Capillary fluid
6. CFP
7. Interstitial fluid
8. Interstitial fluid
9. Osmotic
10. Plasma oncotic
11. POP
12. Protein
13. Interstitial oncotic
14. Protein
15. Filtration
16. Reabsorption
17. CFP and IOP
18. IFP and POP
19. Filtration
20. Reabsorption
21. Edema

EXERCISE 15 • Stages of Tissue Healing

1. Inflammation
2. Pain
3. Secondary edema formation
4. Hematoma organization
5. Fibroblasts
6. Phagocytes
7. Healing
8. Granulation
9. Collagen
10. Stress

GROUP ACTIVITY 1 • Quiz Show

Level 1	Formed Elements	The Vascular Network	Oh, My Heart!	Cardiac Conduction	Pressure and Flow
100	What are erythrocytes?	What is artery?	What is pericardium?	What is right atrium to left ventricle?	What is 120/80?
200	What are WBCs or leukocytes?	What is capillary?	What is the tricuspid?	What is the sinoatrial node?	What is skeletal muscle contraction?
300	What are leukocytes or WBCs?	What is venule?	What is semi-lunar?	What are Purkinje fibers?	What is arterial recoil or rebound?
400	What is hemoglobin?	What is lumen?	What is the left ventricle?	What is the atrioventricular bundle?	What is diastole?
500	What is leukocyte?	What are one-way valves and thinner muscular layer?	What is the right atrium?	What is autorhythmic?	What is systole?

Level 2	Arteries	Veins	Capillary Exchange	Tissue Healing	Potpourri
200	What is brachiocephalic?	What are the vena cavae (inferior and superior)?	Who is Dr. Starling?	What is formation of a platelet plug?	What is hemostasis?
400	What are the subclavian arteries?	The large vein on medial lower extremity and is most prone to the pathology of varicose vein	What are precapillary sphincters?	What is secondary edema?	What is hematopoiesis?
600	What is two fingers superior and left of the umbilicus?	This vein starts in lateral cub-ital and travels full lateral brachium before joining subclavian	What is the arterial side?	What is the subacute or proliferative phase?	What are the globulins?
800	The short artery that connects the femoral to the anterior and posterior tibialis arteries	Unlike most veins, these carry oxygen-rich blood	What is capillary fluid pressure (CFP)?	What is granulation tissue/fibers?	What is the ANS or cardiovascular centers of medulla oblongata?
1000	The artery that delivers blood to the intestines	This vein carries blood into the liver for cleansing	What is plasma oncotic pressure (POP)?	What is collagen remodeling?	What is autoregulation via vasoconstriction and vasodilation?

CHAPTER 11

EXERCISE 1 • Lymphatic System Crossword

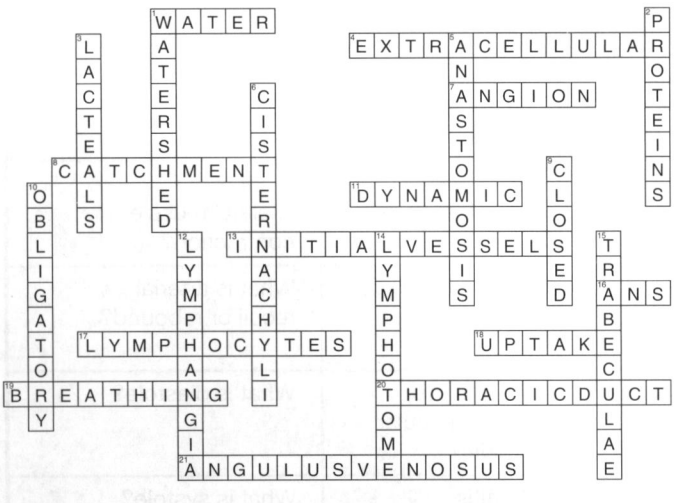

EXERCISE 2 • The Lymphatic Vessels

1. Initial vessels
2. Subepidermis
3. Blind-ended
4. Overlapping epithelial cells
5. Anchor filaments
6. Dermis
7. One-way valves
8. Initial vessels
9. Lymphangia
10. Segments or angions
11. Smooth muscle
12. Collecting capillaries
13. Collecting
14. Major arteries
15. Organ or body region
16. Cisterna chyli
17. Thoracic duct
18. Right lymphatic duct
19. Subclavian vein
20. Left upper and both lower body quadrants

EXERCISE 3 • Structure and Function of a Lymph Node

1. Lymphoid organs
2. Lymphangia
3. Lymph node beds
4. Catchments
5. Filters
6. Dust, pollen, and bacteria
7. Damaged cells and other cellular debris
8. Specialized immune cells
9. Lymphocytes
10. Capsule
11. Trabeculae
12. Sinus
13. Nodule
14. Afferent lymph vessel
15. Efferent lymph vessel

EXERCISE 4 • The Lymphatic Network

1. Submandibular node
2. Right lymphatic duct
3. Axillary node
4. Lymph vessels
5. Inguinal node
6. Cisterna chyli
7. Thoracic duct
8. Cervical node
9. Internal jugular veins
10. Right lymphatic duct
11. Right subclavian vein
12. Brachiocephalic veins
13. Thoracic duct
14. Left subclavian vein

EXERCISE 5 • Edema Uptake Versus Lymphatic Flow

1. EU
2. LF
3. LF
4. EU
5. EU
6. LF
7. EU
8. EU
9. LF
10. EU

EXERCISE 6 • Mechanisms of Lymph Flow

1. Internal mechanisms
2. Siphon effect
3. Contraction of angions
4. Skeletal muscle contraction
5. Compression from adjacent arterial pulse
6. Respiratory pump

EXERCISE 8 • Routes of Lymph Flow

Edema uptake @ anterior thigh: → 1. H → 2. E → 3. F → 4. A → 5. C

Edema uptake @ right medial wrist: → 1. K → 2. D → 3. B → 4. C

Edema uptake @ calf: → 1. J → 2. G → 3. E → 4. F → 5. A → 6. C

Edema uptake @ right ribcage: → 1. D → 2. B → 3. C

Edema uptake @ left lateral elbow: → 1. L → 2. D → 3. B → 4. C

Edema uptake @ anterior ankle: → 1. I → 2. H → 3. E → 4. F → 5. A → 6. C

EXERCISE 9 • Types of Edema

1. Edema caused by dysfunction or failure in the lymphatic system; congenital or genetic defect in lymphatic development
2. Weak or insufficient number of intralymphatic valves; Low ratio of lymphatic vessels per cubic centimeter of tissue
3. Secondary lymphedema
4. Chemotherapy, radiation, infection, parasites (filarial)
5. Chemotherapy, radiation, infection, parasites (filarial)
6. Cardiovascular edema
7. Edema related to dysfunction or disease in the cardiovascular system; dynamic edema
8. Diabetes-related complications, venous insufficiency, or malnutrition
9. The localized and temporary swelling associated with soft tissue injury
10. Sprains, strains, hematomas

CHAPTER 12

EXERCISE 1 • Immunity Crossword

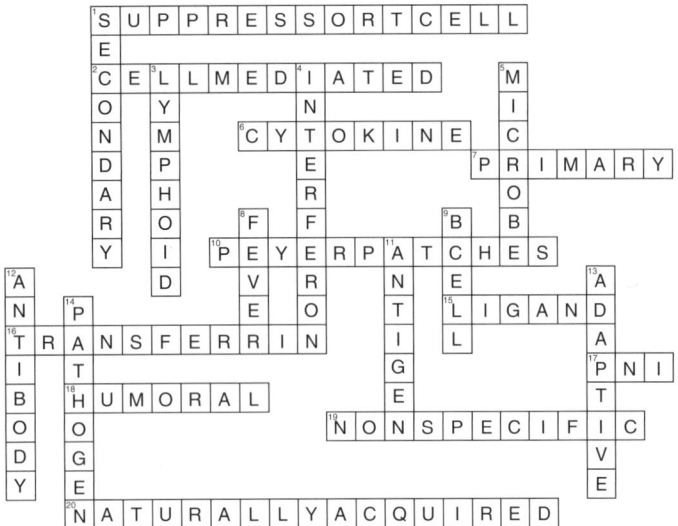

EXERCISE 2 • Lymphoid Tissues

1. P, G
2. S, C
3. S, B
4. P, D
5. S, A
6. S, E
7. S, H
8. S, F

EXERCISE 3 • Nonspecific Immune Defenses

1. Innate
2. Generic or universal
3. Any single type, or any specific kind

Chemical barriers—Chemicals that destroy or discourage the growth and/or spread of microbes, pathogens, and other foreign particles. Include sebum, sweat, tears, gastric juice, saliva, urine, and vaginal secretions.
Internal antimicrobial proteins—Proteins in the body that destroy microbes in a variety of ways such as interferons, complements, transferrins, and antimicrobial peptides
Phagocytes—Cells that eat microbes and cellular debris such as neutrophils and macrophages
Natural killer cells—Roaming cells that kill infected body cells through cytolysis
Inflammation—Physiologic responses that fight and contain infectious agents by increasing vasodilation, capillary permeability, and phagocytosis; prepares tissue for repair
Fever—Elevated body temperature that speeds up metabolism to facilitate tissue repair; kills or inhibits the growth of certain bacteria; increases the effect of interferons

EXERCISE 4 • Specific Immune Responses

Fill-in exercise:

1. Adaptive
2. Exposure
3. B and T
4. Specific
5. Antigen
6. Foreign particle or substance
7. Immune response
8. Antigen
9. Antigen receptor
10. B
11. Antibody-mediated
12. T
13. Cell-mediated

Diagram:

1. Pathogen
2. Antigen
3. APC
4. T cells
5. Cytotoxic T cells
6. Memory T cells
7. Helper T cells
8. Suppressor T cells
9. B cells
10. Plasma cells
11. Antibodies
12. Memory B cells
13. CMI
14. AMI

EXERCISE 6 • Gaining Immunity

1. T
2. T
3. F
4. F
5. T
6. F
7. T
8. T

CHAPTER 13

EXERCISE 1 • Respiratory System Crossword

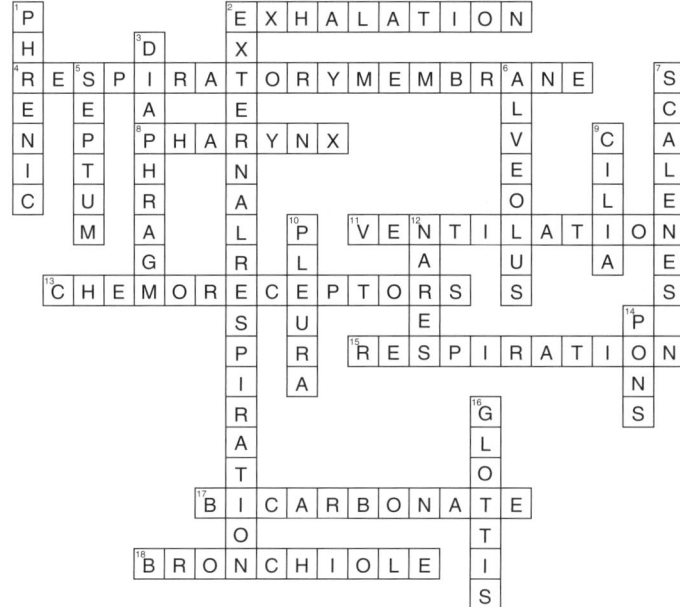

EXERCISE 2 • Respiratory Structures

1. Frontal sinus
2. Nasal cavity
3. Oral cavity (mouth)
4. Pharynx
5. Larynx
6. Trachea
7. Bronchi
8. Bronchioles
9. Right lung
10. Left lung
11. Diaphragm
12. Bronchiole
13. Capillaries
14. Alveoli

EXERCISE 3 • Matching Respiratory Organs

1. D
2. E
3. H
4. A
5. K
6. L
7. I
8. F
9. G
10. C
11. J
12. B

EXERCISE 4 • Upper or Lower Respiratory Tract

1. L
2. L
3. L
4. L
5. U
6. L
7. U
8. U
9. U
10. U

EXERCISE 5 • Muscles of Ventilation

1. External intercostals
2. —
3. Diaphragm
4. —
5. —
6. Rectus abdominis
7. —
8. Internal intercostals
9. Scalenes
10. —
11. Serratus anterior
12. —
13. Pectoralis minor
14. —
15. Sternocleidomastoid
16. —

EXERCISE 6 • Respiration

Fill-in exercise:

1. Oxygen and carbon dioxide exchange
2. Inside the lungs between the alveoli and the blood
3. In the capillary beds throughout the body between the blood and the interstitium
4. Exchange of gases between the alveoli and the blood
5. Internal respiration
6. Diffusion
7. Hemoglobin (Hb)
8. Plasma
9. Oxyhemoglobin (HbO_2)
10. Bicarbonate
11. Carbaminohemoglobin

Diagram:

1. External respiration in the lungs
2. Internal respiration in the body tissues
3. Alveolus
4. Body cells
5. Pulmonary veins
6. Systemic arteries
7. Systemic veins
8. Pulmonary arteries

CO_2 moves out of and O_2 moves into blood during external respiration.

CO_2 moves into and O_2 moves out of blood during internal respiration.

CHAPTER 14

EXERCISE 1 • Digestive System Crossword

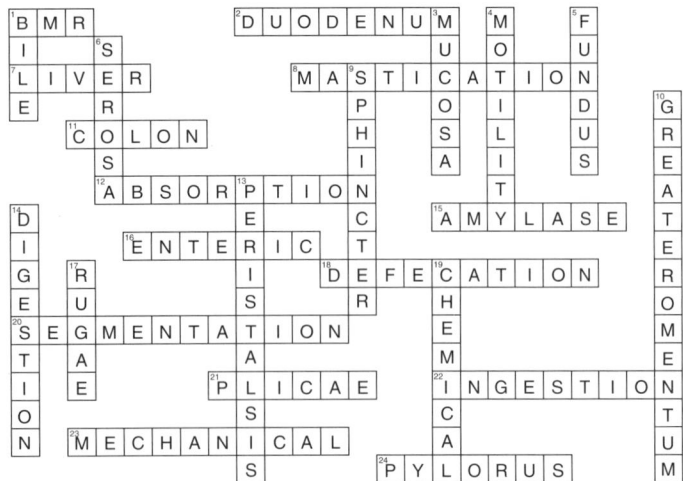

EXERCISE 2 • Gastrointestinal Tract Versus Accessory Organs and Functions

1. GI
2. A
3. GI
4. GI
5. A
6. A
7. GI
8. A
9. GI
10. A
11. GI
12. GI
13. A

EXERCISE 3 • Digestive System Organs

1. Salivary glands
2. Teeth
3. Tongue
4. Mouth (oral cavity)
5. Pharynx
6. Esophagus
7. Stomach
8. Liver
9. Gall bladder
10. Pancreas
11. Small intestine
12. Ascending colon
13. Transverse colon
14. Hepatic flexure
15. Splenic flexure
16. Descending colon
17. Sigmoid colon
18. Rectum
19. Anus
20. Duodenum
21. Jejunum
22. Ileum
23. Cecum
24. Appendix
25. Iliocecal valve

EXERCISE 4 • Layers of the GI Tract

Diagram:
1. Mucosa
2. Peyer patch (MALT)
3. Glands
4. Submucosal plexus
5. Submucosa
6. Longitudinal smooth muscle layer
7. Circular smooth muscle layer
8. Muscularis
9. Myenteric plexus
10. Serosa
11. Mesentery

Matching:
1. G
2. J
3. I
4. B
5. D
6. F
7. C
8. E
9. H
10. A

EXERCISE 5 • Functions of the Digestive System

1. Salivary amylase
2. Swallowing
3. Saliva
4. Peristalsis
5. Hydrochloric acid
6. Pepsin
7. Proteins
8. Pepsin
9. Peristalsis
10. Alcohol
11. Proteases
12. Secretin
13. Mixing via segmentation
14. Segmentation
15. Peristalsis
16. Glucose
17. Triglycerides
18. Mucus
19. Water
20. Vitamin K
21. Bile
22. Concentrated bile made by the liver
23. Amylase

EXERCISE 6 • Diagram the Functions of the GI Tract

1. Mouth (oral cavity)
2. Pharynx
3. Esophagus
4. Stomach

5. Small intestine
6. Large intestine
7. Anus

Ingestion: 1—eating

Mechanical digestion: 1—chewing; 4—churning; 5—segmentation for mixing

Chemical digestion: 1—amylase in the saliva; 4—gastric juices; 5—enzymes and bile from liver, gall bladder, and pancreas, plus enzymes produced by the SI

Motility: 1 and 2—swallowing; 3—peristalsis; 4—peristalsis/gastric emptying; 5—peristalsis; 6—peristalsis

Absorption: 1—sublingual medications, etc.; 4—medications and alcohol; 5—all nutrients; 6—water

Defecation: 7—elimination of feces

EXERCISE 7 • Metabolism and Nutrients

1. Chemical reactions
2. Anabolic
3. Repaired
4. Synthesized
5. Catabolic
6. Produce ATP
7. Macronutrients
8. Glucose
9. Energy
10. Glycogen
11. Fat
12. Lipids
13. Glycerol and fatty acids
14. Adipose
15. Amino acids
16. Liver
17. Protein synthesis
18. Enzymes, receptors, antibodies, hormones, and/or ligands
19. Micronutrients
20. Serving as coenzymes in chemical reactions
21. Minerals
22. Blood and bone
23. Coenzymes that help regulate chemical reactions in the body (similar to vitamins)
24. Water

CHAPTER 15

EXERCISE 1 • Urinary System Crossword

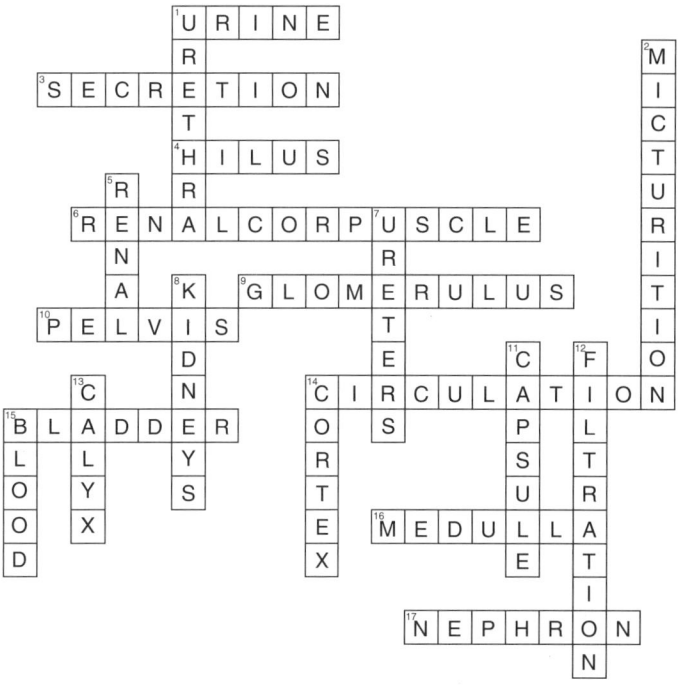

EXERCISE 2 • Urinary System Organs

Diagram:

A. Urethra
B. Bladder
C. Ureters
D. Kidney
E. Diaphragm

Matching:

1. C
2. B
3. D
4. D
5. A
6. B
7. C
8. D
9. D
10. D

EXERCISE 3 • Structure of the Kidneys

1. Renal cortex—Outer region of the kidney
2. Renal medulla—Inner region of the kidney
3. Renal capsule—Large fascial envelope that surrounds each kidney and attaches it to the abdominal wall
4. Renal pyramids—Triangle-shaped bundle of microscopic tubes within the renal medulla that collect urine from a specific group of nephrons

5. Nephron—Microscopic functional unit of the kidney
6. Calyx—Small cup at the bottom of a renal pyramid that collects urine and transfers it to the renal pelvis
7. Renal pelvis—Region of the kidney where urine is collected before being passed into the ureter

EXERCISE 4 • Parts of a Nephron

1. Efferent arteriole
2. Glomerulus
3. Bowman (glomerular) capsule
4. Afferent arteriole
5. Proximal convoluted tubule
6. Venule
7. Peritubular capillaries
8. Loop of Henle
9. Distal convoluted tubule
10. Collecting ducts

EXERCISE 5 • Structure and Function of a Nephron

1. F
2. J
3. A
4. B
5. I
6. C
7. H
8. D
9. E
10. G

CHAPTER 16

EXERCISE 1 • Reproductive System Crossword

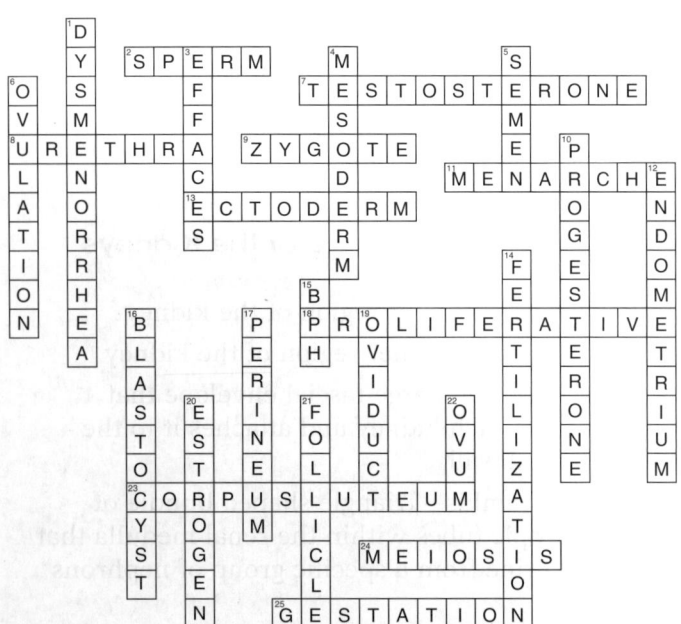

EXERCISE 2 • Mind Map of Common Characteristics

1, 2. M—testes; F—ovaries
3, 4. M—sperm; F—ova
5, 6. M—penis and scrotum; F—vulva
7, 8. M—seminal vesicles, epididymis, vas deferens, ejaculatory duct, urethra; F—fallopian tubes; uterus, vagina
9, 10. M—testosterone; F—estrogens, progesterone
11, 12. M—Leydig cells; F—follicles, corpus luteum

EXERCISE 3 • Male Pelvic Anatomy

1. Bladder
2. Urethra
3. Penis
4. External urethral orifice
5. Testes
6. Scrotum
7. Epididymis
8. Vas deferens
9. Anus
10. Rectum
11. Bulbourethral gland
12. Prostate
13. Ejaculatory duct
14. Internal urethral orifice
15. Seminal vesicle

EXERCISE 4 • Male Reproductive Structures and Functions

1. E
2. I
3. G
4. B
5. A
6. C
7. D
8. F
9. H

EXERCISE 5 • Female Pelvic Anatomy

1. Fallopian tube (oviduct)
2. Ovary
3. Bladder
4. Mons pubis
5. Clitoris
6. Urethra
7. Vaginal opening
8. Anus
9. Vagina
10. Rectum
11. Cervix
12. Uterus

EXERCISE 6 • Female Reproductive Structures and Functions

1. I
2. G
3. F
4. A
5. J
6. E
7. K
8. B
9. C
10. H

UNIT 1 Practice Exam Answers

1. B
2. C
3. A
4. C
5. D
6. B
7. C
8. D
9. A
10. D
11. D
12. B
13. C
14. D
15. A
16. B
17. B
18. C
19. A
20. D
21. D
22. B
23. C
24. C
25. A
26. B
27. D
28. C
29. A
30. D

UNIT 2 Practice Exam Answers

1. C
2. B
3. D
4. D
5. B
6. A
7. B
8. C
9. C
10. A
11. D
12. B
13. B
14. A
15. C
16. D
17. A
18. B
19. C
20. B
21. D
22. C
23. A
24. C
25. B
26. C
27. D
28. C
29. B
30. C
31. A
32. D
33. C
34. B
35. C

UNIT 3 Practice Exam Answers

1. C
2. B
3. A
4. C
5. D
6. B
7. D
8. B
9. A
10. C
11. C
12. B
13. B
14. A
15. C
16. D
17. C
18. C
19. B
20. A
21. B
22. D
23. A
24. D
25. B
26. C
27. C
28. D
29. B
30. C
31. D
32. B
33. A
34. B
35. D

UNIT 4 Practice Exam Answers

1. D	10. A	19. B	28. B
2. B	11. C	20. D	29. B
3. A	12. D	21. A	30. A
4. D	13. B	22. C	31. C
5. C	14. C	23. B	32. C
6. C	15. B	24. D	33. B
7. B	16. B	25. A	34. A
8. A	17. A	26. D	35. D
9. B	18. C	27. C	

UNIT 5 Practice Exam Answers

1. B	8. D	15. B	22. B
2. C	9. B	16. D	23. A
3. B	10. B	17. A	24. C
4. A	11. A	18. C	25. B
5. A	12. D	19. D	
6. D	13. B	20. D	
7. C	14. C	21. B	

UNIT 6 Practice Exam Answers

1. C	10. C	19. C	28. B
2. B	11. D	20. A	29. A
3. A	12. B	21. B	30. C
4. D	13. B	22. B	31. C
5. D	14. A	23. C	32. D
6. D	15. C	24. D	33. B
7. C	16. D	25. A	34. B
8. B	17. A	26. D	35. C
9. A	18. C	27. C	